THE MAKER'S DIET for WEIGHT LOSS

JORDAN S. RUBIN

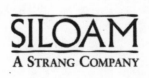

SILOAM
A STRANG COMPANY

Most STRANG COMMUNICATIONS/CHARISMA HOUSE/CHRISTIAN LIFE/EXCEL BOOKS/FRONTLINE/REALMS/SILOAM products are available at special quantity discounts for bulk purchase for sales promotions, premiums, fund-raising, and educational needs. For details, write Strang Communications Book Group, 600 Rinehart Road, Lake Mary, Florida 32746, or telephone (407) 333-0600.

THE MAKER'S DIET FOR WEIGHT LOSS by Jordan Rubin with Bernard Bulwer, MD
Published by Siloam
A Strang Company
600 Rinehart Road
Lake Mary, Florida 32746
www.strangdirect.com

Design Director: Bill Johnson
Cover design by Jerry Pomales, Bill Johnson

Library of Congress Cataloging-in-Publication Data:
Rubin, Jordan.
  The maker's diet for weight loss / Jordan Rubin.
      p. cm.
  Includes bibliographical references and index.
  ISBN 978-1-59979-518-8
  1. Weight loss--Religious aspects--Christianity. 2. Reducing diets--Religious aspects--Christianity. 3. Nutrition--Religious aspects--Christianity. I. Title.
  RM222.2.R8147 2009
  613.2'5--dc22
                              2008039731

Parts of this book were previously published as *Perfect Weight America*, ISBN 978-1-59979-257-6, copyright © 2008.

09 10 11 12 13 — 9 8 7 6 5 4 3 2 1

Printed in the United States of America

CONTENTS

WHAT THE MAKER'S DIET FOR WEIGHT LOSS IS ALL ABOUT

W HEN I RELEASED *The Maker's Diet* in 2004, two things happened that I never expected. One, I could never imagine in my wildest dreams that *The Maker's Diet* would become one of those word-of-mouth publishing phenomena that would propel the book to the *New York Times* best-seller list (in the health category) for forty-seven weeks in 2004 and 2005, with two million copies in print. The overnight success of *The Maker's Diet* led to appearances on *Good Morning America, NBC Nightly News, FOX News, Inside Edition,* and interviews with *TIME, Newsweek,* the *New York Times, Reader's Digest,* and *People* magazine, as well as hundreds of radio stations.

But there was another aspect to *The Maker's Diet* that surprised me, and that was hearing from so many readers who said they used the book to lose weight. This was a fascinating development because, if you remember my story, I was looking for a way to *gain* weight after wasting away to 104 pounds when Crohn's disease, a chronic digestive illness that affects the immune system, nearly claimed my life.

I came closest to dying about eighteen months into my health struggles. One night when I overheard one of my nurses crying outside my hospital room. "This young man is not going to make it through the night," I overheard her telling another nurse. My situation had become *really* serious, and I can remember praying with all my heart, saying, "Lord, I'm ready to go home. I've had a great life so far, but now I just want to be with You. I don't want to be in this body if life is going to be like this."

I fell asleep, not sure if I would wake up in the morning. I opened my droopy eyes to the sight of my morning nurse informing me that I had gained 10 pounds in water weight from intravenous fluids. Now that I had my rally cap on, I needed to put some meat on my bones. I studied hundreds of biblical and historical references about living a healthy lifestyle. I changed my diet to whole foods consumed in biblical times: raw, organically grown whole grains, fruits, vegetables, fermented dairy products, grass-fed beef, and free-range poultry. After gaining 29 pounds in forty days, I was on the right track to regaining my health.

Because I was deeply moved to be alive with restored health, I promised I would dedicate the rest of my life to sharing my health wisdom and transforming the health of this nation one life at a time. I wrote *The Maker's Diet* as a forty-day health experience that would help readers stabilize insulin and blood sugar, reduce inflammation and infections, enhance digestion, and significantly improve overall health.

The Maker's Diet seemed to attract people who had health challenges from all walks of life. Those seeking to shed pounds experienced phenomenal results when using *The Maker's Diet* as a weight-loss tool, but what I found in reading my mail and meeting thousands of people was that the Maker's Diet forty-day health plan was too difficult—or strict. People loved my story, agreed 100 percent with the health principles I laid out, but they could never gain enough traction to stick with the forty-day health plan. In other words, they were defeated before they started because they didn't like the taste of goat's milk, couldn't find buffalo or elk meat, or couldn't afford wild-caught halibut or pastured chicken. Others found the advanced hygiene protocol too daunting.

That's why I've decided to come out with a streamlined sixteen-week program that keeps many of the principles found in *The Maker's Diet* but refines them and makes them more user-friendly and effective. The result is *The Maker's Diet for Weight Loss*, and within the pages of this book, you'll learn about a new way of eating, a new way of thinking, and a new way of living.

The Maker's Diet for Weight Loss is all about giving you the directions you need to make a U-turn in life and get headed in the right direction. Maybe it's been years since you've woken up feeling refreshed or since you attacked the day with some spring in your step. Maybe your life has revolved around innumerable visits to the family doctor and expensive specialists who struggle to find out what's "wrong" with you. Maybe you gulp down powerful drugs to fight off the ravages of hypertension, type 2 diabetes, heartburn, and a host of other ailments—and wonder if the side effects aren't worse than the disease.

If this sounds like your life, then following the health recommendations set forth in *The Maker's Diet for Weight Loss* will hand you the tools to transform yourself in ways you never thought possible. Later in this book, in chapter 7, you will find the four-phase Weight Loss Eating Plan that will tell what foods you should and should not consume during the sixteen-week program. You'll have a road map that you can follow step-by-step to enjoy the optimal health and wellness that you haven't experienced for years or perhaps decades.

You will learn what to eat, when to eat, how to cheat right, which foods can add fat, and which foods can help it disappear. You will discover which foods make you hungrier and which foods keep you feeling full. You will be reminded about the importance of staying hydrated, how to integrate strategic snacking, and how adding superior supplements to your daily regimen will give you that extra edge. You will also read about the benefits of cleansing and detoxification, which you should do seasonally in January, April, July, and October.

An integral part of the Maker's Diet for Weight Loss program is a groundbreaking fitness plan I call FIT—Functional Interval Training. In just twenty minutes you'll strengthen your heart and lungs, build muscle, and ignite your body's fat-burning furnace so you can scorch fat during and after your workout.

In addition, you will learn how to create a toxin-free home to prevent harmful chemical poisons from storing in your fat cells—which will become fewer by the day when you follow this program. You will learn how to put on the Maker's Diet helmet of success to squash all your weight-loss saboteurs. You will be equipped to reduce stress and create the life you've always dreamed of. You will learn the underlying secret to transforming your physical appearance and self-esteem, as well as ways to improve the health of family and friends around you.

WHAT'S DIFFERENT ABOUT THE MAKER'S DIET FOR WEIGHT LOSS?

Please know that *The Maker's Diet for Weight Loss* is not just another diet book. You won't shake off 22 pounds in a hurry like singer Beyoncé Knowles did before playing the role of Deena in the hit film *Dreamgirls*. Beyoncé lost all that weight after embarking on a crash diet that consisted of drinking a mixture of water, cayenne pepper, and maple syrup—and starving herself of regular food. When the supermarket tabloids splashed photos of her newly svelte figure, shoppers made a dash for the maple syrup on aisle 4.[1]

While Beyoncé's "maple syrup diet" may be one of the more outlandish fads to capture attention in recent years, her story is an instructive reminder that millions of Americans are on the lookout for the "next big thing" to lose weight swiftly as well as effortlessly. Fad diets make up a tidy chunk of a multibillion-dollar weight-loss industry that churns out books, CDs, DVDs, shakes, bars, pills, supplements, gym equipment, and infomercials for everything from the latest weight-burning shakes and slimming supplements to bun trainers and abdominal sculptors. Yet, as anyone who's suffered through a crash diet will tell you, weight quickly lost is weight destined to return. Nearly none of these diets can be sustained because these food-restrictive regimens do not deliver a variety of well-rounded, nutritious foods necessary for good health. Nor do they speak to the mental, emotional, and spiritual health of individuals, which is just as important as physical well-being.

The Maker's Diet for Weight Loss addresses all four legs of this stool, which is why this well-rounded program holds its own with many of the diet and exercise books vying for attention on the nation's bookshelves. *The Maker's Diet for Weight Loss* outlines a new lifestyle based on holistic principles that focus on the whole person: physical, mental, emotional, and spiritual. This approach is more in line with the etymology of the word *diet*, which originated from the Greek word *diaita*, meaning "life, lifestyle, way of living."

You're going to be better off jumping in all the way—making a complete lifestyle change—than poking your toes around the edges of the pool. According to a recent study published in the *Archives of Internal Medicine*, smoking, drinking, eating junk food, and getting no exercise are all risk factors for poor health, but tackling all these habits *at the same time* is better than dealing with them one by one in a sequential fashion.[2]

So, if you weigh too much, get tired too easily, live a sedentary lifestyle, or deal with high blood pressure, high cholesterol, and high anxiety, the fact that you're holding this book, *The Maker's Diet for Weight Loss*, tells me that regaining your health is a top priority. You're sick and tired of being sick and tired.

I'm confident that *The Maker's Diet for Weight Loss* will be a great resource for you. You will have to change your American mind-set, though, the one that's dialed into instant gratification. Instead, you'll have to take personal responsibility for the shape you're in.

Once you do that, you must stop listening to yourself. Your nimble mind, which is the essence of your will and determination, loves to capture negative thoughts and spin them around like liquid sugar and pink dye in a cotton candy machine to whip up a confection of doubt and hesitation. Toss those negative thoughts in the trash. Don't listen when your agile mind coughs up one rationalization after another against making a major course correction in life. Shut down your excuse making because at the end of the day, that's all they are—excuses, such as:

- "I'm too busy."
- "I'm too fat."
- "I don't have the energy."
- "I have kids."
- "I have parents to take care of."
- "I'm going on vacation."
- "It costs too much to join a fitness club."
- "I can't get motivated."
- "I don't have the money."
- "Nothing's ever worked before."

The Maker's Diet for Weight Loss calls for an attitude adjustment—fast. The most important attitude you can have is this: "I'm following this program for my health and for those who count on me. The more I put into it, the more I will receive from it. If I give this my best effort, then I can expect the best results."

You'll be following the steady route to successful weight management and a lifetime of extraordinary health. Sure, you'll probably lose a few pounds right away, but the point is that you won't reach your ideal weight in two weeks. You'll certainly be a lot closer, however, after sixteen weeks. Casting off 22 pounds as Beyoncé did is not only unhealthy, but it's also counterproductive in the long run since the elation of losing substantial weight is quickly replaced by despair when the old pounds come right back. Depressed dieters often cope by reverting back to deeply entrenched eating habits, which often leaves them weighing *more* than when they started the quick-loss diet in the first place.

SETTING SAIL

The Maker's Diet for Weight Loss is about making a personal transformation in quantitative categories, such as weight loss and reduction of disease risks, as well as qualitative improvements in mental acuity and physical vitality. Best of all, you will love the eating plan because you will consume an assortment of satisfying and delicious foods as you will discover to your delight in chapter 3, "Eat for Your Ideal Weight." By "ideal weight," I don't mean looking like a runway model in size 0 clothes or a recent exile from the *Survivor* TV show, but a comfortable weight that fits your physique and your age. I'm confident that *The Maker's Diet for Weight Loss* will bring you close to your ideal weight. In the following chapters, you'll learn:

A new way of eating

1. Eat healthy so that you attain and maintain your weight-loss goals.
2. Eat for your individual nutritional type.
3. Optimize your nutrient intake while cutting out unnecessary and unhealthy calories to ensure healthy weight loss.
4. Learn about the nutritional supplements that can make a big difference in your health and vitality.
5. Tap into the Weight Loss Eating Plan, a sixteen-week, four-phase program that offers you approved foods while restricting others.

A new way of thinking

1. Eliminate waste and toxins as you undertake a digestive cleanse.
2. Experience FIT, the exercise program that you can live with.
3. Reduce toxins in your personal environment.
4. Reduce stress and get more rest in order to unlock your health potential.
5. Focus on mental, emotional, and spiritual balance for total body, mind, and spirit wellness.

A new way of living

1. Learn simple steps you can take to live a "green lifestyle."
2. Take weight off the planet, as well as off your body.
3. Incorporate habits that promote sustainability for your health, the health of future generations, and the health of the planet.

I've spoken in a number of churches, and occasionally a heavyset member will ask me, tongue firmly planted in cheek, if he can still enjoy all of his favorite unhealthy foods and snacks and still get past the pearly gates. "Oh, sure, you'll get to heaven," I'll respond. "You'll just get there a lot sooner."

The line is always good for a chuckle, but those who've faced their mortality after a heart attack, debilitating stroke, or cancer diagnosis aren't laughing very loudly. They understand better than most that every minute they have on Earth is precious and should be valued.

If you're married and have children, your family needs you and loves you. Don't you want to stay around for them? Every year you have more to offer, not less, because you have wisdom and experience on your side. Use that wisdom to establish a health legacy for yourself and for your future generations, and you won't live a life of regrets.

Living a long, healthy life matters more than you know. I lost both of my grandfathers way too early. My grandfather on my father's side was significantly overweight and died at the age of sixty-two from a heart attack. My grandfather on my mother's side was overweight as well, and he died of a heart attack at the age of fifty-five. Both of my grandfathers were gone before I turned ten years old. I wish I had known them longer, but I never got the chance.

You may be reading this, however, and thinking, "I've let myself go too far…I can tell when people are staring at me." Well, with *The Maker's Diet for Weight Loss*, you will be empowered to do something about your health and excess weight from this day forward. The question now becomes: What are you going to do about it? Will you take the information and apply it to your life and perhaps those closest to you?

You don't have to die early, as my grandfathers did. You have a wonderful purpose in life—to be there for your loved ones. Chase your dreams, and live life to the fullest. When you have a new way of eating, a new way of thinking, and a new way of living, you will become much more than you ever thought possible.

A LITTLE BIT ABOUT ME

I touched on my story at the beginning of this introduction, but now would be a good time to tell you more about myself. As the eldest of two children born to Herb and Phyllis Rubin, I grew up in South Florida. Dad was a naturopathic physician and a chiropractor. Mom was a homemaker who helped Dad with the office chores.

My parents were born after World War II and came of age in the 1960s. While they weren't exactly hippies, they were definitely countercultural. Not only did they adopt the back-to-nature lifestyle (as it was called back then), but my father also promoted it wholeheartedly during my early childhood, while he attended naturopathic medical school and chiropractic school, and later in his chiropractic practice, where he employed a more natural approach to treating patients who saw him for a variety of aches and pains. Unlike many of my parents' peers in the baby-boom generation, eating healthy was not a fad for them. Their motto was, "The more natural, the better," and they filled their cupboards with raw honey, wheat germ, and granola, and their refrigerator with farm-fresh organic fruits and vegetables.

Kids in my neighborhood didn't exactly flock to our house after school because Mom banned potato chips, cookies, and candy bars. But if they wanted a wheatgrass smoothie or a mason jar of homemade plain yogurt, they came to the right place. You could say that I was a granola kid growing up, but whenever I went to school or my friends' homes, I made a beeline for the junk food. Maybe it was the forbidden fruit syndrome at work. At any rate, I can remember trying to trade baby carrots for chips and cookies during school lunch. I never found many takers, though. Some of my classmates were willing to part with some of their chocolate-covered treats for a quarter, however, so I took them up on their generous offer.

Despite my occasional forays into junk food, I grew into a healthy, athletic teenager. I can't recall anything more serious than a cold or flu keeping me out of the classroom. After high school, I attended Florida State University and earned a spot on the cheerleading squad and a place on the Doak Campbell Stadium floor whenever the 'Noles played at home.

Like someone passing through a buffet line for the first time, I put too much on my plate during my freshman year—literally and figuratively. We were expected to practice every weekday for the FSU cheerleading team; miss a day, and you were cut from the squad. I had a full slate of classes, several books to read each week, intramural football games, and various "functions" at my fraternity, Phi Kappa Alpha. I also was a member of a traveling music group for the college ministry.

I tried to eat healthy on campus, but that was pretty much impossible in those days. Breakfast was a softball-sized blueberry muffin or sugar-laden, fat-free yogurt. During my school day, I fell into a burger-and-fries-and-soft-serve-frozen-yogurt routine. On the plus side, I managed to stay away from the party scene because I didn't drink alcohol or do drugs.

After finishing a hectic first year of college, I went back home and picked up a few dollars by being a counselor at a summer youth camp in the area. It was during that time that I started to experience terrible digestive upsets, painful mouth sores, and weakening fatigue.

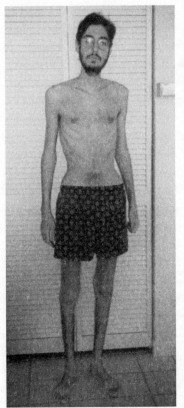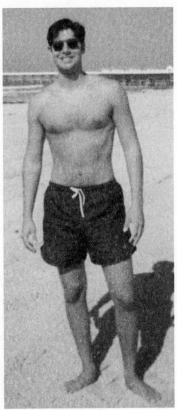

Jordan's experience and results were extraordinary.
Readers should not expect miraculous results.

I hung on as long as I could, but when I couldn't do my job—like helping kids do the ropes course—I knew it was time to see our family doctor. He poked and prodded, then ran a battery of tests. When they came back clean, he shrugged his shoulders and handed me a prescription for two antibiotics. He didn't see any reason why I couldn't return to Florida State in the fall.

If only my body cooperated. The fall quarter was hellacious: 104-degree fevers, listlessness and fatigue, and embarrassing digestive problems. Two months into the football season, I couldn't fool myself any longer. I was really sick.

I called home and described my plight to Mom, who had me fly home the next day. My health steadily worsened over the next six months, including a scary episode with a 105-degree fever that left me speaking gibberish. I was referred to gastroenterologists who felt that my symptoms—vomiting, fever, night sweats, loss of appetite, severe abdominal cramps, and bloody diarrhea—pointed toward a digestive disorder known as Crohn's disease. If I didn't get better soon, one specialist said, I would be a strong candidate for a colostomy, which was the surgical removal of the colon.

At age nineteen, a colostomy sounded like a fate worse than death. In an effort to avoid surgery at all costs, my parents and I embarked on an all-out odyssey to regain my health. Over time, I was seen by seventy doctors and medical practitioners, tried every dietary plan under the sun, and even traveled to Mexico and Germany to seek alternative treatments. My parents tapped into their home equity to cover the $150,000 in medical bills.

Nothing reversed the downward trajectory of my health. My diseases—doctors were also treating me for diabetes, arthritis, anemia, and chronic fatigue syndrome—exacted a heavy toll on my body. After six months, when my weight plummeted to under 110 pounds, I needed a wheelchair to get around the house. How humiliating! I looked like a skeleton after months of wasting away. My lowest point happened when I was hospitalized at Bethesda Memorial Hospital in Boynton Beach, Florida, where I barely survived a harrowing night, as I mentioned earlier.

Nearly two years into the battle for my life, my father happened to have an interesting phone conversation with William Keith, a San Diego nutrition expert. He believed he could help me overcome the chronic digestive diseases plaguing my body—the ones called "incurable" by my doctors.

Intrigued, and figuring I had nothing to lose, Mom and Dad agreed that I should fly out to San Diego and meet with Mr. Keith. My parents purchased a well-used RV so I could get around and have a place to sleep near the ocean. My health rebounded after I began consuming healthy "live" foods that were rich in vitamins, minerals, enzymes, and friendly microorganisms called probiotics—foods that are part of the Maker's Diet for Weight Loss program. Over a forty-day period, I gained 29 healthy pounds and put myself on a path of recovery.

I left San Diego with a renewed sense of purpose and took a job at a health food store that introduced me to the natural health movement. Eager to increase my knowledge, I studied naturopathic medicine and was soon formulating my own nutritional supplements and functional foods. My entrepreneurial spirit prompted me to start a company in my early twenties, and I began formulating and marketing whole-food nutritional supplements, functional foods, and personal care products. In my personal life, I met a beautiful princess named Nicki, whom I married in 1999. After overcoming a two-and-a-half-year stint of infertility, we became the proud parents of Joshua Michael in May 2004. We adopted two newborns in 2008, Samuel and Alexis, so you can see that we're up to our armpits in diapers at the Rubin household.

Today, at the age of thirty-three, I know what my purpose and burning desire is in life: to share my message of health and hope as well as my improbable comeback story. It's a message that I've communicated in *The Maker's Diet* as well as before millions of television viewers and tens of thousands at major conferences throughout the United States, Australia, New Zealand, Malaysia, China, Indonesia, Singapore, South Africa, and the United Kingdom.

All along, my goal has been to impact the health of this world one life at a time, and today that message begins with you. If you are ready for a new way of eating, a new way of thinking, and a new way of living, now's the time to get started.

In our next chapter, we'll talk about how the expansion of American waistlines has been the foreshadowing of all sorts of health challenges today and for the next generation, but before we dive into *The Maker's Diet for Weight Loss*, another introduction is in order.

Introducing Bernard Bulwer, MD

Note from Jordan Rubin: A couple of years ago, I received an e-mail from Dr. Bernard Bulwer, who said he watched several episodes of my half-hour health show on cable TV and liked what I had to say about eating healthy and my prescription for living a long and abundant life. Dr. Bulwer felt we were kindred spirits since he had written a book, *Your Doctor Can't Make You Healthy*, that contained his insights into protecting your health. Dr. Bulwer's book echoed many of the same points I was making.

I soon learned that Dr. Bulwer is a modest man because I practically had to drag out the information that he was an advanced clinical fellow in noninvasive cardiology (echocardiography) at one of the premier teaching hospitals at Harvard Medical School—the Brigham and Women's Hospital. We stayed in contact. After I began writing *The Maker's Diet for Weight Loss*, I felt I needed a medical expert overlooking my shoulder. I wanted to make sure that the science and principles behind this book were medically sound, which is why I asked Dr. Bulwer to review the manuscript and make pertinent observations.

Since I feel it's important for you to get to know Dr. Bulwer, I've asked him to share a little bit about his background.

From Bernard Bulwer

I'm from Belize, Central America, a country the size of Massachusetts, with less than 300,000 inhabitants and English as its official language. My family was large, even by Belize's standards.

My parents had twelve children—and no twins! Though my father and mother never went beyond a basic primary school education, they were exceedingly knowledgeable and intelligent, and they saw eight of their children through to foreign universities across the United States, Europe, Australia, and the Caribbean.

My parents were not "rich" by any stretch of the imagination, but the true wealth they invested in us were those precious things that money can't buy. They taught us the value of hard work, respect for others, and commitment to family. Mom ran a popular restaurant in the neighborhood, and Dad loved farming, but he was best known for the elegant mahogany furniture he built. My father worked hard; two things he despised were laziness and idleness. "The devil finds work for idle hands" was one lesson I learned very early. Today I can say with certainty, and with much gratitude, that these and other lessons have served me well. Included among them is how much I know about food and farming.

Talk about exotic tropical fruits! We didn't have to be coaxed into eating five daily servings of fresh fruit in Belize. Those who've been fortunate enough to experience the tastes and the varieties of our mangoes would know exactly what I mean. If ever a Belize mango could, it would sue an "American mango" for defamation. The call to eat five mangoes in one sitting was normal behavior—indeed too restrictive. So tempting—in both smell and taste—was the local fruit that for many neighbors, the most horrible thing about having fruits in season was that the neighborhood children would not leave their fruit trees alone.

I graduated from high school at age fifteen and pursued premed in zoology, chemistry, and physics, before winning a scholarship to medical school at the regional University of the West Indies in Jamaica and Trinidad. I earned my MD at the age of twenty-four with distinctions in the anatomical and surgical sciences, but I had little desire to spend much of my medical life confined to an operating theater.

Postgraduate studies took me to the University of London at King's College, where I completed a master's degree in nutrition. Specialty training fellowship in diabetes and metabolic medicine (preventive cardiology) in England followed. I had a passionate desire to impart what I learned, so I packed my bags and returned to Belize, where I started the local diabetes association. There, I began educating and empowering the public on how to look after their health. Having served as clinical director of an ambulatory care facility, including being the physician designate for the United States Embassy, I began writing my first book. My activities caught the attention of Dr. David Singer, a visiting Harvard physician, and I was soon invited to pursue fellowship training in Boston in cardiovascular disease.

I finished my U.S. medical licensing exams within months and completed fellowship training in preventive cardiology and later noninvasive cardiology/echocardiography at the Brigham and Women's Hospital, a major teaching hospital of Harvard Medical School in Boston. During this period, I published my first book, *Your Doctor Can't Make You Healthy*—a reflection of my desire to inform readers that their health and health care are two very different things.

The explosion of lifestyle-inflicted diseases that now stalk this nation will not be solved through magical "cures," our preoccupation with prescription drugs, or hospital-based care. Perhaps Don King's "Only in America!" trademark phrase would fittingly describe the frightening scenario of obesity in America, except that obesity does not stop at the water's edge or at the Rio Grande. "When America sneezes, the world catches a cold," goes the saying. Today, people in countries like Belize, and indeed throughout the world, have been seduced into forsaking their traditional organically grown produce in favor of "up market" processed foods. This development has not only upped their waistlines, but it has also upped their medical bills.

Though I am heavily involved in writing medical textbooks and multimedia teaching tools for medical students and doctors for upcoming cutting-edge technologies like ultrasound stethoscope, such cool tools are not the answer to the obesity and heart disease pandemic. The best answers will come when people take more responsibility and better care of their own health.

I made contact with Jordan because he was on the front lines *doing* something—even baring his life's experience and transforming his convictions into what I believe is a pivotal message. This affects people where they live—something that is not the priority at our academic ivory towers. Jordan is doing his part. I hope to do mine, and I sincerely hope you do too. Your health is your biggest investment.

one

Globesity

IN GREEK MYTHOLOGY, Atlas was commonly depicted with a great globe on his shoulders, like some overambitious shot-putter, holding up the world in an agonized asymmetrical position.

If Atlas were holding up the earth today, he'd better truss his loins to lift all of the overweight people inhabiting the planet. For what surely must be a first in the annals of recorded history, demographers have determined that there are more overweight people living among us than those who are undernourished. According to the World Health Organization, one billion adults are overweight (of which 300 million are obese, meaning they weigh at least 50 pounds more than their ideal body weight). At the other end of the spectrum, the number of rail-thin starving and undernourished individuals remains steady at 600 million.[1]

For thousands of years, our forebears eked out an existence that depended upon the sweat of their brows and whether or not nature provided bountiful crops at harvest time. Hunger was their constant companion; famine, their frequent worry. I can't imagine what went through the minds of desperate parents who held their starving, frightened children to their breasts and wondered what they could do to provide something to eat.

The miracle of modernization has taken care of much of that problem, although as someone who supports the relief efforts of Life Outreach and Compassion International, I'm aware that far too many fall asleep each night with gnawing hunger pangs in their growling stomachs. If the World Health Organization's figures are correct, at least one-sixth of the global population has a different dilemma—they're too big from engorging themselves with greasy, high-fat, low-nutrient, chemical-laced, mass-produced foods. The global growth of industry and technology has led to an abundance of cheap, high-calorie meals, unhealthy sugary snacks, and a steep decrease in physical activity, resulting in one of the most blatantly visible, yet most neglected, public health problems in the history of mankind.

The skyrocketing ascent of obesity in both developed and developing regions inspired the World Health Organization to coin a new phrase for this occurrence:

globesity. A nutritional expert for the World Bank warned that if corrective measures aren't taken soon, globesity could become as devastating as malnutrition, especially to the economies of the poorest countries. In other words, the global obesity epidemic could become more harmful to the world community than starvation.[2]

What an astonishing turn of events! I can remember Mom reminding me to clean my plate because of the "starving children in China," but she would have to amend her example if she were raising me today. Ten percent of city-dwelling Chinese children suffer from obesity—a number that's increasing by a shocking 8 percent per year. In Japan, obesity in nine-year-olds has tripled. Twenty percent of Australian adolescents and children are overweight or obese.[3] "The prevalence of obesity in Europe has tripled in the past two decades; half of all adults and 20 percent of all children are overweight," according to an article by the Associated Press.[4]

That's just the tip of a massive iceberg that's threatening to sink the health of young and old from Anchorage, Alaska, to Zurich, Switzerland. The tentacles of globesity reach into every continent and grip every major city in the world. We're seeing hundreds and hundreds of millions who consume Western-like convenience foods shift away from physically demanding jobs in agriculture and devote their growing leisure time to watching TV and surfing the Internet. They're adopting this new lifestyle rather rapidly, unaware that they are putting themselves at risk for chronic diseases that could shave years off of their lives. My colleague Dr. Bulwer says that fast food is everywhere in Belize, where eating "well" means eating like the Americans or the British—the greasy fried foods they see advertised on television.

Another telling example comes from the Japanese, who, after centuries of staying slim on a diet of fish, vegetables, seaweed, fermented soy, and rice, have developed a new millennium sweet tooth for Krispy Kreme doughnuts and Cold Stone Creamery "mix-ins." When the Japanese McDonald's introduced the Mega Mac—a four-patty burger—they sold 1.7 million in four days. The fascination with Yankee junk food is so widespread that the Japanese have coined a phrase—which translates to "in your face food"—to describe their apparent desire to escape the stresses of a pressure-packed society by satiating their stomachs with glazed doughnuts and quadruple-stacked hamburgers.[5]

The Japanese still have a long way to go before they catch up with us, though. Like an Olympic flag bearer, the American contingent is leading the globesity parade. Not only are we the fattest nation on earth, but we're also ballooning to extremely obese proportions at an alarming rate. While most people have heard that two-thirds of American adults aged twenty years and older are overweight (which is defined as having a body mass index, or BMI, of 25 or higher), the number of those who are extremely obese—at least 100 pounds overweight—has *quadrupled* since the 1980s. Twenty years ago, one in two hundred adults were candidates to purchase two seats when traveling on Southwest Airlines; today that number is one in fifty.[6]

If people keep gaining weight at the current pace, U.S. researchers at Johns Hopkins University predict that 75 percent of U.S. adults will be overweight (and 41 percent obese) by 2015, which is just around the corner. "Obesity is a public health crisis," declared Dr. Youfa Wang, who led the study.[7]

HEAVY DEMAND

I haven't met a heavyset person who wouldn't *want* to lose weight, but from my vantage point, many obese individuals harbor attitudes similar to the classic "five stages of grief," as articulated by Elisabeth Kübler-Ross in her seminal book *On Death and Dying*.[8] The five stages are:

1. Denial
2. Anger
3. Bargaining
4. Depression
5. Acceptance

I'm willing to wager that if you're battling your weight, you could place yourself among one of those five descriptions. You could be denying that you're *really* overweight, that all you have to do is set your mind one day to taking off those "extra" pounds on your waist and hips. You could be angry about your lackluster physical condition and appearance, harboring resentment that you've always been heavy or were born into a family that fed you crummy foods growing up. You could be at the bargaining stage, where you'd do anything to lose weight—like undergo expensive gastric bypass surgery or take a pharmaceutical with dangerous and embarrassing side effects. You could be depressed and feel like you have no future and no hope of reaching your ideal weight. Or you could be at the final and most dangerous stage—acceptance, a feeling that you'll always be obese and there's nothing you can do about it.

I'm seeing more evidence that being overweight is a societal norm among the cultural elite. Weight and body image issues are squeezing into college course catalogs as "fat studies" emerge into a growing interdisciplinary field in universities around the country. At Harvard, students can sign up for "Body Sculpting in America," which examines the social and political consequences of being overweight. The University of Wisconsin at Milwaukee offers a course called "The Social Construction of Obesity," which is taught by a human movement sciences professor who challenges the alarmist message about the obesity epidemic in America.

Elsewhere, students on a dozen campuses are organizing groups that focus on promoting "fat acceptance." A San Diego State University graduate student cofounded Size Matters to fight the prevailing attitude that being fat is a moral failure rather than the result of complicated factors. The goal is to get members comfortable with saying, "I'm fat," with a sense of defiance and pride.[9]

I'm all for feeling good about yourself, but for the estimated 72 million dieters in America, a sizable weight-loss industry has stepped into the vacuum. The U.S. weight-loss and diet control market was expected to swell to $58 billion in 2007, according to Marketdata Enterprises, with various options vying for attention:[10]

- Gastric bypass surgery, in which surgeons staple or bind the stomach with an adjustable band. This creates a small pouch able to hold only a few ounces of food. Celebrities such as singer Carnie Wilson, *Today Show* weatherman Al Roker, reality show star Sharon Osbourne, and talk show host Star Jones Reynolds have sung the praises of this potentially dangerous surgery after shedding hundreds of pounds. *American Idol* judge Randy Jackson, who has advised less-than-svelte contestants that they might want to lose some weight, underwent gastric bypass surgery in 2003.[11]

- Commercial chains such as Weight Watchers, Jenny Craig, and NutriSystem, where dieters commit to "customized" diet plans. These structured programs often include "phone meetings" with a trained consultant as well as the consumption of diet meals purchased directly from the company.

- Over-the-counter diet pills such as Xenadrine EFA, CortiSlim, One-A-Day WeightSmart, and TrimSpa, which are heavily advertised on television and radio and in alluring ads in supermarket tabloids. They target the lose-weight-quick crowd with breathtaking copy describing how their "miracle ingredients" and "breakthrough formulas" are "clinically proven" and "guaranteed to work." Anna Nicole Smith, before her untimely death, was a TrimSpa endorser who claimed that she was "hotter than ever" after "just twelve weeks" of taking the diet pill.[12]

- Diet food home delivery, where affluent dieters pay as much as $1,200 a month (per person!) for healthy meals to be delivered daily to their doorstep. A handful of companies such as Chefs Diet, Seed Live Cuisine, and Jenny Direct (part of Jenny Craig) are cashing in on this booming market.

- Weight-loss summer camps for heavy teens, which are a predictable outgrowth of the childhood obesity problem in this country. These types of camps didn't exist in my parents' time because the demand wasn't there. Today, teens seek to turn their lives around at places like Camp La Jolla and Camp Shane.

Adults don't have summer camps, although there are a number of discreet but expensive "fitness spas" that you can check yourself into if you have the time and the *dinero*. In the world of weight loss, anything is possible if you have the money and the opportunity.

Need a Cushy Seat for the Tush?

Talk about a growing market with room for expansion. A host of entrepreneurial companies are marketing products promising to make life comfy and cushy for overweight people. WideBodies Furniture sells oversized sofas, love seats, and chairs. LiftChair.com has introduced recliner chairs that lift and tilt forward so that morbidly obese people weighing as much as 700 pounds can get in and out of them more easily. For those who need a different type of seating, the Big John toilet seat is a full 5 inches wider than the standard 14-inch-wide version—and more receptive to an oversized tush.

Consumer research has helped huge corporations like GM and Ford tailor their products for the growing numbers of overweight people in America. The Detroit automakers have quietly widened seats in their SUVs and light pickup trucks so that heavyset drivers will have "plenty of leg room." You can scroll through Sizewise.com to determine which cars provide the most interior room, but some obese drivers have to take their cars into auto upholstery shops to have seatbelt extenders installed. Those who can't squeeze in behind the wheel have smaller steering wheels mounted at body shops.

Businesses are feeling the weight of heavier customers and employees. Since wide-body jets are carrying a lot of wide bodies these days, the Federal Aviation Administration recently increased its "rule-of-thumb" advisory for calculating the weight of passengers. The airlines now expect male passengers to weigh 184 pounds (a 9-pound increase) and female passengers to weigh 163 pounds (a whopping 18-pound increase).[13] This means the airline industry must top off the tanks with an extra 350 million gallons of jet fuel annually to compensate for the increased "payload."[14] With jet fuel rising to stratospheric heights these days, that's an easy billion-dollar hit to passengers, who must pony up the extra cash to fly. This extra fuel usage hurts not only our economy but our environment as well.

Hospitals, no doubt seeing more obese patients since overweight people are hospitalized more often than the general population,[15] have installed patient hoists in certain rooms. They need the hoists on hand since orderlies cannot lift such large amounts of weight in and out of hospital beds without landing in the hospital themselves—with a hernia.

BEFORE THERE WERE COUCH POTATOES

You could say that we haven't been at a healthy weight for a long time. If I had to pick a date, I would say things started going downhill after 1950. Television, which had been invented, wasn't commonplace, and the term "couch potato" was decades away from joining the American lexicon. *Monday Night Football, Thursday Night*

Football, Super Saturday College Football, Sunday NFL doubleheaders, and Chris Berman had yet to be invented. Fast-forward more than a half-century, and televised sports has exploded, changing us from a nation of doers to a nation of *watchers*.

Football is merely the top dog among a pack of televised sports barking for attention. The others are baseball, basketball, hockey, golf, auto racing, tennis, soccer, and even poker, which is considered a sport by some. Extreme sports like the X Games and Nathan's Famous Hot Dog Eating Contest also compete for eyeballs in a five-hundred-station universe. Women have plenty of shows to keep them occupied as well: *Oprah*, *Rachael Ray*, and Lifetime movies, to name a few.

The U.S. government didn't start keeping records of how much Americans weighed until 1960, when the first National Health and Nutrition Examination Survey was completed. From that baseline, the National Center for Health Statistics says that adult men and women are roughly an inch taller than they were nearly fifty years ago but nearly 25 pounds heavier on average. The average BMI among adults has increased from 25 to 28.[16]

Meanwhile, the average weight for men aged twenty to seventy-four years rose dramatically from 166.3 pounds in 1960 to 191 pounds in 2002, while the average weight for women the same age increased from 140.2 pounds in 1960 to 164.3 pounds in 2002. Though the average weight for men aged twenty to thirty-nine years increased by nearly 20 pounds over the last four decades, the increase was greater among older men:[17]

- Men between the ages of forty and forty-nine were nearly 27 pounds heavier on average in 2002 compared with 1960.
- Men between the ages of fifty and fifty-nine were nearly 28 pounds heavier on average in 2002 compared with 1960.
- Men between the ages of sixty and seventy-four were almost 33 pounds heavier on average in 2002 compared with 1960.

For women, a similar trend occurred:[18]

- Women aged twenty to twenty-nine were nearly 29 pounds heavier on average in 2002 compared with 1960.
- Women aged forty to forty-nine were about 25.5 pounds heavier on average in 2002 compared with 1960.
- Women aged sixty to seventy-four were about 17.5 pounds heavier on average in 2002 compared with 1960.

Meanwhile, the report documented that average weights for children are also increasing:[19]

- The average weight for a ten-year-old boy in 1963 was 74 pounds; by 2002 the average weight was nearly 85 pounds.

- The average weight for a ten-year-old girl in 1963 was 77 pounds; by 2002 the average weight was nearly 88 pounds.
- A fifteen-year-old boy weighed 135.5 pounds on average in 1966; by 2002 the average weight of a boy that age increased to 150.3 pounds.
- A fifteen-year-old girl weighed 124.2 pounds on average in 1966; by 2002 the average weight for a girl that age was 134.4 pounds.

I know that was a ton of statistics to roll out, but the key point to remember is that Americans these days, on the average, carry around 25 to 35 pounds of extra weight. The extra poundage taxes our health and portends all sorts of difficulties, some immediate, some long ranging, and some permanent—like death.

"America's weight problem is rapidly overtaking cigarette smoking as the leading cause of preventable death," according to the Centers for Disease Control.[20] If you're 25 pounds too heavy, you're three times more likely to develop coronary heart disease, two to six times more likely to develop high blood pressure, and three times as likely to get type 2 diabetes. Heavier people are also at higher risk for developing arthritis, gout, gallbladder disease, and the Big C—cancer. (See sidebar on page 20.)

The health risks associated with obesity are formidable. Let's take a closer look from descriptions provided by the Cleveland Clinic physicians behind WebMD .com.[21]

Heart disease and stroke

Heart disease and stroke are the leading causes of death and disability for people in the United States. Overweight people are more likely to have high blood pressure, a major risk factor for heart disease and stroke, than people who are not overweight. High blood levels of LDL or "bad" cholesterol can also lead to heart disease and often are linked to being overweight. Being overweight also contributes to angina (chest pain caused by poor blood flow to the heart) and sudden death from heart attack or stroke without any prior warning signs or symptoms.

Diabetes

Type 2 diabetes reduces your body's ability to control blood sugar. It is a major cause of early death, heart disease, stroke, and blindness. Overweight people are twice as likely to develop type 2 diabetes compared to normal-weight people.

Cancer

Several types of cancer are associated with being overweight. In women, these include cancer of the uterus, gallbladder, cervix, ovary, breast, and colon. Overweight men are at higher risk for developing colorectal cancer and prostate cancer.

Gallbladder and liver disease

Gallbladder disease and gallstones are more common if you are overweight. Your risk of disease increases as your weight increases. Most gallstones are cholesterol-rich. When the cholesterol level in bile (stored in the gallbladder) increases, so does the risk of cholesterol stones. Increased production and excretion of cholesterol by the liver into the bile occurs in obesity.

Osteoarthritis

Osteoarthritis is a common joint condition that most often affects the knees, hips, and lower back. Carrying extra pounds places extra pressure on these joints and wears away the cartilage (or tissue that cushions the joints) that normally protects them.

Cancer and Being Overweight by Bernard Bulwer, MD

We all know that excess pounds raise the risk of heart disease, hypertension, diabetes, stroke, arthritis, and gallbladder disease, but few fixate on the relationship between obesity and cancer. According to the American Cancer Society, obesity is linked to cancer of the colon and rectum, esophagus, stomach, pancreas, liver, kidney, as well as multiple myeloma and non-Hodgkin's lymphoma.[22] These are mainly cancers of the gastrointestinal system, a reflection of what goes into our mouths. In women, obesity increases the risk of death from breast, uterus, cervical, and ovarian cancer. Obese men are at increased risk from prostate cancer. Note that obesity increases the risk of cancers that tend to target our reproductive organs.

Normally, our bodies repair themselves in an orderly fashion, with cell repair and replacement carefully monitored by in-built checks and balances. Excess body fat or adipose tissue, however, is more than just fat that sits idle; it is a major source of harm and mischief. Body fat is a major producer of the female hormone called estrogen. It also obstructs or interferes with the action of insulin—the major hormone regulator of how our bodies handle the food we eat. This spells double jeopardy because your body is suffering at least twice for the same offense. Higher levels of insulin and estrogen, which encourages cell proliferation, may be a time bomb. Unregulated cell growth is the cardinal feature of cancer, with abnormal precancerous or cancerous cells mushrooming into growth that we call tumors or cancer.

Cancer cells have two things in common: (1) they may grow uncontrollably, causing damage where they originate; and (2) worse still, they have the ability to metastasize, or spread to other parts of the body. For example, breast, bowel, or kidney cancer may more likely cause death from being spread to the brain rather than the original cancer itself.

Since cancer, by definition, occurs when damaged or abnormal cells assault the body, researchers have determined that some factors *inhibit* or *promote* the growth of cancer in the body. Examples of *inhibitors* would be nutrients found in fruits and vegetables, as well as properly raised meats and wild-caught fish. Drinking plenty of water allows the kidneys and liver to operate at full capacity and flush waste and toxins out of the body's digestive and urinary tracts, which is where cancer cells tend to congregate.

On the other hand, examples of *promoters* would be smoking cigarettes, eating highly refined high-sugar foods, feasting on fried foods rich in trans-fatty acids, or coming into contact with cancer-causing substances, also known as carcinogens. Tobacco smoke, pesticides, air pollution, and industrial chemicals (such as asbestos) can trigger the initiation of cancer, which can take years to develop into a mass and many more years to detect. This is all the more reason to adopt the principles of *The Maker's Diet for Weight Loss*.

While environmental elements behind cancer are significant, at the end of the day, lifestyle factors are the main causes of cancer. While genetics and family history do play a role (between 5 and 10 percent of all cancers are clearly hereditary), the choices in the food we eat, the amount of time we exercise, the hygiene we practice, the stress we undergo, and the otherwise imbalanced lives we lead account for about 65 percent of cancer deaths in the United States, according to researchers at the Harvard School of Public Health.[23]

Gout

Gout, a disease that affects the joints, is often triggered by high levels of a substance called uric acid in the blood. Obesity causes higher uric acid levels. Uric acid crystals can precipitate in the joints, causing severe joint pain, as well as in the kidney, causing kidney stones and chronic kidney disease.

Sleep apnea

Sleep apnea is a serious breathing condition associated with being overweight. Sleep apnea can cause a person to snore heavily and to stop breathing for short periods during sleep. Sleep apnea may cause daytime sleepiness and even heart failure.

Whether it's one of the big three—cancer, cardiovascular disease, or diabetes—shuffling through life weighing more than you should *will* cut years off your life. A team of University of Illinois researchers recently stated that rising obesity rates could reverse life expectancy gains, which would be the first time this has happened since the U.S. government began keeping track of life expectancy in 1900. Obesity significantly increases the risk of premature death; among the severely obese, life expectancy is reduced by an estimated five to twenty years, according to one government study.[24]

Life expectancy in the United States is now at a high of 77.6 years, but according to a study published in the *New England Journal of Medicine*, that could mean—and I have to emphasize the conditional here—that the generation of my preschool-aged son, Joshua, could live two to five years less.[25] Current trends indicate that the prevalence of obesity will continue to rise and affect ever-younger age groups.

Seven Truths to Think About

According to obesity specialist Gus Prosch Jr., MD, a physician who practiced in Birmingham, Alabama, until his death in 2005, there are seven truths about obesity.[26] Think about each declaration for a moment before moving on to the next one:

1. If you're obese, you have a lifetime disease.
2. Your metabolic processes will always tend to be abnormal.
3. You cannot eat what others eat and stay thin.
4. Anyone can lose weight and stay slim provided the causes of weight gain are determined, addressed, and corrected.
5. Understanding insulin metabolism is the key to losing weight intelligently.
6. There is absolutely no physiological requirement for sugar or processed foods in your diet.
7. You must address all the contributing factors causing obesity.

You cannot lose weight and keep it off successfully by strictly and solely following any special diet, by taking a weight-loss pill, or by following an exercise program. In order to succeed in the fight against obesity, you must realize that losing weight must involve a major lifestyle change.

The good news is that you can *extend* your life by reaching and maintaining the weight that's healthiest for you. Using data from a large federally funded assessment of obesity rates, the researchers calculated how much longer life expectancy would be if everyone who were currently obese were to lose enough weight to obtain an optimal body mass index of 24. Under such a scenario, the authors "conservatively estimated" that the average life expectancy of 77.6 would be extended by four to eleven months longer for white men, four to ten months longer for white women, four to thirteen months longer for black men, and three to nine months longer for black women.[27]

Putting aside life extension for a moment, achieving your ideal weight can begin to reverse the ravages of obesity *now*. These benefits in quality of life—less arthritis pain, lower blood pressure, improved diabetes control, or even reversal, coupled with less dependency on prescription drugs—can occur when you lose weight by following the Maker's Diet program.

TAKING INVENTORY

Most people don't have to guess whether they are at their ideal weight. A glance into a full-length mirror without clothes on usually provides the answer. At the same time, it's helpful to know your body mass index (BMI), the size of your body frame, and what percentage of body fat you're carrying so that you can soberly face the music.

Let's first examine the BMI, a fitness-scale method that has become the measurement of choice for physicians and researchers who study obesity, although the results have to be interpreted with some caution, as I'll explain shortly. The BMI uses a mathematical formula that takes into account a person's height and weight. As a strict formula, the body mass index equals a person's weight in kilograms divided by height in meters squared. For those of you keeping score at home, that's $BMI=kg/m^2$.

You may be saying to yourself, "I haven't done any equations since tenth grade trigonometry, and besides, I don't know my weight and height in the Euro form of measurements."

Have no fear. On page 26 is a converted body mass index chart using inches and pounds. Just find your height in the left-hand column, and then swish your finger over to your weight. The column above your weight (a number between 19 and 40) is your BMI.

The BMI breakdown goes like this:

- 18 or lower: underweight
- 19–24: normal
- 25–29: overweight
- 30–39: obese
- 40–54: extremely or morbidly obese

As an example, someone standing 5 feet 10 inches tall and weighing more than 209 pounds would have a BMI of 30, earning him or her a classification of obese on the body mass index scale. About 30 percent of the U.S. adult population has a BMI of 30 or more,[28] which is why we have an obesity epidemic. Medical experts say that to be "morbidly obese" means having a body mass index, or BMI, of at least 40.

As I hinted at previously, the BMI is not a perfect measurement of where you stand with your weight. I offer myself as an example. I stand a little more than 72 inches tall (that's 6 feet) and weigh 184 pounds. My finger finds number 72 in the left-hand column, slides over to the 184 box, and that tells me I have a BMI of 25.

So am I a tad pudgy with a BMI of 25, which, according to the BMI scale, is borderline overweight? No, because I perform FIT—Functional Interval Training exercises. (You'll learn about this breakthrough exercise program in chapter 9.)

I think you also have to weigh—pardon the pun—the BMI against your body frame size. Some folks are slight of stature; others are flat-out larger than others. Dr. Bulwer says this is the major fault of the BMI. You can have skinny legs and an obese abdomen and still have a normal BMI. On the other hand, a BMI of 25 or 26 ranks you as "overweight" just because you're pear shaped. This, in itself, is not an unhealthy condition.

The simplest—but least accurate—method to calculate your frame size is to grab your wrist with the other hand and try to touch your thumb and index finger where the wrist meets the hand. If your fingers do not touch, you're a big-boned person with a large body frame. If your thumb and index finger just meet, you have a medium frame. If they overlap, you have a small frame.

The more scientific approach involves calculating the ratio of one's height in inches to the circumference of the wrist measured in inches. Yes, I know this sounds complicated, but I'll use myself as an example again. I'm 6 feet, or 72 inches, and my wrist circumference measures 7 inches. By dividing 7 into 72, I come up with a numeral: 10.28. According to the chart below, I have a medium frame, which sounds about right.

Perform this test on yourself. The wrist measurement should be taken where the wrist meets the hand. Divide your height by the wrist measurement. The results:

For women

- 11 or higher: small frame
- 10.1 to 10.9: medium frame
- 10 or lower: large frame

For men

- 10.4 or higher: small frame
- 9.6 to 10.3: medium frame
- 9.5 or lower: large frame

Many people overlook the fact that their skeletal frame dictates the size and shape of their body. If you are genetically predisposed to having a large frame, no matter what diet you follow or how much exercise you do, you will not safely drop your weight below a certain point.

Now that you know what body frame you have, you should apply that knowledge to the following tables calculated by the Metropolitan Life Insurance Company:

FOR MEN				
HEIGHT		FRAME		
Feet	Inches	Small	Medium	Large
5	2	128–134 pounds	131–141 pounds	138–150 pounds
5	3	130–136 pounds	133–143 pounds	140–153 pounds
5	4	132–138 pounds	135–145 pounds	142–156 pounds
5	5	134–140 pounds	137–148 pounds	144–160 pounds
5	6	136–142 pounds	139–151 pounds	146–164 pounds
5	7	138–145 pounds	142–154 pounds	149–168 pounds
5	8	140–148 pounds	145–157 pounds	152–172 pounds
5	9	142–151 pounds	148–160 pounds	155–176 pounds
5	10	144–154 pounds	151–163 pounds	158–180 pounds
5	11	146–157 pounds	154–166 pounds	161–184 pounds
6	0	149–160 pounds	157–170 pounds	164–188 pounds
6	1	152–164 pounds	160–174 pounds	168–192 pounds
6	2	155–168 pounds	164–178 pounds	172–197 pounds
6	3	158–172 pounds	167–182 pounds	176–202 pounds
6	4	162–176 pounds	171–187 pounds	181–207 pounds

FOR WOMEN				
HEIGHT		**FRAME**		
Feet	Inches	Small	Medium	Large
4	10	102–111 pounds	109–121 pounds	118–131 pounds
4	11	103–113 pounds	111–123 pounds	120–134 pounds
5	0	104–115 pounds	113–126 pounds	122–137 pounds
5	1	106–118 pounds	115–129 pounds	125–140 pounds
5	2	108–121 pounds	118–132 pounds	128–143 pounds
5	3	111–124 pounds	121–135 pounds	131–147 pounds
5	4	114–127 pounds	124–138 pounds	134–151 pounds
5	5	117–130 pounds	127–141 pounds	137–155 pounds
5	6	120–133 pounds	130–144 pounds	140–159 pounds
5	7	123–136 pounds	133–147 pounds	143–163 pounds
5	8	126–139 pounds	136–150 pounds	146–167 pounds
5	9	129–142 pounds	139–153 pounds	149–170 pounds
5	10	132–145 pounds	142–156 pounds	152–173 pounds
5	11	135–148 pounds	145–159 pounds	155–176 pounds
6	0	138–151 pounds	148–162 pounds	158–179 pounds

What column do you fall into? The fact of the matter is that you may have to lose less weight than you thought, and that's a good thing. Or you may have to lose more than you thought, based on our next criteria—body fat.

What a Waist!

Did you know that the circumference of your waist, not your overall weight, is one of the leading indicators of mortality related to being overweight? For women, a generally recommended waist size is 32½ inches—with an increased risk of health consequences occurring when the waist size exceeds 35 inches. For men, a generally recommended waist size is 35 inches—with dangerous health consequences increasing when 40 inches is reached and exceeded.

BODY MASS INDEX FOR ADULTS TABLE

	NORMAL						OVERWEIGHT					OBESE									
BMI	19	20	21	22	23	24	25	26	27	28	29	30	31	32	33	34	35	36	37	38	39
HEIGHT (INCHES)	BODY WEIGHT (POUNDS)																				
58	91	96	100	105	110	115	119	124	129	134	138	143	148	153	158	162	167	172	177	181	186
59	94	99	104	109	114	119	124	128	133	138	143	148	153	158	163	168	173	178	183	188	193
60	97	102	107	112	118	123	128	133	138	143	148	153	158	163	168	174	179	184	189	194	199
61	100	106	111	116	122	127	132	137	143	148	153	158	164	169	174	180	185	190	195	201	206
62	104	109	115	120	126	131	136	142	147	153	158	164	169	175	180	186	191	196	202	207	213
63	107	113	118	124	130	135	141	146	152	158	163	169	175	180	186	191	197	203	208	214	220
64	110	116	122	128	134	140	145	151	157	163	169	174	180	186	192	197	204	209	215	221	227
65	114	120	126	132	138	144	150	156	162	168	174	180	186	192	198	204	210	216	222	228	234
66	118	124	130	136	142	148	155	161	167	173	179	186	192	198	204	210	216	223	229	235	241
67	121	127	134	140	146	153	159	166	172	178	185	191	198	204	211	217	223	230	236	242	249
68	125	131	138	144	151	158	164	171	177	184	190	197	203	210	216	223	230	236	243	249	256
69	128	135	142	149	155	162	169	176	182	189	196	203	209	216	223	230	236	243	250	257	263
70	132	139	146	153	160	167	175	181	188	195	202	209	216	222	229	236	243	250	257	264	271
71	136	143	150	157	165	172	179	186	193	200	208	215	222	229	236	243	250	257	265	272	279
72	140	147	154	162	169	177	184	191	199	206	213	221	228	235	242	250	258	265	272	279	287
73	144	151	159	166	174	182	189	197	204	212	219	227	235	242	250	257	265	272	280	288	295
74	148	155	163	171	179	186	194	202	210	218	225	233	241	249	256	264	272	280	287	295	303
75	152	160	168	176	184	192	200	208	216	224	232	240	248	256	264	272	279	287	295	303	311
76	156	164	172	180	189	197	205	213	221	230	238	246	254	262	271	279	287	295	304	312	320

	EXTREME OBESITY														
BMI	40	41	42	43	44	45	46	47	48	49	50	51	52	53	54
HEIGHT (INCHES)	BODY WEIGHT (POUNDS)														
58	191	196	201	205	210	215	220	224	229	234	239	244	248	253	258
59	198	203	208	212	217	222	227	232	237	242	247	252	257	262	267
60	204	209	215	220	225	230	235	240	245	250	255	261	266	271	276
61	211	217	222	227	232	238	243	248	254	259	264	269	275	280	285
62	218	224	229	235	240	246	251	256	262	267	273	278	284	289	295
63	225	231	237	242	248	254	259	265	270	278	282	287	293	299	304
64	232	238	244	250	256	262	267	273	279	285	291	296	302	308	314
65	240	246	252	258	264	270	276	282	288	294	300	306	312	318	324
66	247	253	260	266	272	278	284	291	297	303	309	315	322	328	334
67	255	261	268	274	280	287	293	299	306	312	319	325	331	338	344
68	262	269	276	282	289	295	302	308	315	322	328	335	341	348	354
69	270	277	284	291	297	304	311	318	324	331	338	345	351	358	365
70	278	285	292	299	306	313	320	327	334	341	348	355	362	369	376
71	286	293	301	308	315	322	329	338	343	351	358	365	372	379	386
72	294	302	309	316	324	331	338	346	353	361	368	375	383	390	397
73	302	310	318	325	333	340	348	355	363	371	378	386	393	401	408
74	311	319	326	334	342	350	358	365	373	381	389	396	404	412	420
75	319	327	335	343	351	359	367	375	383	391	399	407	415	423	431
76	328	336	344	353	361	369	377	385	394	402	410	418	426	435	443

BMI Categories

- Underweight = < 18.5
- Normal weight = 18.5–24.9
- Overweight = 25–29.9
- Obesity I = 30–34.9
- Obesity II = 35–39.9
- Obesity III = 40>

Courtesy of National Heart, Lung, and Blood Institute, National Institutes of Health

BODY FAT DISTRIBUTION

It's helpful to know how much body fat your torso contains, because new research is showing that your body fat—not just your body weight or BMI—is a better indicator of how healthy you are. This has generated new terms like apple- or pear-shaped obesity, or scientific terms like the metabolic syndrome or the insulin resistance syndrome. The different terms arose from different ways of measuring or describing mainly the same issue.

We all need some fat on our bodies since fat regulates body temperature, cushions and insulates our organs and tissues, and is the main form of the body's energy storage. However, there is a problem when there is extra fat stored in the body, which translates into extra weight and causes the heart to work harder.

Fat circulates in your blood, and if you were to take a vial of blood and let it sit in a corner, a fatty layer would rise to the top. The difference between what makes you fat or thin is not the amount of fat cells but the size of those cells. The fat globules within each cell increase as you store more fat. Muscles work the same way; you don't make more muscle cells—the muscle cells get larger when you exercise.

Much of the fat absorbed via the intestines gets stored in the *omentum*, which is a fatty apron or curtain that hangs from your stomach. The omentum stores fat that's quickly accessible to the liver but causes bad cholesterol and triglyceride levels to rise. It also takes insulin out of circulation, causing your blood sugar to rise. The more omentum fat present, the more abdominal obesity, high blood pressure, high cholesterol, and other risks associated with coronary artery disease.

Most fitness clubs have skin fold calipers that give a snapshot measurement of body fat by measuring a pinch of skin in several strategic areas of your body:

- Triceps (back of the upper arm)
- Chest (between the arm line and nipple)
- Subscapula (below the edge of the shoulder blade on the back)
- Waist (slight to the right of the navel)
- Suprailium (over the hip bone)
- Thigh (halfway between the hip and knee joints)

At least two measurements should be taken at each site to gain an accurate reading, and some measurements will vary depending upon your sex. If you don't belong to a fitness club, you can go online at find any number of body fat tests that you can take at home. You'll need a cloth tape measure to measure the circumference of your waist, hips, forearm, and wrist.

Once you have a number, compare it to the list on the next page prepared by the American Council on Exercise, which has categorized ranges of body fat percentages as follows:

BODY FAT PERCENTAGE		
DESCRIPTION	**WOMEN**	**MEN**
Essential fat	12–15%	2–5%
Athletes	16–20%	6–13%
Fitness	21–24%	14–17%
Acceptable	25–31%	18–25%
Obese	32%+	25%+

Subcutaneous fat vs. visceral fat

If you're reading *The Maker's Diet for Weight Loss* because you want to do something about the flabby tire around your midsection, then it's time to target the two kinds of fat in your body: subcutaneous fat and visceral fat.

Much of the fat we see in others and ourselves is subcutaneous fat—that jellylike layer of fat found underneath the skin that gives people their pudgy look and men their famous beer bellies. Gender plays a major role in determining where your body stores subcutaneous fat: for most men, it's their bellies; for women, it's the hips and thighs.

Visceral fat, on the other hand, is found deep inside your body in the abdominal cavity, not just under your skin like subcutaneous fat. This type of fat may even infiltrate the internal organs, which contributes to a wide range of health complications. Visceral fat carries a reputation in the medical community as a "killer fat." The pesky cellulite padding on your thighs won't lead to your demise; it's what lies beneath—the visceral fat, which is also known as white adipose tissue.

Golfer Phil Mickelson, whose soft midsection stands out in contrast to flat bellies like Tiger Woods's, thinks he knows the difference between the two types of fat. "The one thing I wish was different about me was that I wish I had visceral fat instead of subcutaneous fat," he told one interviewer.[29]

Actually, Phil should be careful what he wishes for because this deeper, underlying fat, which clamps on vital organs like barnacles, is more likely to increase the risk for heart attacks than subcutaneous fat, according to researchers from Johns Hopkins Medical Institutions.[30] Visceral fat, or white adipose tissue, is also medically linked to various metabolic diseases like diabetes, and it may even present health risks for those who don't appear to have an ounce of fat on their bodies. Often invisible to the naked eye, visceral fat could be more dangerous than the "saddlebag" fat hanging on the frames of the overweight.

Dr. Jimmy Bell, a professor of molecular imaging at Imperial College in London, England, and his team scanned nearly eight hundred people with MRI machines to create "fat maps" showing where people store fat. The results were surprising: those who maintained their weight through diet rather than exercise were more likely to have major deposits of internal fat.[31]

Researchers at the Duke University Medical Center found that energetic exercise can significantly reduce your visceral fat. Lead author Dr. Cris Slentz said that the more people exercised, and the higher the intensity, the faster they lost their excess visceral fat.[32] Short, intense workouts, not low-impact walks through the neighborhood or light steps on a treadmill, are foundational to my fitness plan described in chapter 9. I've followed a program called Functional Interval Training (FIT), with a heavy emphasis on short spurts of intense exercise, followed by rest periods, that will burn both peripheral (subcutaneous) and visceral fat during and after your workout. As for those with the more noticeable subcutaneous fat, this book's dietary approach, with its emphasis on eating foods from organic sources and staying away from processed, high-sugar treats, will do something about the fat that everyone sees because of the reduction in caloric intake and the increase in fiber and nutrients.

GET ON BOARD

The point of this discussion about the BMI, body frame size, and body fat is that no "ideal weight" can be applied across the board. God created everyone differently, and our bodies change shape as we grow older. While I don't think anyone can tell you what your ideal weight should be, the Pew Research Center reports that dieters say they are 29 pounds heavier than they would like to be.[33] If that number sounds like it's in your ballpark, then embarking on the Maker's Diet for Weight Loss program—and sticking to it—will move you much closer to your weight-loss goals, help you feel much better about yourself, and even change the world around you.

I want to help you lose weight, but before embarking on any decision to get healthier and shed pounds, you should have a whole host of support around you. Begin with your health professional, especially if you have a family history of heart disease or other medical illnesses. Be sure to include your family as well as friends and co-workers who seek only the best for you. You do *not* need critics or negative people to be included in your network. They will only drag you down.

So how can you lose that weight? In a nutshell, here are three guidelines for doing so—which are expanded upon in the rest of this book:

1. Maximize food; minimize nonfood

Losing weight is not necessarily eating less; it's about eating more intelligently—more of the "right" foods. Our bodies were designed with a biological instinct of how our bodies originally looked and functioned best. Knowledge and application of this fact is key to successful weight loss.

2. Maximize life; minimize life drainers

The plan for attaining and maintaining your ideal weight is individualized, even though it is important to include accountability and collaboration during this endeavor. You can't discuss weight issues without exploring the reasons why your individualized brain, hormones, and emotions may drive you to overeat. Take responsibility for your body—love it and then lose the weight—by yourself *or* with the help of others.

3. Maximize care; minimize carelessness

You need to understand how and why the body naturally stores fat—to protect itself in times when it needs to provide energy in the absence of food. The balance of nutrition and eating times and intervals, as well as types of foods, all figure into successful and sustained weight management.

Eating right (and frequently) with consistent functional integrative exercise is key to successful and sustained weight management. *The Maker's Diet for Weight Loss* can work in ways that will teach your body to eat and work smart—resulting in "trimming the fat." Beginning in chapter 3, you will find out the foods you should be eating so that you can live a leaner and healthier life.

Losing weight does not have to be a complicated, difficult, and starvation-like experience that becomes drudgery and causes you to lose hope instead of weight. You will learn that your diet and exercise program can be easily integrated into your life and be easily sustained. Your DNA is not necessarily your destiny in determining your weight and health. In fact, through diet and exercise, you can once and for all win the battle against chubbiness.

Before we get into specifics of the foods you should eat, the nutritional supplements you should take, and the sustainable lifestyle you should lead, we should talk about why many diets don't work, the often-untold drawbacks of gastric bypass surgery, and how the media shape our perceptions, which we'll do in our next chapter, "What Are You Failing For?"

The Maker's Diet for Weight Loss Recap: Globesity

1. If present trends continue, the percentage of overweight American adults will increase from 67 percent to 75 percent by 2015, portending profound effects on individuals, families, and even the nation's public health.
2. Many who have been overweight for years or decades exhibit attitudes mirroring the five stages of grief: denial, anger, bargaining, depression, and acceptance.
3. Since 1960, American adults weigh—on average—between 25 to 30 pounds more than they did in 1960.
4. Scientific researchers fear that rising obesity rates could mean that children born in this decade could see their expected life expectancy drop by two to five years.

5. The body mass index (BMI) is the standard measurement for determining whether you're overweight or obese, but it's important to submit to other criteria such as body frame size and body fat.
6. There are two types of fat in the body: subcutaneous fat and visceral fat. The fat you can't normally see—visceral fat—can actually be more dangerous to your health than the fat you can see around people's midsections—subcutaneous fat.

two

What Are You Failing For?

S TOP ME IF you've heard these clichès before.
- You have to eat a sensible diet and start exercising.
- Eat less and move more.
- Make healthy food choices and join a fitness club.

It's not difficult to decode most diet books. Many work on the principle of cutting 500 calories a day and burning another 500 on the treadmill. Keep that up for seven days, and the deficit of 7,000 calories results in the net loss of two pounds per week.

No one will argue with the admonition to get your buns moving, but simply cutting calories doesn't work for long. Continuous calorie restriction almost always backfires because your body thinks it's starving to death, so your brain sets off a chain of chemical processes, including the slowing down of the body's metabolic rate. A sluggish metabolism, however, allows the body to become *more* efficient at storing fat. When you stop eating rabbit food—or whatever the "special" diet calls for—and resume the consumption of your favorite edibles, your much slower and inefficient metabolism can't keep up. Bottom-line result: you gain the weight back even faster, even though you may be eating less than you were before you embarked on the diet.

"You can initially lose 5 to 10 percent of your weight on any number of diets, but then the weight comes back," said Traci Mann, a UCLA associate professor of psychology who analyzed thirty-one studies that followed people on diets for two to five years. In fact, said Ms. Mann, several studies found dieting was a consistent predictor of *future* weight gain. When asked what overweight people should do, Ms. Mann replied, "Eating in moderation is a good idea for everybody, and so is regular exercise."[1]

I disagree with this simplified, two-front approach, as you'll see in later chapters of *The Maker's Diet for Weight Loss*. But since it is universally agreed upon that 95 percent of all diets fail,[2] which only keeps overweight people in bondage and despair, what's the biggest reason why mainstream diets are so universally unsuccessful?

I think it's because dieters get too hungry.

The primal urge to open our mouths and receive sustenance is a survival instinct that materializes from physiological and psychological needs. For example, when the clock says it's noon, many people salivate like Pavlov's dog and automatically become hungry. Hunger is also triggered by our senses, like the smell of frying potatoes or an alluring TV advertisement promoting a grilled chicken panini sandwich. Whatever the reason, the brain's thalamus in the limbic system—the seat of human motivation and emotions—converts the sensory information into a palatable craving. Depending on how hungry you become, that longing can range from "I think I'll snack on something" to "I'm hungry! I've got the munchies!" Very few can resist the siren call of food, glorious food, as Oliver Twist and his orphan colleagues sang.

No matter how hard you try to be "good," no matter how much you watch what you eat, satiating the appetite will overwhelm every instinct you have (except the will to live, of course). That's why simply slashing calories doesn't cut it and is doomed to failure. Physiologically speaking, hunger begins in the brain when the limbic system determines that the body is low in blood sugar, or glucose. Most of the food you eat is converted into glucose, much of which is converted by the liver into fat for later use. When glucose levels are low, the liver sends signals to the hypothalamus— the small but vital gland at the base of the brain below the thalamus—that blood sugar levels have dipped precipitously. The hypothalamus, in turn, triggers stomach contractions or hunger pangs, demanding a fill-up. When nothing happens, nasty growling noises ensue. The hunger cravings can drive you batty, making you feel light-headed and irritable. An oft-quoted proverb says it well: *The spirit is willing, but the flesh is weak.*

Scientists have known that the hypothalamus plays a key role in regulating food intake and body weight since the 1940s, but it's only been in recent years that they've discovered how a pair of "hunger hormones" secreted by the body—leptin and ghrelin—also reduce *or* spike hunger pangs. The hormone leptin, which is generated by fat cells, sends crucial signals to the brain's "satiety center" to stop eating when the stomach is full, kind of like a yellow light at an intersection. The trouble is that many with weight problems have conditioned their bodies to ignore the internal cautionary reminder to stop grazing at the buffet table. With each additional bite, they speed past the intersection of appropriate satisfaction, which is the epicurean equivalent of running a red light—and just as foolhardy and dangerous.

As overweight people build up a resistance to the appetite-suppressing effects of leptin, levels of leptin continue to drop, which makes them even *hungrier*, says obesity expert Mary Dallman, PhD, from the University of California at San Francisco. This is another explanation for why many dieters eventually regain all the weight they lost.[3]

On the other hand, the hormone known as ghrelin *increases* appetite. Released primarily in the stomach, ghrelin levels rise dramatically before you eat, then plays a leading role in determining how quickly hunger strikes back after noshing on a snack or meal. When your stomach feels empty, ghrelin levels spike again, which explains why you're ready to raid the refrigerator at midnight. Those who maintain a deprivation diet dial up the intensity of their hunger pangs, which prompts the body to secrete even *more* ghrelin. Any remaining willpower to "be good" melts in the face of such a hormonal onslaught.

All is not lost, however. Of the two hormones, leptin—the appetite suppressor— appears to be the bigger player in our bodies' energy balance. While one of leptin's duties is to inform the brain that the body has enough energy stores such as body fat, for some reason, many obese people don't respond to leptin's signals even though they have higher levels of leptin because they are desensitized or resistant to its effects. Those who need to lose the most weight are often the ones with the biggest appetites. Life becomes a vicious circle: as overeating causes weight gain, the body's ability to regulate its hunger hormones is reduced even more.

The most important thing you can do is recognize the body's yellow caution signals and take your foot off the gas when your stomach feels just right—satiated. Consciously ask yourself, "Am I full yet? Have I had enough to eat?" When you feel a sense of satisfaction, set the knife and fork on the plate and take a break. It will take time—as well as discipline—to become aware of the yellow caution lights. It may mean allowing yourself only one pass through the buffet table or saying no to seconds when offered at a dinner party. You must stop eating when you feel satisfied.

Word Play

Readers of the *Washington Post* newspaper are asked each year to participate in its annual "neologism" contest, where contestants are asked to supply alternate meanings for common words. Sample: *balderdash* (n.), a rapidly receding hairline. Here are two entries that relate to what you may be feeling:

1. flabbergasted (adj.), appalled over how much weight you have gained
2. abdicate (v.), to give up all hope of ever having a flat stomach

---

BETTER PLAN

People often follow the path of least resistance when hunger strikes by reaching for something convenient—a bag of salty potato chips or a bowl of candy—even though they know deep down that processed snacks and chocolate-coated treats will set them back. Reaching your ideal weight will involve *choosing something better* to eat rather than a quick fix to squelch hunger pangs.

The quick fix is the staple of today's 24/7 broadcast and print media—television, radio, and magazines, as well as the Internet. Not only are the mainstream media famous for having all the answers in a thirty-second sound bite or a "how-to" article, but also TV talk shows and women's magazines love promoting whatever's new in the weight-loss world—especially if a celebrity author is flacking a "new" diet.

Listen, I would appreciate any media attention for *The Maker's Diet for Weight Loss*, although I'm not convinced that the media's short attention span will "get" what we're trying to accomplish here. They certainly haven't shown us why low-fat and low-carb diets—the two biggest dietary regimens of the last fifteen years—are ultimately destined to fail.

Back in the early 1990s, the conventional wisdom in the media was that foods containing *any* fats were to be avoided. If you were a teenager back then (as I was), you probably read influential articles in *People* and *Parade* magazines about how bad fat was for you. Your supermarket dairy case was public enemy number one: no butter, no eggs, no whole milk.

Media coverage at the time planted the notion that if you wanted to lose weight, then eating foods without fat would do the trick. Young girls took that advice to heart, believing they would be as thin as the supermodels taking flight down the runways of Milan and Paris if they eliminated fat from their diets. In a demonstration of the law of unintended circumstances, however, low-fat diets led to an unprecedented leap in anorexia and bulimia among weight-conscious teen girls.

One of the media darlings behind the low-fat craze was an over-the-top woman with a platinum buzz cut named Susan Powter. Her mantra could be summed up in two sentences:

- "Stop the insanity!"
- "It's fat that's making you fat!"

Taking their cue from Ms. Powter, scores of magazine articles and newspaper features sang the praises of a low-fat, high-carbohydrate diet. Impressionable high school girls nodded their heads in agreement and gobbled up anything with the magic words *fat free* or *reduced fat* printed on the packaging: cheese, crackers, cookies, yogurt, and ice cream. In high school, I can remember the cheerleaders studying the labels on packets of salad dressing to detect the presence of fat grams. Food manufacturers responded to this fascination with low-fat foods by flooding supermarket aisles with thousands of reduced-fat and nonfat products. Restaurants revamped their menus with low-fat entrees to suit the changing tastes of health-conscious consumers.

Did a low-fat diet make us any thinner? No, I'm afraid not. The problem with reduced-fat cookies and fat-free cream cheese was more than their low taste: these convenience foods had nearly the same amount of calories as the "full-fat" versions. People would eat more reduced-fat cookies because they thought they could, not knowing that food makers often replace the fat in snack foods with extra sugar, flour, and other waist-bulging ingredients.

After low-fat diets fizzled, the media was ready to pounce on the next get-thin-quick idea. They waited until the summer of 2002, when reporter Gary Taubes wrote a lengthy article in the *New York Times Magazine* about Robert Atkins, a Manhattan cardiologist who authored *The Atkins Diet Revolution* in 1972. The thrust of the *New York Times* article was that American doctors who recommended eating less fat and more carbohydrates—in other words, the essence of the low-fat diet—had it all wrong. Instead, it was low-carb diets that worked. Like a lone voice in the wilderness, "the unrepentant Atkins was right all along," Taubes declared.[4]

That was all that editors at the country's largest women's magazines—who live in the Big Apple and read the *New York Times* religiously—needed to jump on the Atkins bandwagon. Overnight, *Glamour, Redbook,* and *Cosmopolitan,* as well as NBC's *Dateline,* CBS's *48 Hours,* and ABC's *20/20,* cranked out features extolling the benefits of a low-carbohydrate, high-protein, high-fat diet. Readers and viewers learned that increasing their intake of protein from sources such as meat, fish, and dairy and reducing their intake of carbohydrates like bread, pasta, and rice would cause their bodies to burn excess body fat for fuel. Many dieters thought they had died and gone to heaven because they could gorge themselves with steaks, lobster, bacon, cream sauce, cheese, and eggs to their heart's content.

Overweight folks definitely lost weight following the Atkins diet, but they could never sustain a low-carbohydrate regimen. They got too hungry—the Achilles' heel of many a diet—and when they fell off the Atkins bandwagon, they fell hard. Many binged on carb-heavy junk foods and gained all the weight right back—plus a few pounds more. That didn't stop the unquestioning media from changing its generally positive coverage of *Dr. Atkins' New Diet Revolution* as well as two other low-carb diets: *The South Beach Diet* by Miami cardiologist Arthur Agatson, MD, and *The Zone* by Barry Sears, PhD. It wasn't until Atkins Nutritionals, a company founded by the late Dr. Atkins that produced a line of low-carb convenience foods, snacks, and condiments, filed for bankruptcy protection in 2005 that the bloom fell off the low-carb rose.

UNREALISTIC EXPECTATIONS

Unwittingly or not, feature stories and airbrushed advertisements set unrealistic expectations of what your ideal weight should be by highlighting celebrities and fashion models with tiny waists, large breasts, and great legs. Thin is in and has been for a long time. Wallis Simpson, the Duchess of Windsor and fashion icon from the 1930s, is famous for saying, "You can never be too rich or too thin."

With PhotoShop these days, digital photos are routinely manipulated to accentuate the positive, like the time a *GQ* cover shot of "healthy-sized" actress Kate Winslet was digitally altered to lengthen her legs and flatten her stomach. (The British film star was not pleased. "Like it or lump it, I'm not a twig and refuse to be one," she said.[5]) Another criticism leveled at today's advertising is the portrayal of unobtainable body images. We are so accustomed to seeing shirtless hunks with chiseled abs and bikinied women with knockout figures that we feel inadequate because we don't resemble them at all.

Consider these facts:

- By the time a girl is seventeen, she has seen more than 250,000 messages about what she is supposed to look like.
- Twenty years ago, the average model weighed 8 percent less than the average American woman. Today, the average model weighs 23 percent less.
- The average American woman is 5 feet 4 inches tall and weighs approximately 165 pounds. The average American model is 5 feet 11 inches tall and weighs 117 pounds.
- A survey of college-aged women found that those who read magazines and watched television programs glamorizing thinness were more likely to have an eating disorder.
- Twenty-seven percent of girls openly admit that the media pressure them to have a perfect body.
- A Harvard University study showed that up to two-thirds of underweight twelve-year-old girls considered themselves too fat.
- By age thirteen, at least 50 percent of girls are unhappy with their appearance. As many as 10 million females and 1 million males are currently struggling with an eating disorder in the United States alone.
- Forty percent of newly identified cases of anorexia are in girls aged fifteen to nineteen.
- Fashion models are 25 percent thinner today than models forty years ago.[6]

To achieve their ultra-skinny state, fashion models binge, purge, use laxatives, smoke, drink diet soda, and overexercise. These activities trigger a cascade of molecules in their blood to help them rebound from their severe diets, which causes them to overeat all over again. Thus they binge, purge, and diet even more rigorously. This turns into an ugly cycle that works in opposition to their body's natural chemical construction.[7]

Maybe Susan Powter's catchphrase—"Stop the insanity!"—needs to make a comeback. Fashion shows from Milan and Paris to London and New York are grappling with whether or not they should ban stick-thin models with BMIs less than 18.5 from the catwalk. Spanish officials in Madrid passed an ordinance doing just that after the eating-disorder deaths of two young models, Luisel Ramos, of Uruguay, and Ana Carolina Reston, of Brazil. Ms. Reston, who was 5 feet 8 inches tall and 88 pounds when she died, reportedly lived on a diet of apples and tomatoes in the weeks before her death.[8]

The point of these stories is that *no one* is satisfied with their weight when they focus on media-driven standards of appearance. Wherever you are on your journey to a healthier weight, it's more important to take control of your health than worry about what others think of how you look.

ADVERTISING FOR DOLLARS

The media stay in business by selling advertising, and advertising works. Pizza delivery companies aren't stupid: on football weekends, they stack their cheesy ads in the first half and wait for the orders to pile in. Domino's typically sells more than one million pizzas on game days.[9]

Advertising foods to kids is like shooting fish in a barrel. Have you ever wondered why your kids pester you into buying something they want? A Federal Communications Commission task force made up of FCC officials; members of the food, television, and advertising industries; and consumer health experts began studying the link between viewing habits and childhood obesity in 2007. It will be interesting to read the final report. Since the FCC estimates that children watch between two and four hours of TV per day and view a barrage of 40,000 TV ads every year—most of them for sugary cereal, candy, and fast food—I'm not sure what conclusion could be rendered except for the obvious: a barrage of junk food ads spurs sales of junk food.[10]

Soft drink makers, cereal makers, and candy makers target kids because they want them to become "brand loyal" consumers who will stay with the brand for their entire lifetimes. So billion-dollar titans square off like it's *Wrestlemania*: Pepsi vs. Coke or McDonald's vs. Burger King. Your kids are not the winners. Studies show that:

- American kids consume more than one-third of their daily calories from soft drinks, sweets, salty snacks, and fast food.
- Ads targeted to kids twelve and under lead them to request and consume high-calorie, low-nutrient products.
- A preschooler's risk of obesity jumps 6 percent for every hour of TV watched, 31 percent if the TV is in their bedroom.[11]

The reason junk food advertisers saturate the airwaves is because they're aware that children have "pester power," a unique ability to nag their parents into buying something they want. If your children are not at a healthy weight, you should limit their exposure to junk food advertising. Whether or not you're nodding your head in agreement, it's my contention that children aren't eating healthy because their *parents* aren't eating healthy.

Did I strike a nerve?

MY BIG FAT GREEK FRIEND

Another topic receiving favorable media coverage is gastric bypass surgery, where you'll read nary a contrary word. To illustrate my concern with gastric bypass surgery, let me tell you about Nick Yphantides, MD, a San Diego family physician and author of *My Big Fat Greek Diet*.

One evening as we ate dinner together, he regaled me with a remarkable story of how he lost 270 pounds—and it wasn't by having his stomach stapled.

His story begins when Dr. Yphantides (a Greek name pronounced *ee-FAHN-tee-dees*) would treat indigent patients—mainly Hispanics—at a community health clinic in his hometown of Escondido. After a long day of office visits, he liked to reward himself by driving through his favorite fast-food joint, one that had a cultlike following in California—In-N-Out Burger. His order was always the same: a "4 x 4," large fries, and a Coke.

The "4 x 4"—four hamburgers and four slices of American cheese stacked in a hamburger bun with all the sauce and trimmings, plus the deep-fried fries and a 16-ounce soft drink—contained 1,400 calories and 100 grams of fat, but that didn't bother Dr. Nick a bit. In his mind, the drive-through forays were just a snack, something to eat *before* dinner.

Dr. Nick had been gaining mounds of weight ever since medical school in the early 1990s, when he fortified his late-night study sessions with snack cakes and heaping bowls of rocky road ice cream. During interminable forty-hour shifts as an intern, he continually raided the hospital break room, where someone had set out a plate of sweets to be shared by the attending staff.

When Dr. Nick entered the public health arena as a family physician, he could be charitably described as "corpulent." He couldn't tell you how much he weighed, though, because he had stopped weighing himself. His expanding girth actually turned into an occupational blessing: his patients viewed Dr. Nick as a larger-than-life advocate for the poor, the big man with a big heart who cared for his community in a big way.

Overweight patients *loved* Dr. Nick because they knew they would receive tea and sympathy from someone who also shopped at the "big-and-tall" sections of department stores. From a doctor's perspective, he was always gracious with those who struggled with their weight. More than a few times, he looked a heavyset woman or large fellow in the eye and said with a smile, "Do as I say, not as I do."

Shortly after he turned thirty years of age, however, Dr. Nick began experiencing declining health and a host of unusual symptoms that led him to a doctor's examination room. A week later, he learned the bad news: he had testicular cancer. (Remember how I talked about the link between cancer and obesity in the previous chapter?)

The surgical excision of the right testes and aggressive radiation over twelve weeks saved his life—and caused some soul-searching. The way Nick saw it, he had dodged the cancer bullet, but there was another round in the chamber: his gargantuan weight had to be causing incredible amounts of stress on his organs—heart, lungs, and liver—as well as his skeletal frame. He wondered how much stress he was putting on his knees, which were bearing such a severe load.

One day, Nick planted his feet on two scales—one for each leg. Each needle came to rest on "233½." A fourth-grader could do the math: Dr. Nick Yphantides, the jolly doc with the Santa Claus-like image, weighed in at a hefty 467 pounds.

Nick was scared. His cancer had forced him to face his mortality, and now he was sure that each bite of a burger brought him one swallow closer to the grave.

Something needed to be done. Nick was tired of dressing in XXXXL T-shirts. Tired of booking uncrowded red-eye flights so that he wouldn't have to buy a second seat. Tired of gawkers staring at his monstrous midsection in restaurants. Ahead of him was a future filled with high blood pressure, high cholesterol, and debilitating diabetes—unless he made a radical lifestyle change and lost a ton of weight. Well, maybe not a ton, but 200 pounds would be a good start, he figured.

In April 2000, Nick gave notice that he would be stepping down and leaving the Escondido Community Health Center for one year. Then he began formulating a game plan. Since he wasn't going to work, he needed something to do—a diversion to keep his mind off being so hungry. That's it! Nick loved baseball, so he decided to drive around the country and visit all thirty major league ballparks and watch baseball games. He calculated that he had been consuming 5,600 calories a day to maintain his weight. To lose weight slowly but surely, he would embark on a liquid diet—drinking a protein meal supplement offering just 800 calories a day, which is not exactly the eating plan recommended in *The Maker's Diet for Weight Loss.*

On April 1, 2001, Nick sailed off in a used RV, a vehicle he christened the USS *Spirit of Reduction*, with the intention of becoming half the man he used to be. His father rode shotgun as an accountability partner. Going cold turkey from food gave Nick the shakes, just like any junkie coming down off a high. "I was so hungry at the ballpark that I would have eaten a cigarette butt dipped in mustard," he said.

At first, the pounds melted off Dr. Nick like a snowman standing in the Sahara Desert—17 pounds in the first week. After that initial surge of encouragement, his weight loss went from a gusher to a steady drip-drip as he continued to drink his protein shakes. He settled into an average of 1.1 pounds lost per day.

When Nick returned home in time for Thanksgiving, his mother was shocked by his appearance. Some of his nieces and nephews didn't even recognize him. Nick, now weighing 269 pounds, had shed nearly 200 pounds. He ate his first solid food in nearly eight months on Thanksgiving Day: some vegetables and a baked potato.

He continued to lose weight as he returned to solid food and his medical practice, and at one point, he was down to a svelte 197 pounds—270 pounds less.

When I met Dr. Nick, he looked great. His weight had settled in at 220 pounds. To this day, though, Nick said he still meets colleagues and acquaintances who casually ask him, "So, how did the surgery go?"

How did the surgery go?

They automatically assume that the only way Nick could have lost all that weight was by submitting to gastric bypass surgery, which is a radical form of "stomach reduction" or "bariatric" surgery. Such surgeries are aimed at either reducing the stomach size (by gastric banding or stapling) or bypassing the stomach altogether (gastric bypass).

In the last decade, hundreds of thousands of overweight people have barged down the doublewide doors of surgical centers in major cities around the country and had their stomachs stapled. Gastric bypass procedures have increased rapidly since 1998, when 14,000 were performed,[12] to a whopping 177,000 in 2006, according to the American Society for Bariatric Surgery.[13]

The reason for the explosive growth has been the development of laparoscopic surgical techniques, which have made the invasive procedure less risky to the body. Gastric bypass surgeons staple the stomach—or bind it with an adjustable band—so that a small pouch is created to hold two or three ounces of food. This restricts food intake and interrupts the normal digestive process. People experience the sensation of being full after a few bites of food; if they eat any more, they often become nauseated.

A normal stomach can hold three pints of food or twenty-four ounces of food, which is a large plate of food. Gastric bypass surgery reduces the stomach to one-tenth of the size it used to be, so you'll lose weight because you can't eat any more. You don't have to be a brain surgeon to figure out that you're going to feel full very quickly.

The concept behind gastric bypass and gastric banding certainly sounds good: since most overweight people don't have the self-control they need to eat the way they should, let a team of doctors do some surgical rearranging of the stomach's gut to help them out. Several aspects to gastric bypass surgery, however, greatly concern me. I've met plenty of folks who've undergone the procedure, and I can see desperation written all over their faces. Their stories are almost universally the same: after losing a modest amount of weight, the pounds are coming back and they don't know what to do. They are like the baseball manager who's already used his last relief pitcher, but his team's getting shelled and there's no one left in the bull pen to call into the game. It's the same with gastric bypass: once you shrink-wrap your stomach, you're out of medical options.

THE NEXT STEP

Following the principles outlined in *The Maker's Diet for Weight Loss* will give you a greater chance to reach your ideal weight than submitting to an uncertain medical procedure. Beginning with the next chapter, I'll get into specifics for:

- What you should eat
- What you should drink
- What you should snack on
- The importance of regular cleansing
- The key role of nutritional supplements
- Embarking on a FIT exercise program—Functional Interval Training
- The role of emotions and eating
- Ways to take weight off your world by adopting simple sustainability

A CLOSING THOUGHT

Remember, the aim of *The Maker's Diet for Weight Loss* is not to look like Kate Moss or even Kate Winslet. The goal is to reach a weight that makes you look and feel good about yourself and that will promote good health for the rest of your life.

I probably don't have to remind you that the way you view yourself—your self-image—has a profound effect on your weight. Your self-image is a combination of all the ideas you have formed about yourself over the years. Ever since childhood, you have developed a set of beliefs about who you are, what you look like, what you are worth, and what you deserve. These beliefs, over time, became part of your subconscious and help define who you are today.

The way you view yourself can be influenced by your self-talk and/or beliefs dictated by others, but only if you allow them to be. Thankfully, your self-image and the subconscious mind can be reprogrammed, as Dr. Nick told me. Over time, the subconscious mind will accept any thought you regularly think about yourself. Therefore, if you start to have positive thoughts, your self-esteem rises, and you feel better about who you are.

Next time you look in the mirror, don't zero in on the negative things you see. Find something you like and focus on that. As you begin to lose weight, say positive things to yourself like: "I can see the weight coming off, and I feel good about my results so far."

I've spoken with people who have reached their ideal weight but still had a negative view of their body and themselves. Self-worth is not equated with what the scales say; it is more about who you are. Your self-worth is measured in terms of the positive things you bring to people and events around you.[14] So find out what motivates *you* and be about it!

If there were an easier way to lose weight and change your life, someone would have found it by now. Losing weight should make you feel better about yourself, but don't forget the health benefits that come from a reduced risk of heart attack, diabetes, stroke, and cancer. Acting upon the information contained in *The Maker's Diet for Weight Loss* will likely improve your chances of living a longer, healthier, and, hopefully, happier life.

The Maker's Diet for Weight Loss Recap: What Are You Failing For?

1. The standard diet-book advice to cut calories and walk on a treadmill like a hamster rarely works over the long haul because dieters get too hungry. When they go back to their old comfort foods, the pounds—and then some—always seem to come back.
2. Low-fat diets don't work because these foods often have the same amount of calories as their "regular" versions.
3. Thanks to advances in laparoscopic surgical techniques and a growing population of overweight candidates, gastric bypass surgery—also known as "stomach stapling"—has become a viable option for the obese. The procedure has its risks, and some lose a modest amount of weight before the pounds start creeping back.

Section I

MAXIMIZE FOOD AND MINIMIZE NONFOOD

three

Eat for Your Ideal Weight

OLEDO, OHIO'S, FAVORITE son—and biggest homegrown celebrity—is Jamie Farr, who played the comical role of cross-dressing Corporal Klinger on the hit TV show *MASH*. Often clothed in a spring dress with pumps and pearls, the otherwise dutiful orderly with the 4077th Mobile Army Surgical Hospital unit perpetually angled for a Section 8 discharge.

One of the inside jokes was that Corporal Klinger was a Lebanese-American from Toledo, just like the real-life Jamie Farr. In several *MASH* episodes, Klinger rhapsodized about the chili-and-hot-pepper hot dogs found at Tony Packo's Cafè, located in the Hungarian/Polish neighborhood of East Toledo. Another Toledo restaurant, though, had an even more special place in Jamie Farr's heart, as he described in the coffee-table book *Toledo: Treasures and Traditions*. Here's what the famous Hollywood actor wrote in the introduction:

> And who could forget one of the favorite meeting—and eating—places for the young and old, Chili Mac's. For a quarter, you could get the greasiest chili (or, some said, the chilliest grease) served on a mound of spaghetti and lined with the stalest soda crackers anywhere. You'd leave the joint with the worst heartburn—but with the best taste and best bargain in town. It always reminded me of one of Will Rogers' lines: about how chili was the world's most economical food because you eat it once and enjoy it for three days. Sadly, Chili Mac's is now but a memory.[1]

Although I haven't arrived at an age where I can appreciate nostalgia, I chuckled when I read Mr. Farr's reminiscences—and grimaced at the same time. His story demonstrates that dining out hasn't changed much in fifty years: you can serve the general public just about anything, and they'll eat it as long as it tastes good going down and is easy on the wallet.

What *has* changed, though, is the restaurant scene. Beginning in the 1950s, greasy spoons like Chili Mac's closed down in droves after they couldn't compete with a new innovation—the fast-food restaurant and its assembly-line menu. When

Ray Kroc opened the first McDonald's in 1955, he set the stage for a massive overhaul in the way Americans eat. "Great-tasting food at a reasonable price in a clean environment" became the mission statement of the fast-food industry. The success of McDonald's sired a stampede of imitators and matured into a colossal industry that collected $142 billion—that's *billion*—in 2006, according to the National Restaurant Association.[2]

Just in my parents' lifetime, fast-food restaurants have become as common as streetlights and exist as destination points on every main boulevard and thoroughfare in America. From the crack of dawn to late-night runs, between 20 and 25 percent of the U.S. population regularly passes through a drive-through lane or lines up at the counter to order something quick and tasty.[3] With 250,000 quick-serve restaurants to choose from, Americans fork over more money on burgers, burritos, and bacon-topped sandwiches each year than what we spend on higher education, new cars, and computers combined.[4]

Commuters start their day with an Egg McMuffin, a Krispy Kreme doughnut, or an Einstein bagel. At noontime, they'll join their work colleagues at Burger King or Taco Bell for a "value meal." For dinner, they'll sit down with their families and share a Papa John's deep-dish pizza delivered to their doorstep. These mundane, everyday examples demonstrate how much eating out—and ordering in—has become entrenched in our culture. A little more than half of our "food dollar"—the money budgeted to feed us and our family—is tossed away on restaurant food, compared with 25 percent in 1955.[5]

Our fast-food nation is hooked on greasy fried foods, captivated by sugar and sweets, and relatively clueless about what's healthy to eat. This obliviousness has exacted a heavy toll on our national health. The scientific research on obesity is unanimous on this, but a casual stroll through a crowded stadium on a Sunday afternoon would confirm that America, land of the free and home of the brave, has a star-spangled obesity problem.

Frankly, we are an unhealthy people who haven't learned to discern. We traipse down supermarket aisles, pulling colorful and enticing boxes off the shelves and dropping them into the cart without a second thought—or a first thought regarding where the products came from, what the ingredients are, or how healthy they are to eat.

Brightly lit, gleaming supermarkets are the end product of something I call the food-industrial complex, which is patterned after the term "military-industrial complex," an expression coined by President Dwight Eisenhower in his farewell address. Just as the phrase *military-industrial complex* referred to the close and symbiotic relationship between the nation's armed forces, private industry, and political interests in Washington, today's food-industrial complex is comprised of big agriculture, mammoth food production companies, media advertising and tie-ins (one example: the Tostitos Fiesta Bowl college football game), and a sophisticated retail network that works together to grow, harvest, produce, market, and sell fresh, frozen, and processed foods to 300 million Americans every day.

The good news is that we don't have a major hunger problem in this country, thanks to this interlocking economy. The bad news is what the food-industrial complex has wrought: homogenized, highly processed, and manufactured "products" of modern food science that are peddled to the masses for as cheaply as possible and to last on the shelves for as long as possible, thanks to chemical preservatives. More than 300,000 different processed foods and beverages compete for our food dollars in this country—and 116,000 of those have been introduced since 1990.[6] It seems like every one of those 300,000 foods and drinks is on display whenever I step into a convenience store to pay for a gas fill-up.

No wonder our national taste buds have been manipulated by zillions of sweet and salty foods ready to be eaten or heated up in a microwave oven. Just about anything that comes in a box or a bottle is sweetened with sugar or high-fructose corn syrup or soaked in sodium. The strategy has worked: we're hooked on greasy foods high in calories, high in fat, high in sugar and salt, and—as a young Jamie Farr believed—high in taste. We're exiting convenience stores, supermarket checkout lines, ice cream stands, and fast-food restaurants with palate-pleasing foods pumped up with excess calories, and that's a root cause of our national health problems.

Making a Lifestyle U-Turn

I know what you may be saying: "But, Jordan, I don't want to go on a diet—diets don't work."

Here's the deal: if I followed you into a grocery store, shopping trip after shopping trip, week after week, month after month, I would see you purchasing the same thirty to fifty foods over and over again. The same milk. The same cereal. The same bread. The same meat. The same TV dinners. The same soft drinks. The same snacks. The same frozen vegetables, and the same occasional fruit and salad.

Each day you and your family eat the same things over and over again. In other words, you're already on a diet, and yours just stinks.

When it comes to a dietary strategy for winning the battle of the bulge, the most important step you can take is a lifestyle U-turn in what you choose to eat. You do that by following two fundamental principles for losing weight. They are:

- Eat what God created for food.
- Eat foods in a form healthy for the body.

Eating foods that God created means shopping for foods as close to the natural source as possible. I'm talking about:

- A wide array of organically grown fruits and vegetables
- Healthy dairy products like yogurt, cheese, and butter
- Healthy red meats like organic grass-fed beef, lamb, venison, and bison
- Cold-water fish caught in the wild
- Pastured or free-range chicken
- Whole grains like wheat and barley
- Nuts and seeds

These foods are part of the Weight Loss Eating Plan, which I share in chapter 7. This sixteen-week plan has four phases and involves a comprehensive yet simple eating plan that will march you toward your weight-loss goals. That information, combined with a personal hydration program, proactive snacking, nutritional supplements, and a breakthrough exercise program comprise the total Maker's Diet for Weight Loss program.

As you can probably guess, I'm a proponent of natural foods grown organically and sustainably. Organic means the fruit or vegetable was grown without the use of most synthetic and petroleum-derived pesticides and fertilizers, antibiotics, genetic engineering, irradiation, and sewer sludge for three consecutive years. Organic meats must come from animals that eat 100 percent organic feed without any animal by-products; for dairy cows, the whole herd must have eaten organic feed for the previous twelve months. As for the term *sustainably*, this refers to a system of farming that maintains and replenishes soil fertility without the use of toxic and persistent pesticides and fertilizers. Livestock are pasture raised and grass fed, and fish are not pulled from the ocean faster than they can reproduce or caught in ways that destroy other sea life or undersea habitats.

The U.S. Department of Agriculture set standards that producers and handlers must follow in order to be certified organic. The green-and-white USDA seal stamped "100% Organic" means just what you think it would: the food or product is comprised of 100 percent organic ingredients. A simpler "Certified Organic" designation means that the product is comprised of at least 95 percent organic ingredients, while a "Made with Organic Ingredients" label means at least 70 percent of the ingredients must be organic; the remaining 30 percent cannot include any biotechnological crops that have been genetically modified, meaning that scientists fiddled with the plant's genetic composition to boost crop yields or resistance to certain pests. Genetically modified grains (called GMOs since they come from genetically modified organisms) have been a source of international controversy because of questions about their environmental safety, so stick to organic as much as possible.

Organic is the popular buzzword these days as word gets around that there's a much healthier option to eating processed foods and meals-on-the-go. Sales of organic groceries have skyrocketed at an astonishing rate of nearly 20 percent annually for the last seven years, and industry experts are forecasting continued rapid growth in the next decade.[7] Progressive markets like Whole Foods, Wild Oats, Bristol Farms, Sprouts, and Sun Harvest have sprouted up like spring mushrooms in downtown storefronts and suburban malls to meet the surging demand for organic foods.

Beware of Frankenfood

If you pull a box of breakfast cereal off the supermarket shelf, there's a strong chance you would see that the grains came from genetically modified (GMO) crops, which are created in the laboratory by taking genes from one organism and inserting them into another to make them grow higher, larger, denser, and more resistant to insect infestation. While this is a laudable goal, the problem is that scientists are adding a gene to a food that wasn't originally part of that food, which is unnatural and changes the DNA character of the crop. "You just can't get an elephant to mate with a corn plant," said Margaret Mellon of the Union of Concerned Scientists. "Scientists are making combinations of genes that are not found in nature."[8] My friend Jeffrey Smith, author of the groundbreaking book *Genetic Roulette*—which I highly recommend— quipped that GMO should stand for "God, Move Over."

While the science behind this technology is breathtaking, it's also stunning how quickly GMO crops have made it into the food chain. U.S. acreage has grown substantially in the last decade: today, 89 percent of soybeans, 83 percent of cotton, and 61 percent of corn are genetically engineered to resist weed-killing chemicals or help the plants make their own insecticides.[9]

While you won't find many GMO whole fruits or vegetables in your local supermarket—watch out for seedless watermelon and seedless grapes, however—it's estimated that 75 percent of the processed foods in this country (breakfast cereals, baked goods, vegetable oils, and so on) contain a potpourri of genetically modified ingredients.[10] I find this to be an amazing development because GMO crops such as corn, soybeans, and potatoes have only been around since the mid-1990s. I wouldn't be surprised if 100 percent of processed foods are made with GMO elements a decade from now.

As an aside, you can determine if your produce is GMO by looking at the sticker plastered on the fruit or vegetable. These little stickers contain different PLU codes that tell you whether the fruit was conventionally grown, organically grown, or genetically engineered. (PLU stands for Price Look Up and is a standard number in the United States, Canada, Europe, Australia, and South Africa.) The PLU code for conventionally grown fruit consists of four numbers, organically grown fruit is five numbers prefaced by the number 9, and GMO fruit is five numbers but prefaced by the number 8.

For example:

1. A conventionally grown PLU would be 4446
2. An organically grown PLU would be 94446
3. And a genetically modified PLU would be 84446

Proponents of GMO foods believe they are riding the wave of the future, but I'm worried that we may be unleashing a form of "agricultural asbestos" on the American public. Genuine concerns about GMO foods have been raised worldwide, particularly in Europe, where they refuse American GMO imports. I will not purchase, or knowingly eat, foods produced from genetically modified ingredients until we have a solid body of research regarding the short-term and long-term effects of eating GMO foods— and that doesn't look like it's happening any time soon. Until then, my family and I will sit on the sidelines and continue to shop for organic fruit, vegetables, grains, and meats. Besides, just on taste alone, organic foods have genetically modified crops beat by a country mile.

Nicki and I do the bulk of our food shopping at two places: Nutrition S'Mart, a small chain of Florida health food stores, and Whole Foods, a luminous 39,000-square-foot natural foods market that's packed with organic fruits, vegetables, dairy products, breads, cereals, canned soups, frozen pizza, ice cream, tortillas, chips, and dip—everything a regular supermarket would stock. The notable difference between a Whole Foods and a regular grocery store is that the former only sells products, for the most part, that are either natural or organic.

Americans are increasing their consumption of organic foods for a variety of reasons. More than half of the respondents to a major poll said they believe organic foods are better for the environment (58 percent) and better for their health (54 percent). Almost one in three Americans (32 percent) believes organic products taste better, and 42 percent believe organic foods are better quality.[11] Americans also cite health as a key motivation in food purchases, declaring that they are eating healthy food to avoid illness later in life.

Good and Healthy vs. Bad and Unhealthy

Eating healthy, organic whole foods will give you the most nutritious, healthy fuel you need to attack the day *and* reach your ideal weight.

Consider these points:

- Good, healthy foods satiate you, are nutrient dense, make you feel and look younger, decrease inflammation in your body, and help put an end to yo-yo dieting.
- Bad, unhealthy foods make you hungrier, are nutrient deficient, prematurely age you, increase your body's inflammation levels, and perpetuate the yo-yo dieting pattern.
- Good, healthy foods are nutritional gold mines and contain no refined or processed carbohydrates and no artificial sweeteners.
- Bad, unhealthy foods are nutritional wastelands and contain genetically modified ingredients, unnatural additives, and potentially dangerous preservatives.
- Good, healthy foods come from natural and organic sources and are raised humanely and sustainably.

- Bad, unhealthy foods are produced by assembly-line workers in white lab coats or teens in hair nets, manning fast-food kitchens.
- Good, healthy food takes time to prepare.
- Bad, unhealthy food is prepared in a hurry and often subjected to ionizing radiation.

Food Additives and the Chinese Connection

China exports a lot more than cheap toys and plush animals to the United States. In the last decade, China has become the world's leading supplier of food flavorings and preservatives. China exported $2.5 billion of food ingredients to the United States and the rest of the world in 2006, a staggering 150 percent increase from just two years earlier.[12] The reason? Because they're cheaper, which fattens the bottom line of mega-huge U.S. food makers.

Here's a look at three of the most common food additives imported into the United States from China:

1. Citric acid, used to give foods a tart taste and enhance fruit flavors, is used in soda, fruit-flavored beverages, candy, and flavored syrups.
2. Sorbic acid, a preservative that inhibits the growth of mold and yeasts, is used in cheese, baked goods, and wine.
3. Vanillin, an ingredient often made from wood pulp, is used in chocolates and cookies as an artificial vanilla flavor.

Foods that God created and in a form healthy for the body contain far fewer calories, and calorie restriction with optimal nutrition is an important component of the Weight Loss Eating Plan in chapter 7. As a way of example, you consume only 60 calories when you eat one of these foods as a snack, according to the Mayo Clinic:[13]

- One small apple
- One-half cup of grapes
- Two plums
- Two tablespoons of raisins
- One and one-half cups of strawberries
- Two cups of shredded lettuces
- One-half cup of diced tomatoes
- Two cups of spinach
- Three-fourths cup of green beans

On the other hand, a Cold Stone Creamery treat—a medium-sized mocha ice cream with Reese's Pieces and Oreo cookies mixed in and topped with pistachio nuts—comes out to a whopping 1,150 calories, or *twice* the amount of calories contained in *all* the fruits and vegetables I just listed!

"But, Jordan," you may be saying, "if you're telling me to just eat more fruits and vegetables to lose weight, it can't be this simple." Well, just so you know, I'm not advocating a diet of strictly low-cal fruits and vegetables, which doesn't provide the body with the full slate of nutrients that it needs. What I'm saying is that too many of us—when given the choice—will choose ice cream for dessert rather than a bowl of fresh strawberries. I guess it's true what Irish dramatist and novelist Oscar Wilde said years ago: "I can resist anything but temptation."

Eat Less and Live Longer?

These days, I'm intrigued by a concept called "calorie restriction with optimal nutrition," or CRON. The idea is that reducing the intake of calories by 20 percent to 40 percent will improve health and extend your lifespan.

It's a concept that's been studied since the 1930s in laboratory settings. One of the researchers, Dr. Roy Walford of the UCLA pathology department, conducted experiments in which laboratory mice were given less and less to eat—but always enough to live on. Surprisingly to Dr. Walford, the deprived mice lived longer than their well-fed counterparts.

Dr. Walford then wondered if the same theory held true for humans. Offering himself as a human lab experiment, the research scientist voluntarily chose to eat very little for more than twenty years. His search for the fountain of youth led to a dietary regimen that consisted of small servings of low-fat milk shakes, vegetable salads, fish, and baked sweet potatoes. His daily calorie count of 1,600 was about half the 3,000 calories per day consumed by most Americans.

Dr. Walford, who was widely featured in the *New York Times* and *Newsweek*, and on newsmagazine shows like *Dateline* and *Nightline*, was the author of *Beyond the 120-Year Diet: How to Double Your Vital Years*. Unfortunately, he didn't make it to 120 years of age. Dr. Walford died in 2004 at the age of 79 following a battle with amyotrophic lateral sclerosis, commonly known as ALS or Lou Gehrig's disease.

Scientific research has yet to support or refute whether a CRON diet extends life for humans. Julian Dibbell, writing in *New York* magazine, said that following the CRON diet meant living "as close to the brink of starvation as your body can stand."[14] I don't think God, who gave us wonderful foods to eat from His creation, wants us to go through life hungry. Neither does He want us to abuse our bodies by stuffing our mouths with junk food.

A happy medium must be found, but the idea of trimming the caloric sails a bit could make for a longer passage through life. It is my hope that by following the eating principles behind *The Maker's Diet for Weight Loss*, you will not only live longer, but you will also live better.

I want to help you discover—or rediscover—foods found in nature, as well as to retrain your taste buds. Do you have to think hard to remember the last time you bit into fresh raspberries, scooped up a handful of raisins, or supped on lentil soup? These listed foods are nutritional gold mines and contain no refined or processed carbohydrates and no artificial sweeteners. A diet based on consuming whole and natural foods fits within the bull's-eye of eating foods in a form healthy for the body. The basic components of a healthy diet include the right amount of:

- Protein, which is found in fish, meat, poultry, dairy products, eggs, and beans
- Fat, which is found in animal and dairy products as well as nuts and oils
- Carbohydrates, which are found in fruits, vegetables, whole grains, beans, and other legumes
- Vitamins such as vitamins A, B, C, D, E, and K
- Minerals such as calcium, potassium, and iron[15]

You'll see how all these nutrients come together in the Weight Loss Eating Plan, but the CliffsNotes version on reaching your weight-loss goals means that you will:

1. Eat foods low in sugar and refined carbohydrates, which will lower your daily glycemic load
2. Add more omega-3 fats from wild-caught fish, grass-fed beef and game, and wild plants
3. Try to balance your consumption of protein, fat, and slowly absorbed carbohydrates during your main meals
4. Consume an abundance of vitamins and minerals from foods and whole-food nutritional supplements
5. Eat foods high in alkalizing minerals, such as vegetables, which will prevent your blood from becoming too acidic
6. Lower your intake of sodium
7. Consume a high amount of antioxidants from foods, snacks, and whole-food nutritional supplements
8. Eat foods with a high fiber content

This last point needs to be circled in red because fiber is a natural appetite suppressant that curbs the appetite and keeps your cholesterol and blood sugar at optimal levels and your bowels functioning smoothly. High-fiber foods give you the biggest bang for your caloric buck because they pack a high volume of content into a low-calorie package. The reason you feel satiated when you eat fiber-rich foods is because fiber interacts with a gastrointestinal hormone called cholecystokinin—or CCK for short—that is secreted by the small intestine to signal the body, "Hey, we're getting full down here!" High-fiber foods promote and prolong the elevation of CCK in the blood, which in turn allows you to feel full for longer periods of time.[16]

Increasing your levels of CCK throughout the day will make it easier to decrease your caloric intake and still feel satisfied. Fiber also has a "flushing" effect on the bowels, which is why I recommend eating high-fiber foods during quarterly ten-day, detoxifying cleanses described in chapter 8. Not only do the water and fiber in food flush toxins out of the body, but fiber also reduces the absorption of calories from food that you've already consumed.

How does this happen? People who eat diets high in fiber excrete more calories in their stool for the simple fact that fiber is not digestible. (A random thought, but how would you like to be a lab tech given the chore of determining the amount of calories in a stool sample?) The "flush effect" means that when you go to the bathroom, you are eliminating 7 calories per gram of fiber that exit the body, unused.

You will have to up your intake of fiber-rich foods to get there. Here's a list that you can draw from, but keep in mind that scientists haven't been able to ascertain the exact total content of fiber in foods, especially fruits and vegetables, because of their complexity.[17]

FRUITS	SERVING DESCRIPTION	FIBER
Apples	One medium	4.0 grams
Blackberries	Half-cup	4.4 grams
Figs	Three	10.5 grams
Oranges	One large	2.4 grams
Peaches	One medium	2.3 grams
Pears	One medium	4.0 grams
Red raspberries	Half-cup	4.6 grams
Strawberries	One cup	3.0 grams

VEGETABLES	SERVING DESCRIPTION	FIBER
Broccoli	¾ cup, fresh and cooked	7.0 grams
Carrots	Half-cup	3.4 grams
Corn	One medium ear	5.0 grams
Green peas	Half-cup, fresh	9.1 grams
Spinach	Half-cup, cooked	7.0 grams
Yams	One medium, cooked	6.8 grams

MISCELLANEOUS FOODS	SERVING DESCRIPTION	FIBER
Black beans	One cup, cooked	19.4 grams
Lentils	⅔ cup, cooked	5.5 grams
Pinto beans	One cup, cooked	18.8 grams

Other high-fiber sources include:

- Most berries
- Barley
- Cauliflower
- Celery

- Sprouted nuts and seeds
- Oat bran
- Oatmeal
- Brown whole-grain rice
- Vegetables with edible skins

Besides its "flushing" effect, fiber performs many important functions in the body. Fiber protects the health of the intestinal tract by increasing stool bulk and decreasing transit time, which minimizes the contact of carcinogenic and harmful elements with the intestinal lumen. Be aware that there are two kinds of fiber, soluble and insoluble. Water-soluble fibers are the slippery type found in grains such as oats, seeds, legumes, and pectins that make up part of the edible portions of seeds, vegetables, and fruits. Insoluble fibers are cellulose and lignin, found in the bran of wheat and other whole grains, and hemicellulose, found in whole grains, nuts, seeds, fruits, and vegetables.[18] This is the type of fiber Grandma calls "roughage."

Fiber helps with weight loss by satisfying your hunger so that you're not tempted to fill up on fatty and sugary foods. Good sources of fiber are nuts; seeds; beans; whole-grain sprouted breads; whole grains such as quinoa, amaranth, buckwheat, millet, and brown rice; green peas; carrots; cucumbers; zucchini; tomatoes; and baked or boiled unpeeled potatoes. Green leafy vegetables like spinach and fresh fruit are also fiber rich.

You will see that I include generous amounts of fiber-rich foods in the Weight Loss Eating Plan in chapter 7. In practical terms, this means upping your consumption of vegetables with your meals and eating fruits for dessert. Fiber is like a sponge that soaks up fat and sugar in your gut and both slows and prevents some of their absorption, which helps you lose weight.[19] Fiber in your diet is a miracle ingredient when it comes to losing weight.

Forget About the Food Pyramid

With a huge media splash, the United States Department of Agriculture released its first food pyramid in 1992, which quickly became the basis of school lunch programs, hospital and nursing home menus, and all federally funded institutions that served food. After the government-sponsored food pyramid was introduced, this country reduced its intake of fat; increased its consumption of bread, rice, pasta, and cereals; and doubled its rates of obesity.[20] Not coincidentally, I might add.

The primary purpose of the USDA is not *your* health. It is to promote American agriculture—meaning Big Food. Experts on this subject, like Walter Willett, MD, and chairman of the Department of Nutrition at the Harvard School of Public Health, and professor Marion Nestle, PhD, have indicated in their books and writings that no food advice ever gets told to the American public that directly challenges the bottom line of the American food industry. Nutritional advice always gets yanked or watered-down by special interests. The end result: you lose. Marion Nestle, in particular, has been a recipient of a number of letters and threats of lawsuits clearly designed to silence her or wear her down. Who writes these letters? They come from the food-industrial complex, of course—like Big Sugar.

Case in point: the original USDA food pyramid, which was terribly misleading as well as fundamentally flawed, according to Dr. Willett, who says that we're still trying to recover from the damage done by the media. The following axioms have been trumpeted in the mainstream media since the food pyramid's introduction more than fifteen years ago:

1. All fats are bad.
2. All complex carbohydrates are good.
3. Protein is protein.
4. Dairy products are essential for calcium intake.
5. Potatoes are good for you.

In addition, the food pyramid made no recommendations regarding exercise or taking vitamins. After Dr. Willett and his team thoroughly researched those declarations, the Harvard professor shot them down like clay pigeons. His findings:

1. All fats are bad.

Not true, said Dr. Willett. While trans fats are bad for your health, monounsaturated and polyunsaturated fats, as well as fats from fish, nuts, olive oil, and grains, are good for you.

2. All complex carbohydrates are good.

Not true, again. Besides, the food pyramid's recommendation to eat six to eleven servings of carbohydrates daily was way too much, Dr. Willett declared. The original food pyramid did not differentiate between refined carbohydrates (such as commercial pasta) and healthy carbohydrate foods (fruits, vegetables, whole grains, and whole-grain bread).

3. Protein is protein.

Again, the Harvard doctor disagreed. Some sources of protein are better for you than others. For example, red meat is a high-quality protein that's high in saturated fats, and wild-caught salmon is rich in heart-healthy omega-3 fatty acids.

4. Dairy products are essential for calcium intake.

According to Dr. Willett, this is also not true. He insists that there is not a calcium crisis in the United States. "In reality," he said, "there are studies that suggest that too much calcium can increase a man's chances of getting prostate cancer or a woman getting ovarian cancer."

5. Potatoes are good for you.

This claim didn't make any sense to Dr. Willett, who pointed out studies showing that eating a baked potato increases blood sugar levels and insulin faster and higher than an equal amount of calories from pure table sugar.

Finally, according to the Harvard professor, a healthy diet without exercise is counterproductive and adding vitamins and minerals to your diet is important.[21]

The USDA issued a revised set of food guidelines in 2005, but the new food pyramid was only a mild improvement, remarked Mark Hyman, MD, author of *Ultrametabolism: The Simple Plan for Automatic Weight Loss.* "Rather than educating about the dangers of refined carbohydrates and sugars, they [the USDA] meekly advised us to 'choose carbohydrates wisely,'" stated Dr. Hyman.[22]

WHAT NUTRITIONAL TYPE ARE YOU?

While boosting the amount of fiber in your diet is an important first step to losing weight, you need to understand that the nutrients in our food—proteins, fats, and carbohydrates—are like putting fuel in your car's gas tank. When you eat the right foods, you should notice an improvement in your energy level, an uptick in your mental agility, a stabilization of your emotional well-being, and an overall feeling of satisfaction. But if you finish a meal and notice your energy level dropping, or you're as grumpy as an airport security screener, then you have eaten an improper combination of proteins, carbohydrates, and fats.

Since we're born with different metabolisms, it stands to reason that certain foods can affect you in different ways, which, in turn, can positively or negatively influence your digestion, your mood, and, ultimately, your weight. The idea of eating for your unique metabolism is a concept called "metabolic typing," which was introduced by William Kelley, DDS, in the 1960s and today is championed by several health experts, including Dr. Joseph Mercola, author of *Take Control of Your Health*, and researcher William L. Wolcott, author of *The Metabolic Typing Diet*.

Wolcott believes you can determine how well your body processes macronutrients—the proteins, the fats, and the carbohydrates—and use that information to make specific dietary recommendations.[23] He says people fall into three general metabolic types:

1. Protein types burn, or oxidize, carbohydrates quickly and must eat protein and fat to slow down this process. Protein types tend to be frequently hungry and often feel edgy and anxious.

2. Carb types have generally weak appetites, love sweets, have problems keeping weight off, and are often hooked on caffeine.

3. Mixed types generally have average appetites, no huge cravings for sweet and starchy foods, keep their weight under control, but tend to feel fatigued, anxious, and nervous about life.

Shortly, I'll present a simple test—although it's not foolproof—to determine what metabolic type, or what I prefer to call "nutritional type," you are. Before we get there, however, let me give you some more background information on protein and carbohydrates and how these nutrients impact your body.

THE POWER OF PROTEIN

Proteins, one of the basic components of foods, help you feel fuller than do carbohydrates or fats, so along with eating more fiber, you will need to eat adequate amounts of lean protein to control your hunger and food intake.

Proteins are the worker bees: they provide for the transport of nutrients, oxygen, and waste throughout the body and are required for the structure, function, and regulation of cells, tissues, and organs. Consuming meals rich in high-quality protein—chicken, beef, lamb, dairy, eggs, and so on—will leave you feeling full and satisfied, which supports weight loss.

The best and healthiest sources of protein are organically raised cattle, sheep, goats, buffalo, and venison. Grass-fed beef is leaner and lower in calories than grain-fed beef. Organic beef is higher in heart-friendly omega-3 fatty acids and important vitamins like vitamins B_{12} and E, and way healthier for you than meat from hormone-injected cattle eating pesticide-sprayed feed laced with antibiotics.

Even better, as it relates to weight loss, is that grass-fed beef is high in conjugated linolenic acid (CLA), a fatty acid that appears to modestly reduce body fat while preserving muscle tissue, according to researchers at the University of Wisconsin School of Medicine. Those participating in the study who took 3.2 grams of CLA each day had a drop in fat mass of about 0.2 pound per week, or around a pound a month, compared to those given a placebo.[24] Grass-fed animals have three to five times more CLA than grain-fed animals.

Fish with scales and fins caught from oceans and rivers are also lean sources of protein and provide essential amino acids. Supermarkets are stocking these types of foods in greater quantities these days, and, of course, they are found in natural-food stores, fish markets, and specialty stores. Consuming fatty fish—wild salmon, mackerel, and sardines—comes with additional benefits. They provide the healthy omega-3 fats described earlier.

Protein is important when trying to lose weight for these reasons:

- Chicken, beef, fish, beans, and other high-protein foods slow the movement of food from the stomach to the intestine.
- A stomach that slowly empties means you feel fuller longer and get hungrier later.
- Protein's gentle, steady effect on blood sugar avoids the quick, steep rise in glucose levels that occurs after eating a rapidly digestible carbohydrate like white bread or baked potato.[25]

So If You're a Vegetarian...

That complicates things, especially if your nutritional type is skewed toward protein. Lacto-ovo vegetarians can get along fine if they consume lots of high-quality protein sources such as organic eggs and cultured dairy, but strict vegetarians will have a more difficult time meeting their protein needs on the Weight Loss Eating Plan. You will need to substitute other foods for your protein needs, such as nuts, seeds, legumes, and cereal grains. Since these foods are only decent protein sources, however, you should seek the advice of a nutritionist who can offer nutritional guidance.

Many vegetarians, due to the nature of vegetarianism, eat an excess of carbohydrates and not enough proteins and fats. This is why you can be overweight while being a "perfect" vegetarian. A vegetarian diet of cereals, pastas, breads, and sweets is not helpful—for reasons aforementioned.

A good vegetarian diet should emphasize coconut, chia, avocado, tempeh (fermented soybean loaf), seeds, legumes, nuts, and whole grains such as amaranth, buckwheat, millet, and quinoa to get all the protein you need. A good vegetarian diet also provides healthy fats from extra-virgin coconut, olive, and flaxseed oils. You will find it necessary to mix and combine foods to get the needed nutritional balance at every meal. While being a vegetarian demands more planning and work to pull off, you can still achieve your weight-loss goals.

KILLING THOSE CARBS SOFTLY

If protein and fats don't cause people to get fat, what's left?

You're right—carbohydrates. Too many carbohydrates, especially those from refined sources, are the culprits. Pigging out on refined carbs forces the body to convert any excess carbohydrates into body fat, which keeps pounds resting on the midsection.

You won't lose weight and keep it off when your diet is heavy in refined carbohydrates. Refined foods, a process in which fruits, vegetables, and grains are stripped of their vital fiber, vitamins, and mineral components, will never match up to the nutritional power of fresh produce and grains. Examples of common refined foods are Pop-Tarts, Post Raisin Bran cereal, Hot Pockets sandwiches, Jell-O pudding, Kraft Macaroni and Cheese, and Hamburger Helper.

At the same time, carbohydrates are the body's chief source of energy. Carbohydrates are necessary for the digestion and assimilation of other foods, and they help regulate protein and fat metabolism. Fats require carbohydrates to be metabolized in the liver. We need carbohydrates. We just don't need the carbs from refined foods.

In response to the intake of too many carbs, your body is forced to produce extra insulin in order to prevent large spikes in blood sugar. Dr. Bulwer says this spike in insulin levels can overcorrect and cause blood sugar to transiently go too low in the short term—a state called hypoglycemia. This typically causes hunger pangs and a headache and leads to craving for more sweets. "Clearly, this leads to weight gain," he said. "A state of habitual high carb intake and progressive obesity leads to a state of hyperinsulinemia, where circulating insulin levels may increase two- or threefold."

If there's too much insulin in the bloodstream, which often happens when you eat highly refined, high-carb foods like rolls, pastas, and sweets, the body stores the extra sugar as fat. Cutting way back on refined carbs, however, will reduce the insulin and blood sugar roller coaster and cut down on fat production.

Apart from dietary fiber and sugar sweeteners, the other main carbohydrate form is starch, which is found in plant-based foods such as rice, potatoes, corn, and grains. When starchy foods are eaten, the digestive tract breaks down these long-chained starches into simpler sugars and finally into glucose (blood sugar), which is a source of immediate energy. If these calories are not expended, however, the body stores them as fat, which becomes a weighty problem—and is why high-starch foods should be eaten judiciously.

How fast the body turns these starches into blood glucose is a measure of the glycemic index, known as GI. The glycemic index is a ranking of foods based on their immediate effect on blood sugar levels as well as a measurement of how quickly the carbohydrates in food are digested. Carbohydrate foods with a high glycemic index, such as white breads, starchy potatoes, and sugary desserts, raise your blood sugar levels dramatically.

Carbohydrate foods with a low glycemic index, such as certain fruits, vegetables, salads, and organic whole-grain products, take your blood sugar to levels right where they should be. "Entry of glucose into the bloodstream occurs more slowly and smoothly," said Dr. Bulwer. "One thing that should not be forgotten is that the *quantity* of carbohydrates you eat is perhaps even more important than *what* you eat in terms of the degree of spike in blood sugar. This has given rise to the term that some prefer: glycemic load."

As I mentioned in chapter 2, diets that generally strike carbohydrates from your eating plan are doomed to failure. The human body, especially the brain, needs a constant supply of glucose because glucose levels that drop too low can result in weakness and fatigue. It's better to eat small, frequent meals that focus on fresh fruits and vegetables, whole grains, seeds, nuts, legumes, and healthy dairy foods. These foods that God created will help stabilize insulin and blood sugar levels. This doesn't mean that you should be nibbling all day long, however. Even too much of a good thing isn't good for you.

You will have to be careful about the type of carbs you eat. It's always best to consume proteins, fats, and foods lower in carbohydrates, like fresh vegetables, before eating any high-starch carbohydrates like potatoes, rice, grains, and bread. I know when you go out to a neighborhood trattoria it's tempting to fill up on the delicious Italian panini and butter before the chicken cacciatore arrives. That's the absolute wrong way to eat, however. Leave the bread and rice or potatoes until the end of the meal, or, better yet, leave them out altogether if you're feeling satisfied.

The Skinny on Fats

Fat—along with protein and carbohydrates—is the third major nutrient found in food. If you recall from our last chapter, it's not fat that's making you fat, so there's no need to remove fat from your diet. Actually, we need to eat *some* fat: fats are a concentrated source of energy and source material for cell membranes and various hormones, have a protective effect against heart disease, play a vital role in the health of your bones, protect the liver from alcohol and other toxins, and guard against harmful microorganisms in the digestive tract. All fat-soluble vitamins—A, D, E, and K—need fat in the diet for their absorption and utilization.

Misconceptions are hard to overturn, however. For decades, the media have reported on studies that vilified fats, especially saturated fats, for those experiencing cardiovascular disease. The researchers conducting these trials, however, totally ignored the evidence that their subjects were carbo-loading on pasta, bread, cereal, muffins, doughnuts, Danishes, and desserts while failing to exercise; they were also drinking too much alcohol, which prolonged high insulin levels. Because insulin influences the biochemical processes that lead to atherosclerotic plaque formation in arteries, these subjects had higher rates of heart disease.

The Holy Grail of the "diet-heart" connection is the Framingham Heart Study, which began in 1948 when researchers recruited 5,209 men and women between the ages of thirty and sixty-two from the town of Framingham, Massachusetts. The study conducted extensive physical examinations and lifestyle interviews with participants in a search of common patterns relating to cardiovascular disease development.[26]

In the Framingham study, researchers found that those who consumed more saturated fat and cholesterol in their diet actually weighed *less* and had a *lower* risk for heart disease, yet the Framingham study is often cited by the media as proof that fat and cholesterol are harmful. Now, other voices are being heard. One of them is the physician who was the associate director of the Framingham study for three years, George Mann, MD, who edited a book called *Coronary Heart Disease: The Dietary Sense and Nonsense*. In that volume, Dr. Mann provided powerful evidence that saturated fat is *not* the cause of heart disease.[27]

Another author, Diana Schwarzbein, MD, who wrote *The Schwarzbein Principle: The Truth About Losing Weight, Being Healthy, and Feeling Younger*, states that eating the right fats causes you to lose body fat and reach your ideal body composition.[28] The "right fats" are healthy saturated fats, omega-3 polyunsaturated fats, and monounsaturated (omega-9) fatty acids. You can find these fats in a wide range of foods, including salmon, lamb, goat's and sheep's milk and cheese, coconut, walnuts, olives, almonds, and avocados.

"My clinical experience with thousands of people has shown that eating saturated fats is not the culprit!" Dr. Schwarzbein exclaimed. "On the contrary, the patients I have followed, who have increased their consumption of saturated fats (as well as all other good fats), have improved their cholesterol profiles, decreased blood pressure, and lost body fat, thereby reducing their risk for heart disease. Eating saturated fats should be part of your balanced diet while, at the same time, your focus should be on reducing all the factors that increase insulin levels."[29]

The more healthy fats you eat, the healthier you'll become. Did you know that the inhabitants of the Greek isle of Crete, whose intake of fats was almost 50 percent of their total daily calorie intake (as noted by the famous Keys Seven Countries Study in the 1950s and 1960s), showed the lowest rates of heart disease? They consumed loads of extra-virgin olive oil. The Inuits ate a lot of fats—mainly omega-3 and saturated fats from fish, seals, reindeer (caribou), and whales, including their fatty blubber. They have traditionally enjoyed very low rates of heart disease.

Below is a list of saturated, monounsaturated, and polyunsaturated fats that are good for you, along with some of the foods and where they are found. Within this list, be sure to shop for "pure cold-pressed" oils. The cold-pressing process, used to extract oil from natural sources, does not damage the fat. When heat processes are used to extract sunflower oil from sunflower seeds, for example, that damages the fat. This is an important point because your body cannot easily metabolize damaged fat.

Saturated fats (saturated fat oils are best for cooking)

1. Butter
2. Cheese
3. Coconut and palm oils (look for extra virgin, as they are healthier than refined)
4. Cream, dairy only
5. Beef, venison, buffalo, and lamb fat (when found within the meat and raised organically)
6. Eggs
7. Ghee (clarified butter)
8. Sour cream
9. Chicken, duck, and turkey fat (when found within the meat and raised organically)

Monounsaturated fats (these oils can also be used for cooking but are less preferable to saturated oils)

1. Avocados (they contain almost as much healthy monounsaturated oleic fats per gram as olive oil—a whopping 70 to 75 percent)
2. Almond oil
3. Grapeseed oil
4. Peanut oil
5. Extra-virgin olive oil (best if used on salads; should *not* be heated)
6. Keep in mind that not all olive oils are the same: olive-pomace oils, from the last dregs after pressing, are highly refined, chemically treated, and not recommended.

Polyunsaturated fats (for polyunsaturated fat oils, use only those that are cold pressed; they are not to be used for cooking purposes since heat damages these fats)

1. Flaxseed oil
2. Chia seed oil
3. Hemp seed oil
4. Sunflower oil
5. Safflower oil
6. Cod liver oil

7. Herring oil
8. Menhaden (fish) oil
9. Salmon oil
10. Sardine oil
11. Sesame seed oil
12. Wheat germ oil[30]

In addition, your diet should be rich in healthy fats from the following sources:

1. Omega-3, free-range eggs
2. Grass-fed red meat
3. Free-range chicken
4. Wild fish
5. Nuts and seeds

Polyunsaturated fats are made up of high levels of omega-3 fats and omega-6 fats, known as essential fatty acids (EFAs). Omega-3 fats can improve cardiovascular health and help balance insulin and inflammation levels. Wild-caught fish, free-range eggs, walnuts, and flaxseeds are excellent sources of these important omega-3 fatty acids. The types of fats you *really* want to run away from are trans fats, which have been vilified in the mainstream media for the last few years—and rightfully so. These horrible, artery-clogging fats are produced by heating liquid vegetable oils in the presence of hydrogen to make them solid at room temperature—a process known as hydrogenation. Food conglomerates routinely utilize hydrogenated oil inside their manufacturing plants, which means that trans fats are found in nearly all of our processed foods. The reason food producers employ so much chemistry in the hydrogenation process is because it allows them to produce a more competitively priced product with a longer shelf life. The list of foods containing trans fats is endless: vegetable shortening, frozen pizza, ice cream, processed cheese, potato chips, cookie dough, white bread, dinner rolls, snack foods, doughnuts, candy, and salad dressing. The worst offender is margarine, even those touted in "heart healthy" tubs. Commercially prepared fried foods, like french fries and onion rings fried in polyunsaturated vegetable oils, also contain gobs of trans fat. Anything deep-fried in polyunsaturated oils—chicken, steak, or fries—contains higher-than-average trans fat levels.

Mark my words: trans fats are horrible for your health, and that's the reason why they are in the crosshairs of politicians these days. City officials in Tiburon, California, an exclusive enclave on the San Francisco Bay, successfully coaxed the city's eighteen restaurants to voluntarily stop using trans fats in their cooking oils in 2004. News of Tiburon's voluntary trans fat prohibition prompted cities like Philadelphia and New York City to pass laws banning restaurants from serving foods cooked or fried with oils that contain or produce trans fats. Eateries in both major cities were given until the summer of 2008 to be in compliance. Metropolises such as Boston, Chicago, and Los Angeles may soon join them, and at least thirteen states are considering a trans fat ban, including a bellwether state, California. This will be interesting to watch unfold.

In Europe, the Danes are way ahead. Denmark passed laws effective in 2004 restricting the use of industrial trans fats to a maximum of 2 percent of the fat in any food product. American multinationals like McDonald's and KFC had to comply with new oils in their fryers, so it *is* possible.

Beware of the Trans-Fat Gimmick! by Dr. Bernard Bulwer

Question: Can you explain how it's possible—since the passage of legislation requiring the amount of trans fats to be listed on food labels—that products with hydrogenated or partially hydrogenated fats (the source of bad trans fats) can still splash their packages with phrases like "Trans Fat Free" or "Zero Trans Fat"?

Answer: Because of the verbal gymnastics allowed by government loopholes. Even though the packaging says the food is trans fats free or has zero trans fats, manufacturers can still put dangerous trans fats in your food—as long as they ensure there's less than 500 milligrams of trans fat per serving.

The problem is that when you multiply 500 milligrams by the amount of servings you consume, then eat many different foods that play the same tricks with their labels, you're consuming trans fats when you thought you were being "good" and staying away from these menacing compounds.

Now you understand the deception, and it's all legal. Read your ingredient labels, and if you see the words *hydrogenated* or *partially hydrogenated* listed, figure that you'll be ingesting some amount of trans fat, no matter what the colorful label promises.

WHAT'S YOUR NUTRITIONAL TYPE?

Now that you have a better understanding of protein, carbohydrates, and fats, what nutritional type are you? Instead of categorizing people as protein, carb, or mixed types, I've simplified things by coming up with two categories:

- Meat types, for their need to eat a higher-protein diet
- Potato types, for their need to eat a diet higher in carbohydrates

You can determine, generally speaking, your nutritional type by answering the following questions adapted from Dr. Mercola's book *Total Health Program*, which will give you a broad idea of whether you are a meat type or a potato type:

1. When you eat or snack on high-carb foods like bread, cereals, fruits, grains, or vegetables, are you satisfied, or do you want to eat more?
   a. I'm generally satisfied after eating these high-carbohydrate foods.
   b. I'm in the middle—not satisfied but not hungry for more.
   c. I'm still hungry.
2. When you eat red meat regularly, do you lose or gain body weight? Do you feel slimmer?
   a. The bathroom scale confirms that I've gained weight.
   b. Eating red meat doesn't affect my weight either way.

      c. I actually lose weight when I eat red meat.

3. Do you think about food all the time? Are you one of those persons who live to eat?
      a. No, I'm not hung up on food.
      b. I'm in the middle: not hung up on food or crazy about it.
      c. I can't wait to chow down again.

4. What is your appetite like at breakfast?
      a. I'm not hungry at all.
      b. I can eat, but I'm not super hungry.
      c. I'm definitely hungry.

5. What is your appetite like at lunchtime?
      a. I'm not hungry at all.
      b. I can eat, but I'm not super hungry.
      c. I'm definitely hungry.

6. What is your appetite like at dinnertime?
      a. I'm not hungry at all.
      b. I can eat, but I'm not super hungry.
      c. I'm definitely hungry.

7. Does eating something higher in fat and/or protein (macadamia nuts, yogurt, whole milk, cheese, and guacamole) within an hour or two of bedtime help you sleep better?
      a. No, not at all.
      b. Eating those foods just before bedtime doesn't affect me one way or another.
      c. I sleep like a log when I snack on those foods.

8. Do you need to eat frequently, or can you eat three square meals and not feel the need to snack in between?
      a. I only need to eat one or two times a day, including snacks.
      b. Three square meals is all I need.
      c. I have to snack in between meals; otherwise I won't make it.

9. How much do you enjoy eating fermented foods like pickles, sauerkraut, or beets?
      a. I love them.
      b. They're OK, but I'm not a huge fan of fermented foods.
      c. I can't stand them.

10. When the Thanksgiving turkey is being carved, are you a white meat or dark meat type of person?

a. I always eat the breast—white meat.

b. I like both kinds of meat.

c. I always go for the dark meat.

Add up your score of a, b, and c answers. If most of your answers were in the "b" and "c" categories, you're a meat type, someone who should be eating more protein foods. If most of your answers were in the "a" category, you're a potato type, someone who should consume a diet higher in carbs.

Meat types, as you would expect, do better eating higher protein and lower carbohydrate foods that include plenty of the "good" fats. Meat types burn fuel quickly, which is why they are known as "fast oxidizers." My experience has been that meat types like sweets but perform better on healthy protein foods. They have big appetites and also tend to crave salty and fatty foods, burning carbohydrates quickly. Eating more protein and more fat will slow this process.

Potato types feel bullish about the world when they're eating a lot of carbohydrates. They feel best when their plates are filled with carbohydrate foods like breads, grains, and vegetables. The danger is that this type of diet can increase fat storage. Pigging out on too many carbohydrates, especially those from refined sources, forces the body to convert any excess carbohydrates into body fat, which keeps pounds resting on the midsection. Potato types are also "slower oxidizers," meaning their bodies don't burn proteins and fats as efficiently. This explains why potato types tend to struggle when they go on a low-carb Atkins-type program—their bodies demand more carbs.

You should start by paying attention to the amount of proteins, carbs, and fats in your diet, and then adjust the proportions according to your taste and appetite. See how you feel as you go about your day. If you do not react optimally to your meal, you can change the ratios the next time around and analyze your reactions, fine-tuning each meal to the ratios of proteins, carbs, and fats that are just right for you.

Let's say you have a bland chicken breast with salad for lunch. If within an hour or two you feel absolutely famished, you probably need more fat in your salad. Next time, add an extra tablespoon of healthy salad dressing, extra-virgin olive oil, cheese, avocado, or almonds, and see if your mid-afternoon cravings disappear. Generally speaking, you should feel terrific for at least one hour after you eat. If you are still having food cravings or a noticeable dip in energy level, these are clues that you're probably not eating appropriately for your nutritional type.

I've designed eating plans for meat and potato types that can be found in chapter 14.

THE CONCEPT OF FOOD COMBINING

There's another aspect to eating that I want you to be aware of: the concept of "food combining," which encourages separating specific foods and eating certain ones together. A New York physician, William Howard Hay, MD, introduced the food-combining concept nearly a century ago when he suggested that certain foods, when broken down, leave an acid pH, and other foods leave an alkaline pH. Translated into plain English, Dr. Hay believed food combining means not eating carbohydrates and protein at the same meal.[31]

Medical research has not been able to support Dr. Hay's food-combining theories, and no scientific proof asserts that foods digest better when carbohydrates and protein are eaten separately. I believe digestive systems were created to handle a variety of nutrients coming down the pike at the same time. If you happen to eat carbohydrates like grains, breads, pasta, cereal, fruits, and veggies with certain proteins like meat, fish, poultry, beans, and nuts, but don't appreciate the way your stomach feels afterward, feel free to experiment. You may find that nonstarchy green vegetables like broccoli, mushrooms, and zucchini work better with lean meats, eggs, and cheeses.

Some people say that combining fruit with any other food delays digestion and causes gas and bloating to occur. We know physiologically that fruits stay in the stomach for only a short time—twenty to forty-five minutes. For myself, I've found that I need to be careful about the fruits I eat and when I eat them. I've always remembered an old expression about melon that Dad used to say when I was growing up: "Eat it alone, or leave it alone." Since melons are comprised of 90 percent water, he said, they leave the stomach faster than other foods, including other fruits. That's why I eat melon alone as a snack. You may find that sweet fruits like bananas, dates, and figs aren't compatible in your stomach when consumed with acidic fruits like grapefruit, pineapple, or oranges. While I'm not totally on board with the principles of food combining, it never hurts to listen to your body.

Along these lines, I recommend consuming fiber and fat with every meal and not eating your carbohydrates naked. Fiber and fat slow the absorption of sugar into the bloodstream, which keeps insulin levels in check.

EAT YOUR COLORS

Have you noticed the lack of color in a McDonald's value meal? Once you get your sandwich out of the wrapper, a Quarter Pounder and medium french fries is monochromatic beige. Same thing over at the Colonel's, where a plastic plate of KFC extra-crispy chicken, mashed potatoes, gravy, and corn are mainly lighter and darker hues of brown with a dash of pale yellow.

You usually don't find many colorful foods in fast-food restaurants, unless you order a salad. Contrast this with a visit to the produce department at a Whole Foods or Wild Oats, where fruits and veggies with vibrant reds, greens, oranges, purples, and yellows are on display. Whether you're cooking at home or ordering out in a restaurant, you'll never go wrong eating foods exhibiting the pulsating, radiant colors of the rainbow. At one of my favorite restaurants, P. F. Chang's China Bistro, I'm partial to the Oolong Marinated Sea Bass entrèe that's broiled and served with sweet ginger soy, baby corn, and spinach. Since we eat with our eyes first, this type of meal just *looks* better and healthier.

Many of the vivid colors in fruits and vegetables come from phytochemicals like anthocyanins, phenolics, lutein, indoles, flavonoids, and carotenoids like lycopene. These nutrients help the body maintain memory function, cardiovascular health, and a healthy weight. Pigments with health-promoting properties color every fruit and vegetable, and their benefits are unique to each color. For instance, blueberries—my favorite berry—are colored by the phytochemical anthocyanin. Green vegetables owe their pigment to chlorophyll. Another phytochemical known as lycopene is the reason why tomatoes and watermelon are red. The nutrient fucoxanthin is a pigment that makes brown seaweed brown. All these phytochemical pigments offer antioxidant protection as well as other health benefits.

Being mindful of adding color to your plate at a place like a Chili's-type restaurant means ordering a spring salad instead of french fries to go with your sandwich. When you're making a sandwich for work, add a leaf of lettuce and a thick slice of tomato to your turkey, tuna, or chicken. Shredded carrots bolster the look of tuna salad, and fruit salad with green grapes, red raspberries, and white banana add a pleasant ending to any meal.

What color has your diet been? For some of you, it's been beiges and browns, the colors of restaurant food and frozen dinners. You should illuminate your diet with the following colors:

- Red: tomatoes and tomato sauces, raspberries, apples, strawberries, pomegranates, cherries, peppers, radishes, and watermelon
- Purple-blue: plums, grapes, prunes, blueberries, blackberries, red cabbage, beets, and eggplant
- Orange: oranges, sweet potatoes, cantaloupe, carrots, winter squash, apricots, peppers, and mangoes
- Orange-yellow: tangerines, oranges, peaches, papayas, pineapples, peppers, and nectarines
- Yellow: corn, lemons, peppers, and yellow squash
- Green: salad greens, kiwi, broccoli, avocados, brussels sprouts, chives, green onions, parsley, cilantro, green beans, spinach, peppers, Swiss chard, and kale
- White-green: celery, asparagus, honeydew, and pears

- White: mushrooms, onions, cauliflower, garlic, leeks, shallots, bananas, artichokes, and bamboo shoots

That's just a partial listing of all the colorful foods in God's creation, but the next time you sit down for a meal, regard what's on your plate or in your hand, and you'll find your dietary true colors.

The Five Tastes

The ten thousand taste buds on your tongue can detect five tastes: sweet, sour, salty, bitter, and umami. The latter one, umami (pronounced *oo-MAH-mee*) is a meaty, savory taste that's responsive to free glutamates—like monosodium glutamate (MSG)—as well as the savory tastes of Parmesan and Roquefort cheese. Since we were created with five distinct tastes, it's important to consume foods and beverages that supply *all* these tastes, not just the sweet and salty foods that define much of the American diet. Exposing yourself to all five food tastes will open your palate to a wider variety of foods and the beneficial properties they impart to the body.

Given a little time, you could have a hankering for venison, goat's cheese, and kefir—three of my personal favorites!

EATING WITH THE SEASONS

My grandmother Rose, the youngest of seven children, grew up on a Polish farm the first thirteen years of her life. Her father owned a mill where they pressed poppy seeds and flaxseeds into oil during the fall harvest. She and her brothers and sisters loved gathering the pressed seeds and patting them into hard cakes, which were dipped into *schmaltz*, the rendered fat from chicken soup.

When autumn gave way to the inevitably harsh winter, the Catz family consumed only cooked foods, save for the barrel of sauerkraut they kept in the cellar as a source of veggies. They ate what was in season because they had no other choice.

The same could be said of celebrity chef Wolfgang Puck, who grew up in Unterbergen, Austria, following the war. His parents never stocked cans in their pantry. Instead, the Puck family ate summer fruit in the summer and winter vegetables in the winter, just as nature intended, he said.[32]

Today, thanks to hulking container ships the size of football fields and fleets of interstate truckers, we can shop for fresh fruits and vegetables year-round: table grapes from Chile, ruby red strawberries from New Zealand, Haas avocados from Mexico, and pineapple and papaya from Costa Rica. Even though we can shop for great-tasting produce any day of year, should we?

Not necessarily. Traditionally throughout history, people have eaten the foods that were available in season, just as Grandma Rose did when she was a young girl. While it's not the end of the world if you snack on a bowl of Chilean grapes while watching the snow pile up outside your living room window, it makes more sense to eat warm foods when there's a blizzard outside—just as it's common sense to consume mouth-watering fruits during a heat wave. I know that Nicki instinctively craves homemade chicken soup when Florida winter nights turn cool, and I could eat watermelon all day long when our summer heat feels like an inferno. In traditional Chinese medicine, it is believed that cooked foods impart warming properties to the body and raw foods impart cooling properties.

Many Americans who suffer from metabolic or thyroid issues have a low basal body temperature, so consuming cold, raw foods during the middle of winter makes things worse. That's why someone living in Bozeman, Montana, in the month of January should consume mostly cooked vegetables, plenty of nourishing soups, cooked healthy meats, and whole grains cooked with healthy oils. Those living in West Palm Beach in the month of July should consume lots of raw fruits, salads, and juices.

If you've never given the concept of "eating with the seasons" a thought, then begin paying attention to what you eat based on the time of year and the temperature outside. Speaking in general terms, here's how I see the ratios breaking down:

- In winter, try to eat 75 percent cooked foods and 25 percent raw foods. Eat warming foods like fish, chicken, beef, lamb, and venison. Potatoes, onions, and garlic fit well, as do eggs.
- In spring, try to eat 50 percent cooked foods and 50 percent raw foods. This time of year, tender, leafy vegetables are popping up in stores: Swiss chard, spinach, romaine lettuce, fresh parsley, and basil.
- In summer, try to eat 25 percent cooked foods and 75 percent raw foods. Peaches, cherries, watermelon, strawberries, pears, and plums are in their seasonal glory.
- In fall, try to eat 50 percent cooked foods and 50 percent raw foods. Look for more warming foods like root vegetables, sweet potatoes, onions, and garlic.

Here's a guide to when certain fruits and vegetables are at their peak:

- **Spring:** asparagus, blackberries, green onions, leeks, lettuces, new potatoes, peas, red radishes, rhubarb, spinach, strawberries, and watercress.
- **Summer:** apricots, blueberries, cherries, eggplant, fresh herbs, green beans, hot peppers, melon, okra, peaches, plums, sweet corn, sweet peppers, tomatoes, and zucchini.
- **Fall:** apples, broccoli, brussels sprouts, cauliflower, collards, grapes, kale, pears, persimmons, pumpkin, winter squash, and yams.
- **Winter:** beets, cabbage, carrots, citrus fruits, daikon radishes, onions, rutabagas, turnips, and winter squash.

Eating with the seasons is a concept that's been forgotten in this country, thanks to modern-day shipping, but the seasons form a natural backdrop for eating and a source for diversity. When you buy foods produced from distant areas, this weakens the market for locally grown food and dampens regional economic viability. This is a truly green concept since when you shop locally for local produce, you reduce fuel consumption by shipping and trucking, and hence greenhouse gases, while supporting local enterprises.

THE DIRTY DOZEN

No matter what time of year, you will be stealing from your future *and* robbing your health if you eat any of these foods that I call the "Dirty Dozen."

I wouldn't be surprised if some of these are among your favorite foods to eat. Nor would I be surprised if you find my list of "Dirty Dozen" foods to be controversial. When you eliminate these foods from your shopping list and/or toss out what's left in your cupboards and refrigerator, however, you will take a major step toward excellent health and reaching your ideal weight.

The following "Dirty Dozen" items should never find a way onto your plate or into your hands:

1. All pork products

Did you just sit up in your chair? I'm sure I got your attention because America *loves* pork. Fast-food establishments have watched their earnings sizzle by topping every hamburger and chicken sandwich in sight with strips of salty bacon; they go by names like Bacon Mushroom Melt, Big Bacon Classic, Cravin' Bacon Cheeseburger, Mesquite Bacon Cheeseburger, and Arch Deluxe with Bacon. America's favorite pizza toppings are pepperoni (a pork product) and Hawaiian (pineapple and Canadian bacon). Only the Chinese, who have four times our population, consume more pork meat than we do.

I've met people who have told me they have an emotional attachment to bacon for breakfast and pork chops with mashed potatoes and gravy for dinner. That was how they were raised, and maybe you feel the same way. Marketed brilliantly as "the other white meat," pork chops and pork ribs are usually the most inexpensive meats on display at the supermarket. Many folks eat pork three times a day: ham and eggs in the morning; a "BLT" sandwich—bacon, lettuce, and tomato—or a bacon-topped burger for lunch; and pork "barbecue" or pork tenderloin for a hearty supper. Others love snacking on pork rinds—the cooked skin of pigs. (I think I'm going to lose my lunch.)

So what's my beef with pork? My aversion to sowbelly is partly based on a pig's physiology. A pig's fast-acting physiological makeup and instinct allow them to eat any swill thrown at their muddy feet. Well, maybe swill isn't the right word. Actually, I'm thinking about the old saying: *Happy as a pig in slop.*

Yes, pigs will chomp on pails of you-know-what and not be bothered in the least. They will derive nutrition from human excrement dredged from a latrine pit, eliminating a sanitary problem for their rural masters. Even their own waste tastes fine to them. Although it's anecdotal, I heard the story about the pig farmer who stacked ten pigs in individual wire cages, one on top of another. All the farmer had to do was feed the pig in the penthouse cage and let trickle-down economics prove itself. As I'm fond of saying in my seminars, "Remember, if you eat the meat of animals, you are not just what you eat; you are what they ate!"

As for their physiology, pigs have a simple stomach arrangement. Whatever a pig eats goes straight into a simple stomach, where's it's rudimentarily digested and pushed out the back end. Total transit time: four hours.

Now compare the pig's digestive tract to animals that are OK to eat, such as cows, goats, sheep, oxen, deer, buffalo, and so forth. These animals put their vegetarian diet—they usually chomp on grasses, alfalfa, and hay—through a "wash and rinse cycle," thanks to a stomach and a secondary cud receptacle available for the task. Instead of a speedy four hours to digest and eliminate their waste, these animals take a more leisurely twenty-four hours.

Another reason I don't eat pork is my Jewish background. In Leviticus and Deuteronomy, two of the first five books of the Torah (if you're Jewish) or the Bible's Old Testament (if you're Christian), God forbade the Hebrew people to eat swine: "You shall not eat any detestable thing. These are the animals which you may eat: the ox, the sheep, the goat, the deer, the gazelle, the roe deer, the wild goat, the mountain goat, the antelope, and the mountain sheep. And you may eat every animal with cloven hooves, having the hoof split into two parts, and that chews the cud, among the animals. Nevertheless, of those that chew the cud or have cloven hooves, you shall not eat, such as these: the camel, the hare, and the rock hyrax; for they chew the cud but do not have cloven hooves; they are unclean for you. Also the swine is unclean for you, because it has cloven hooves, yet does not chew the cud; you shall not eat their flesh or touch their dead carcasses" (Deuteronomy 14:3–8).

The Scriptures used Hebrew words that can be translated as "foul," "polluted," and "putrid" to describe these "unclean meats" that were to be banished from their diets. What were God's reasons for doing so?

It wasn't because the Israelites didn't have refrigerated trucks following them from Egypt to the Promised Land to keep ham, bacon, or baby back ribs in a cool environment and "safe" for consumption. No, God scratched pork from their meal plan because He knew all about their physiology, and He created them to be nature's garbage cleaners.

If you decide to strike pork from your diet, I'm predicting that you won't miss sausage, bologna, salami, bacon, and butchered cuts from the hog at all. I promise you there are great alternatives.

Some of you will feel that swearing off pork completely is too drastic—too radical given your attachment to Easter ham and *carnitas* burritos. If that's the case, remember that every time you choose beef, chicken, or fish—especially from organic sources—you are taking a fantastic leap forward in your health, but each time you take a bite of crisp bacon, grilled sausage, and shredded pork, you are falling further behind.

2. Shellfish and crustaceans

You may have been blown away by my recommendation to strike pork from your diet, but I'm not done yet. Shrimp and lobster, two of the most popular foods in America, are, in my opinion, extremely unhealthy to eat and should also be avoided, even if chains like Red Lobster and Olive Garden delectably advertise entrees like breaded shrimp or scampi with pasta.

Invariably, whenever I take out my wife, Nicki, for our anniversary dinner at an expensive seaside restaurant in South Florida, a waiter with a French accent will approach our table and say, "Monsieur et Madame, ze special tonight is pork tenderloin ringed with Alaskan crab and drizzled with a lobster sauce."

But that's not what I heard. His description sounded more like this: *Monsieur et Madame, ze special tonight is fresh garbage, ringed with raw sewage and drizzled with solid waste.*

Stay with me here. Shellfish and crustaceans, as well as fish without fins and scales (such as catfish, shark, and eel), were also declared to be "detestable" back in Moses's day. The reasons are similar to those that make pigs out of bounds: lobsters, crabs, shrimp, and catfish are bottom-feeders. They troll along the seabed or lakebed, sustaining themselves with fish waste. The physiology of crabs, clams, and lobsters means that whatever they consume goes straight into their system, which is why scientists can measure water pollution by checking the flesh of shellfish and crustaceans for toxin levels. While all this "clean up" is great for water quality and one of nature's ways to scrub the aquatic environment, eating shellfish and crustaceans is not good for your bodies or your health.

3. Processed meats and hydrolyzed soy protein

The quintessential processed meat of all time is Spam, a syllabic abbreviation of "**Sh**oulder of **P**ork and h**AM**." Actually, Spam's name should be an acronym for "**S**pecially **P**rocessed **A**merican **M**eat," because it deserves Hall of Fame status in the pantheon of faux foods. Spam is one of those mystery meats—along with breakfast links, frankfurters, salisbury steaks, bologna, sausages, and salami—where you have *no* idea what part of the steer or pig was used. You can figure, though, that you're eating ground-up stomach, snout, intestines, spleens, edible fat, and even lips.

One thing you can be sure of is that processed meats contain nitrates to convey flavor, give meats their bloodred color, and resist the development of botulism spores. Nitrates can convert to nitrites, which have been studied for decades in public and private settings and found to cause cancer and tumors in test animals.

While we're on this unpleasant topic, I would also steer clear of processed turkey and chicken luncheon meat for the same nitrate reasons.

You may be wondering what hydrolyzed soy protein is all about. Have you ever substituted imitation crab for the real stuff when making a pasta dish for the family? Sprinkled imitation bacon bits on their salad? Ordered inexpensive sushi at a restaurant? All these foods, which are not part of the Maker's Diet program, are forms of hydrolyzed soy protein.

Hydrolyzed soy protein usually contains a significant amount of genetically modified soy as well as compounds that closely mirror the dangerous monosodium glutamate, or MSG. Hydrolyzed soy protein is also a known excitotoxin, which means it has the potential to cause neurological disturbances. It's not fish or fowl, and it's not real food.

4. White flour

One major reason why we have an obesity epidemic is because the standard American diet is weighted way too heavily with sketchy foods containing refined grains where the wheat has been stripped of wheat germ, bran, and half of the healthy fatty acids during the milling process. The end result is something called "enriched white flour," but the only reason why enriched flour is bright white is because the wheat stalks are rinsed with various chemical bleaches that sound like a vocabulary test from a high school biology class: nitrogen oxide, chlorine, chloride, nitrosyl, and benzoyl peroxide. The "enriched" adjective comes from the millers adding a few isolated and synthetic vitamins and minerals back into the nutritionally stripped flour, but that's like dressing an American Girl doll in tattered clothes.

Enriched flour, the main ingredient in nearly all the bread and buns on supermarket shelves as well as a zillion other food items baked in commercial bakeries, is easy to spot on the list of ingredients: it's usually the first item listed. The healthy alternative is purchasing or making your own whole-grain bread from unprocessed whole-grain flour.

5. Hydrogenated oils

Pick up a loaf of white bread at the supermarket, and you will notice that hydrogenated oils or partially hydrogenated oils are usually recorded right after enriched white flour on the ingredient list. If you see any words with the "hydro-" prefix or "partially" on a package or box, don't buy it. If a friend offers you a packaged doughnut or cupcake, don't eat it.

During the hydrogenation process, hydrogen gas is injected into the oil under high pressure to make the oil solid at room temperature and prevent the oil from becoming rancid too quickly, but as mentioned earlier, this hydrogenation process produces an ugly stepchild: trans fats. Research shows that trans fats by far are the most dangerous for your heart. They lower the good HDL cholesterol, increase the bad LDL cholesterol, and increase triglycerides as well as another dangerous fat called lipoprotein (a).

As mentioned earlier, if the ingredient list includes the words "shortening," "partially hydrogenated vegetable oil," or "hydrogenated vegetable oil," then the food contains trans fat. Even if the ingredients label says "zero trans fat," that doesn't mean what you think it does; the FDA allows food manufacturers to have any amount less than 0.5 grams of trans fat in the food (per serving) and still legally say "zero trans fats" on the packaging.

It's a good idea when you're eating in a restaurant to ask the server if the kitchen is using partially hydrogenated oil for frying, baking, or cooking their dishes. Ask about salad dressings as well.

6. Pasteurized, homogenized skim milk

When it comes to dairy products, the conventional wisdom in the diet world can be summed up in this way: whole milk, bad; skim milk, good.

Whole milk is loaded with fat and calories, right? But removing the fat to make 2 percent or skim milk makes the milk less nutritious and less digestible as well as causes allergies. Yes, whole milk has more calories, but I've seen research suggesting that the mix of nutrients found in milk, such as calcium and protein, may improve the body's ability to burn fat, particularly around the midsection. Besides, the thought of a cow naturally delivering reduced fat or fat-free milk is "udderly" ridiculous, but I'm going to milk this topic for all it's worth because milk does a body good. (End of cliché alert.)

The richest food sources of calcium are milk and milk products, but I don't recommend drinking any commercially homogenized and pasteurized milk. The pasteurization process alters vital amino acids, which reduces your ability to access the proteins, fats, minerals, and great vitamins like vitamin A, vitamin B_{12}, vitamin D, and folic acid found in raw, unpasteurized milk. The homogenization process may be even more dangerous as it alters the fat globules and creates a compound known as XO, or xanthine oxidase, which is believed by some to cause damage to the arterial walls and may lead to an increased risk for cardiovascular disease.

I recommend drinking unpasteurized milk from grass-fed animals instead of homogenized, pasteurized milk. Unfortunately, raw milk can be dangerous if it comes from a farm that lacks sanitary practices, which is why it's not available in many states. The next best thing is finding cultured or fermented dairy whole-milk products, such as yogurt and kefir, which are produced from pasteurized, non-homogenized milk.

If you can get used to its "goaty" smell and taste, goat's milk is naturally homogenized, less allergenic, and more rapidly absorbed in the digestive tract. Goat's cheese, which has become widely available in the last few years, is very healthy, as is cheese made from raw cow's milk. My favorite dairy products are made from sheep's milk, which are easy to digest and more nutritious than dairy products made from cow's or goat's milk. I find the creamy taste wonderful. Look for sheep's milk yogurt and cheese at your local natural foods grocery.

You've probably noticed that major supermarkets as well as warehouse clubs sell organic milk. I don't believe commercial organic milk is the answer, however. Some companies with organic brand names you would recognize produce pasteurized and homogenized milk.

7. White sugar

I'll bet you that any food with enriched flour also contains sugar or one of its sweet relatives—high-fructose corn syrup, fructose, and sucrose. You'll find these sugars among the first ingredients listed in candy bars, pastries, snack cakes, cookies, and ice cream. You will also find plenty of sugar in foods you might think are healthy, like "natural" breakfast cereals, energy bars, raisin bagels, certain whole-wheat breads, hot dog buns, salad dressing, steak sauce, ketchup—the list is endless.

Sugar is so omnipresent that most people don't realize they eat sugar with every meal: their breakfast cereal is frosted with sugar; break time is soda or coffee mixed with sugar and a Danish; lunch has its cookies and treats; and dinner could be sweet-and-sour ribs, sweet potatoes covered with marshmallows, a garden salad doused with artificially sweetened dressing, and a sugary parfait for dessert. Talk about adding a sweet exclamation point to the day! A United States Department of Agriculture study revealed that we eat an average of *31 teaspoons* of sugar daily—with 17 teaspoons coming from high-fructose corn syrup, and 14 teaspoons coming from cane or beet sugar (sucrose).[33] This adds up to more than 500 calories daily.

If you're looking for a guilty party to blame for the bellies hanging over beltlines, then look no further than King Sugar, which takes sugarcane or sugar beets from the fields and processes it 99.9 percent before it's dumped into 5-pound bags of bleached white sugar. (I'm sure research scientists are working overtime to remove the last one-tenth of 1 percent in sugarcane that's healthy.)

According to Ann Louise Gittleman, author of *How to Stay Young and Healthy in a Toxic World*, "Sugar is not an innocent substance that gives us pleasure and causes no harm. Quite the contrary; there is perhaps nothing else in the diet that promotes disease and aging more over the long term than excess sugar."[34] She says that more than sixty ailments, ranging from allergies to vaginal yeast infections, have been associated with this dietary demon.

"Without a doubt the biggest change in our diets has been our sugar consumption...refined white sugar known as sucrose, brown sugar, corn sweeteners, high-fructose corn syrup, dextrose, glucose, lactose and maltose," said Ann Louise Gittleman. "Over the past two centuries, we have literally shocked our bodily systems with outrageous and ever-growing amounts of nutrient-robbing sugar. At the end of the 1700s, sugar consumption was less than 20 pounds per person per year. By the end of the 1800s, sugar consumption had risen to 63 pounds annually. Now, 100 years later, the average American eats over 170 pounds of sugar each year."[35]

Attention: all that sugar makes for a pounding headache when you cut it from your diet. When you change your diet and cut out drastic amounts of sugar, you can expect to experience withdrawal-like symptoms like less energy, gyrating mood swings, and monster cravings.

8. Soft drinks

A 12-ounce, sugar- or high-fructose corn syrup–sweetened beverage contains nearly 9 teaspoons of sugar and 150 calories—empty calories that provide little or no nutritional value. If you drink one can of soda per day and don't change anything else about your diet or exercise regimen, you will consume 55,000 extra calories in one year, which adds up to fifteen pounds of weight gain.

Soft drink manufacturers know that once teenagers leave the adolescent years, they become more health conscious, or at least more aware of how bad sweetened soft drinks are for them, so that's why they try to hook 'em young. Nicki swore off soft drinks during her senior year of high school, but not because she wanted a better fit in her prom dress. Her epiphany came after conducting an experiment in her science class. One day her teacher informed the class that they were going learn about acidic reaction. He dramatically dropped a galvanized construction nail into a glass of Coke to see what would happen overnight. The nail didn't dissolve—that was an old wives' tale—but the red rust encrusting the galvanized nail blew Nicki away. She hasn't had another soft drink since then.

9. High-fructose corn syrup

High-fructose corn syrup, or corn sweetener, is more than plain bad for you—it's horrible for your health and the worst form of sugar. Americans receive some 200 calories daily, mainly from soft drinks. High-fructose corn syrup is a major contributor to weight gain because foods with fructose may not turn off your hunger signals. You get hungry *after* eating a snack containing high-fructose corn syrup because you're not satiated. Your appetite is saying, "Nice try, but I'm still famished!"

With such a highfalutin name, you'd think that a sweetener with the word *corn* in it wouldn't be as bad for you as regular white sugar, but it is. With high-fructose corn syrup (HFCS), research scientists invented an enzymatic processing method that begins with milling corn to produce cornstarch, which is then made sweeter by chemically converting some of the glucose to fructose. The more fructose in the end product, the sweeter it is. A widely used variety of HFCS, known as 55-

HFCS, consists of 55 percent fructose and 42 percent glucose. Thanks to a system of price supports and sugar quotas that have been in place for twenty-five years, importing sugar into the United States has become cost-prohibitive, which has opened up a huge market for American companies manufacturing high-fructose corn syrup.

Coca-Cola and Pepsi dumped the sugar from their carbonated soft drinks back in 1984, substituting cheaper HFCS in its place. These days you'd be hard-pressed to walk into a 7-Eleven and find a soda pop sweetened with sugar. The only holdout I could find was Goose Island sodas, although Jolt Cola did use sugar one time with the following marketing slogan: "All the sugar and twice the caffeine." But the makers of Jolt Cola reformulated their product with high-fructose corn syrup, no doubt to make the product less expensive in the stores. I'm sure the opportunity to lower costs is the reason why high-fructose corn syrup has become the principal sweetener in fruit juices, baked goods, canned fruits, dairy products, cookies, gum, and jams and jellies.

So what makes high-fructose corn syrup such an unhealthy, fat-promoting form of sugar? The body handles fructose differently than it does other sugars. For starters, the body metabolizes fructose into triglycerides more than other sugars, which raises blood triglycerides significantly and increases the risk of heart disease. (Triglycerides are the body's storage form for fat and are found in fat tissues.) Unlike glucose, fructose does not stimulate leptin, the hormone that tells you "I'm full," but reduces ghrelin hormone levels, which tell you "I'm still hungry." Consumption of fructose from corn sweeteners comes with no enzymes, vitamins, or minerals, so it cheats the body of micronutrients. HFCS is different from the natural fructose found in whole fruit because with fruit, the body gets the enzymes, vitamins, and minerals to help with digestion and utilization of the fructose.[36]

The liver cannot handle fructose very well. When fructose reaches the liver, says Dr. William J. Whelan, a biochemist at the University of Miami School of Medicine, "the liver goes bananas and stops everything else to metabolize the fructose." The fructose propels the liver into a fat-promoting mode by activating the formation of enzymes that lead to elevated levels of "bad" cholesterol and triglycerides.[37]

The consumption of high-fructose corn syrup in beverages—about two-thirds of all HFCS consumed in the United States is in beverage form—has certainly left its fingerprints vis-á-vis our nation's obesity epidemic. The consumption of high-fructose corn syrup increased 1,000 percent between 1970 and 1990, far exceeding the changes in intake of any other foods or food group.[38] Juice drinks like Minute Maid's Hi-C are among the worst offenders: despite flavors like Blazin' Blueberry and Orange Lavaburst, Hi-C lists pure filtered water and high-fructose corn syrup as its first and second ingredients. At least they're filtering the water!

King Corn

I like to pick up a freshly cooked ear of fresh, organic corn and dig in at a summer picnic, but I'm having some trouble digging up some sympathy for this simple vegetable—or grain. (Corn should be considered a vegetable when consumed raw and a grain when cooked.) Economists say that we can blame corn for the sharp spike in grocery prices in the last year, and that's likely to continue as the American food economy—especially ethanol production for gasoline—becomes more and more dependent on corn. The price of corn rose 46 percent during 2007,[39] which carries all sorts of implications since corn is the main building block for much of the American food supply.

What's happening is that an ever-increasing amount of corn is being diverted to make ethanol to mix with gasoline. Ethanol now gobbles up 18 percent of the domestic corn supply, up from 10 percent in 2002.[40] This is set to escalate further. As corn prices move up to meet the demand for ethanol, this raises production costs for all sorts of foods: dairy cows eat corn to make milk, hens consume corn to lay eggs, and cattle, hogs, and chickens are fattened on corn before slaughter. I've already detailed how corn syrup is the main sweetener of soda pop and thousands of other food items.

Future outlook: look for King Corn to tighten its grip over its subjects.

10. Artificial sweeteners

Dieting and artificial sweeteners go together like…ham and eggs? *Mea culpa* for the jarring simile, but the huge demand for low-calorie and sugar-free foods and beverages by those seeking to consume fewer calories has created a $6 billion market for artificial sweeteners. Aspartame, saccharin, and sucralose are found in umpteen thousands of foods as well as in blue, pink, and yellow packets of Equal, Sweet'N Low, and Splenda found on restaurant tables.

I will fully address the safety of artificial sweeteners in chapter 10 (sneak preview: they're toxic and dangerous), but if you have always thought that artificial sweeteners will help you lose weight, you might want to rethink your position. Researchers at Purdue University say these sugar substitutes could interfere with the body's natural ability to count calories based on a food's sweetness. In other words, drinking a diet soft drink instead of the full-octane sugar version will reduce your caloric intake, but it could also trick the body into thinking that other sweet items don't have as many calories either. This sort of thinking gives weight-conscious people another mental alibi for overindulging in sweet foods and beverages.[41]

I understand the rationale behind drinking low-cal or no-cal drinks—lower total caloric intake—but sipping artificially sweetened drinks is not the solution. Sweeteners like aspartame are addicting. Read this edited exchange between skeptical Bill O'Reilly, host of *The O'Reilly Factor*, and Shari Lieberman, PhD, a certified nutrition specialist:[42]

Bill O'Reilly, host: In the "Back of the Book" segment tonight, Americans drink billions of gallons of diet soda a year. It's incredible how much we consume. And some believe millions of Americans are addicted to the stuff. They have to have it.

With us now is Dr. Shari Lieberman, a certified nutrition specialist here in New York City.

All right. So it's—ten billion cases of soda sold every year in the USA, and 30 percent of that, approximately, is diet soda, and I know people who walk around all day long drinking diet soda. What is that all about?

Shari Lieberman, PhD, certified nutrition specialist: It's unbelievable. It is such an addicting substance. You have the aspartame, the Nutra-Sweet, combined with the caffeine. You're basically getting a rush all day. It actually messes with your brain chemicals, Bill.

O'Reilly: Does it really?

Lieberman: It really does. You know, aspartic acid actually makes what we call excitatory neurotransmitters. Imagine we have a balance of ones that calm us down and ones that hype us up. So, if you're drinking something that's going to make the ones that are excitatory or making us hyper all day long, that's why there are so many side effects associated with NutraSweet, such as irritability and anxiety…

O'Reilly: Now is this physically addicting, do you believe, or is it psychological?

Lieberman: I believe it's physically addicting. You know, we know that caffeine is. So you've got a ton of caffeine in the diet sodas. Then you actually have a substance [artificial sweeteners] that's affecting neurotransmitters. So they're really getting a double whammy, and, of course, we're talking about people that are drinking it all day long.

O'Reilly: Yes, and they think that, well, I can drink it all day long because there's no calories in it, I'm not going to get fat. Go ahead.

Lieberman: I have to tell you something about that. If you look at the research, people that drink diet sodas are oftentimes eating more calories than people drinking regular sodas.

I already made the last point, but I'd like to make another: as bad as sugar and high-fructose corn syrup can be for your body, I'd rather you consume them than artificial sweeteners. They're that bad for you.

11. Artificial flavors and artificial colors

The dictionary definition of *artificial* refers to something not made by human beings or a copy of something natural. Since the goal of *The Maker's Diet for Weight Loss* is to eat natural foods, anything containing artificial flavors or artificial colors will be naturally unhealthy as well as increase the toxic load on the body.

Take the recipe for Waldorf-Astoria Red Velvet Cake—please! The cooking instructions for this ooh-la-la confection, which originated at the iconic Manhattan hotel, calls for squeezing two bottles of FD&C Red No. 40 into a mixing bowl filled with the requisite shortening, flour, eggs, and sugar. Pastry chefs say they have to wear gloves to keep the shameful dye off their skin or rub nail polish remover if any red spots appear on their double-breasted white jackets.

"Why should a dose of Red No. 40 turn Betty Crocker into Hester Prynne?" asked Slate.com writer Daniel Engber, referring to the fictional colonial woman forced to wear a scarlet letter "A" for committing adultery. "Ask a gourmand, and you're likely to hear three specious answers. First, Epicurean: *Artificial color tastes bad.* Second, Hippocratic: *It's bad for your health.* And third, Platonic: *It makes food unnatural.*"[43]

Don't purchase foods that list artificial flavors and colors on the packaging. These additives have been linked to behavioral problems in children and increase the body's toxic load. They have also been associated with allergies and skin rashes.

12. Beer, wine, and alcoholic drinks

If you like to watch a football game with a beer in hand or dine with a glass of fine wine, I have some troublesome news for you: during the first three phases of the Weight Loss Eating Plan in chapter 7, I'm asking you not to drink any alcohol.

Although I'm a teetotaler who may enjoy a glass of organic wine a couple of times a year, I recognize that there have been studies pointing out the benefits of drinking modest amounts of red wine for cardiovascular health. The "French Paradox," so called for the observation that the French typically suffer low rates of heart disease despite having a diet rich in saturated fats, was attributed to alcohol and olive oil intake. The "French Paradox" is only a paradox if you assume that saturated fat is the cause of obesity and heart disease—something I point out in the next section. No wonder the French—eating all kinds of real food to their hearts' content and toasting family and friends with a glass of *vin rouge*—have that certain *joie de vivre*. (I've now officially used up all the French I know.)

So, you're welcome to open a bottle of nice wine in Phase IV of the Weight Loss Eating Plan, but I balance alcohol's benefits against the downside of excessive drinking, which damages family relationships as well as every organ in the body (especially the liver), promotes depression, causes digestive ailments (ulcers, gastritis, and pancreatitis), and impacts fertility. Alcohol adds weight, a full 7 calories per gram, almost twice that of protein or carbs. That's a significant reason why we see beer bellies in this world.

If you are a regular drinker, see how you feel after you've jumped on the Maker's Diet for Weight Loss bandwagon. I'm not saying that you should never have another adult beverage or savor a fine glass of wine with an exquisite meal again, but you may realize that drinking has become a weight-inducing habit that needs to be trimmed back.

THE TOP HEALING FOODS

As part of the Maker's Diet for Weight Loss program, the following top healing foods should find a way onto your grocery list.

Grass-fed meat

Let me make another case for staying away from commercially produced beef and chicken and purchasing organic, grass-fed, and pastured cuts of meat. Michael Pollan, author of the excellent book *The Omnivore's Dilemma*, says it's not necessarily our food that's making us sick but what we feed our food.[44] Commercially raised livestock are raised on corn, pumped full of antibiotics, and fattened as fast as possible to get them to market quickly. Seventy-five years ago, steers were four or five years old when they were led into the slaughterhouse. The age fell to two or three years in the 1960s. Today, "production" cattle are fattened up in fourteen to sixteen months before being carved up into roasts, steaks, and hamburger.

"Without cheap corn, the modern urbanization of livestock would probably have never occurred," said Pollan. "We have come to think of 'corn fed' as some kind of old-fashioned virtue; we shouldn't. Granted, a corn-fed cow develops well-marbled flesh, giving it a taste and texture American consumers have learned to like. Yet this meat is demonstrably less healthy to eat since it contains more saturated fat—up to 40 percent. Compare this to the 2 or 3 percent fat found in venison, caribou, or bison.

"A recent study in the *European Journal of Clinical Nutrition* found that the meat of grass-fed livestock not only had substantially less fat than grain-fed meat but that the type of fats found in grass-fed meat were much healthier," Pollan continued. "A growing body of research suggests that many of the health problems associated with eating beef are really problems with corn-fed beef. In the same way ruminants have not evolved to eat grain, humans may not be well adapted to eating grain-fed animals. Yet the USDA's grading system continues to reward marbling—that is, intermuscular fat—and thus the feeding of corn to cows."[45]

I would like to encourage you to step out of your comfort zone and sample grass-fed buffalo, bison, lamb, and venison. These meats are not "gamy" but rather have delightfully clean, subtle tastes that will please your palate. One of Nicki's signature dishes is a spinach-and-goat-cheese lasagna with ground buffalo meat she cooks whenever we have guests over. Another Rubin family favorite is Nicki's venison meat loaf. My mouth is watering as I type these words.

Grass-fed veal is another meat worth trying. I know that veal has been out of favor ever since the Humane Farming Association spearheaded a national veal boycott back in the 1980s. They purchased full-page magazine ads picturing a frightened calf chained inside a twenty-two-inch crate so small that it could not turn around. The formula-fed veal calves were administered an anemic diet so that the distinctly white meat would retain a mild flavor that epicureans prize.

Seemingly overnight, factory-farm veal was about as socially acceptable as fur coats. Back in the 1960s, Americans ate four pounds of veal on average, but these days the per capita consumption has leveled off to only half a pound per year.[46]

Lately, however, veal has been making a comeback as farmers got the message and made changes in the way they raised their herds. "Unfortunately, I was a sinner," said John Holloway of Misty Morning Farm in Cherry Tree, Pennsylvania. "I did raise factory veal—all the chemicals, antibiotics, steroids I used. We wouldn't let our friends eat what we used to raise." Now all of Holloway's veal is pastured and organic and sold in stores with "Certified Humane" stickers.[47]

Fine meat purveyors and celebrity chefs like Wolfgang Puck say they've noticed the difference: organic veal is more flavorful because it's been allowed to walk around pastures. "If we feed the animals better, treat them better, we will have a better product and a healthier product," said Wolfgang Puck.[48]

Eat More Lamb

It's a shame that Americans don't enjoy the taste of lamb. Our annual per capita consumption of lamb stands at a measly four-fifths of a pound, not much more than one grand meal a year—Passover or Easter—when you figure a five-pound leg serves eight people.

I love lamb, and it doesn't have to be a special holiday occasion for lamb to be served at our dinner table. There's something about the golden brown skin and moist pink flesh that resembles beef but is accentuated with a distinctive but pleasing gamy taste. The way to my heart is to serve a lamb roulade—a deboned leg of lamb filled with herbed pesto and crumbled goat cheese, topped with a red wine reduction.

Lamb is high in vitamin B_{12}, which supports the production of red blood cells and allows nerves to function properly. The tender meat is also an excellent source of zinc, a mineral critical to immune function and wound healing. Carnitine is great for the heart. We've become big lamb eaters in the Rubin household because of its wonderful flavor. We love all the cuts, especially roasts and barbecued lamb chops. The chops come from the loin muscle, which gets very little exercise and is naturally tender. We also use ground lamb for burgers, meatballs, and meat loaf.

Better yet, more than half of the lamb sold in the United States is imported from Australia and New Zealand, where herds are raised on dewy grasses found in valley meadows. American lambs are "finished" on grains, which means they're not grass-fed raised like the little lambs from Down Under and New Zealand.

We've got some catching up to do: Aussies and Kiwis eat more than fifty pounds of lamb per year.[49]

Wild-caught fish

Fish aren't tethered inside crates like calves, but much of the fresh fish sold these days—salmon, trout, and tilapia—is "farm-raised," which means they spend their lives lazily circling around concrete tanks, fattening up on pellets of dubious man-made chow. These "feedlot" fish don't taste as good or pack the same nutritional punch as their cold-water cousins that streak through the ocean or ford mountain streams sustaining themselves on small marine life. Fish caught in the wild provide a richer source of omega-3 fats, protein, vitamins, and minerals.

Many popular diets include canned tuna and salad as a lunchtime or dinner staple. I must note, though, that there's canned tuna, and there's *canned tuna*. What I mean is that much of the canned tuna on supermarket shelves comes with something else inside the 6-ounce tin: mercury. You should shop in health food stores for a low-mercury, high-omega-3 tuna that's extremely healthy and safe to consume. For recommended brands, check out the resource guide in the back of the book.

Fermented/cultured dairy products

Fermented? As in fermented cabbage or sauerkraut? Sort of, but not exactly. Dairy products like yogurt, kefir, cottage cheese, and cultured cream (also known as crème fraîche) are examples of lacto-fermented foods and have been around for centuries.

Fermentation, also known as culturing, preserves dairy products for longer periods of time. Dairy products are usually stricken from most conventional diets because of the perceived "fat" they contain, but as I've been saying, natural and organic whole-milk dairy products—especially those made from sheep's milk and goat's milk—contain the right fats. I'm also a big fan of strained Greek yogurt, which is high in protein.

I recommend the following dairy products in chapter 7:

- Whole-milk plain yogurt
- Sheep's milk yogurt
- Goat's milk yogurt (plain)
- Whole-milk cheese
- Soft goat's milk cheese
- Sheep's milk hard cheese
- Goat's milk hard cheese
- Feta cheese (sheep's milk)

- Full-fat plain kefir
- Full-fat cottage cheese
- Ricotta cheese
- Full-fat sour cream
- Plain almond milk
- Goat's milk protein powder (substitute for dry milk)
- Buttermilk

Fruits and veggies

Besides being low-calorie foods, fruits and veggies should be eaten in abundance anyway because of all the rich vitamins, minerals, and antioxidants they supply to the body. The government bureaucrats behind the food pyramid came up with a "5 a Day" motto, but that recommendation has fallen on deaf ears as Americans swarm fast-food and sit-down restaurants. Except for salads—which are usually tossed with a chemical-laden dressing to deliver a satisfying "mouth feel"—people don't order many entrées with vegetables. If the main meal does come with any veggies, it's often a few twigs of overcooked and unappetizing broccoli. And fresh fruits just aren't sold in restaurants; the proprietors would rather pad their profits by enticing you to order *mousse au chocolat* or apple pie à la mode.

Rather than counting servings of fruits and vegetables, I would adopt a mindset that says a meal is not complete without eating some fruits and/or vegetables. I've already mentioned one of my favorite foods—berries. Blueberries, blackberries, raspberries, and strawberries are nutritional powerhouses: low in calories and among the highest antioxidant-containing foods on the planet. I seem to recall that some scientific evidence suggests that blueberries prevent age-related memory loss, but I forget where I heard that. (Just teasing.) Seriously, berries are the unsung heroes of good nutrition.

Figs, whether eaten fresh or dried, are a good source of fiber and potassium, a mineral that helps control blood pressure. If you've had blood work done recently, there's a good chance that you'll have a potassium deficiency, which is a sign that you're not eating enough fruits and vegetables and consuming too much sodium found in processed foods. Upping your intake of organic fruits and veggies will turn these numbers around in a heartbeat.

Also, don't overlook cultured and fermented vegetables such as sauerkraut, pickled carrots, beets, and cucumbers, which are some of the healthiest foods on the planet. If you're not a big fan of sauerkraut or pickled beets, try adding pickled relish atop broiled fish. Fermented foods are excellent sources of digestion-enhancing probiotics and enzymes.

Soups and stocks

There's nothing better than zesty soup made from scratch with fiber-rich vegetables such as celery, carrots, onion, and zucchini, especially when it's freezing outside. (For more on eating with the seasons, see page 71.)

My Grandmother Rose, being of European Jewish heritage, was big on homemade chicken soup, which she called "Jewish penicillin." Countless times she delivered containers of her homemade chicken soup to my bedside when I was hospitalized after those horrible illnesses afflicted me as a college student.

The recuperative effects of chicken soup date as far back as the twelfth century when the Jewish physician and philosopher Moses Maimonides recommended its use for the treatment of respiratory infections. When you're hacking away and battling a cold, chicken soup acts as an anti-inflammatory, meaning that sipping chicken soup reduces the inflammation that occurs when coughs and congestion strike the respiratory tract. In addition, chicken soup keeps a check on inflammatory white blood cells, also known as neutrophils, which are produced by the onset of cold symptoms.

While a hearty soup is good for the soul when there's a raging blizzard outside, I've found that I like a hot soup during Florida's frigid months, like when the highs barely get into the sixties. Seriously, when a cold snap sweeps through, I like to roll up my sleeves and make a soup from scratch. My specialty is Thai Coconut Chicken Soup, a spicy hot soup that dazzles the palate with subtle flavors. The unsweetened coconut milk is a flavorful counterbalance to the Thai chilies and stalks of lemon grass.

Thai Coconut Chicken Soup, like many soups, starts with a stock, which is also called broth. Stocks are extremely nutritious and swimming with minerals, cartilage, collagen, and electrolytes. Meat, fish, chicken, and turkey stocks also contain generous amounts of natural gelatin, an odorless, tasteless substance extracted by boiling bones and animal tissues. Easy to digest, gelatin aids in overall digestion. So, the next time you bake a whole chicken or serve a holiday turkey, don't throw those bones in the trash. Use them to make a healthy stock that can form the basis of many great soups.

Extra-virgin coconut oil

Speaking of coconuts, organic extra-virgin coconut oil can be a wonderful ally in your quest to lose weight. Extra-virgin coconut oil has been the recipient of some great press the last few years for its ability to help balance the thyroid, aid in metabolism, and help the body with energy production. Some experts recommend that people with thyroid and weight troubles should consume as many as 2 to 4 tablespoons of coconut oil per day.

A balanced thyroid plays a vital role in your metabolism. Mary Shomon, author of *The Thyroid Diet*, says that certain foods high in tyrosine assist the body in the production of the thyroid hormone T3, which helps you utilize more oxygen and burn more calories.[50] Besides extra-virgin coconut oil, foods high in tyrosine are cottage cheese, egg whites, safflower seeds, and meats such as turkey, antelope, quail, and buffalo.

One way to add coconut oil to your diet is to add some to a saucepan whenever you cook scrambled eggs; need to glaze diced onions, peppers, or other vegetables; or heat up leftovers. When I make smoothies, I often add a teaspoon of extra-virgin coconut oil among the ingredients. Coconut oil is one of those healthy fats that provide satiety and slow the absorption of sugar into the bloodstream, thereby keeping blood sugar and insulin levels on an even keel.

HOW TO BE A GOOD SHOPPER

I know what you're thinking: "All those top healing foods sound fantastic, Jordan, but I can't afford to buy them."

The cost of organic foods is a barrier for many. It does cost more to shop in natural-food stores, a 20 percent to 200 percent bigger bite out of the family food budget. The situation should improve as market forces and increasing consumer demand drive down prices. But here are some steps you can take in the interim:

- Realize that eating organic food prepared at home is far cheaper than taking the family out to eat at a sit-down family restaurant or even a fast-food joint. If you're a family of four, it costs anywhere from twenty dollars for burgers and fries to thirty dollars or more for an Applebee's-type dining experience. For those amounts, you can eat *really* well at home for the same amount if you cook for yourself and your family.
- Eating the foods recommended in the Weight Loss Eating Plan (see chapter 7) cost half as much as following a special diet or dietetic meal plan like Jenny Craig, NutriSystem, or Weight Watchers.
- Keep in mind that those "convenience" foods—frozen pizza, Lunchables, Dove ice cream bars—are more expensive than you think. A fresh peach is cheaper than peach low-fat yogurt. A banana is cheaper than a candy bar.

Build family dinners around:

- Healthy salads (romaine lettuce, radicchio, escarole, and endive) with tomatoes, celery, red onions, peppers, and avocados
- Healthy grains like amaranth, millet, buckwheat, and quinoa
- Healthy vegetables like spinach, broccoli, cauliflower, onions, sweet potatoes, and white potatoes

- Grass-fed meat, free-range chicken, and wild-caught fish, all served as a vital ingredient, not necessarily the main course

Look for deals when you shop—and stock up. Even the natural foods stores have "loss leaders" designed to get you in the store, where they figure you'll do the bulk of the family grocery shopping that week.

WHERE WE GO FROM HERE

Phew! This was our longest chapter, but eating the wonderful foods found in nature in a form healthy for the body is the key linchpin undergirding *The Maker's Diet for Weight Loss.* In our next chapter, we'll turn our attention to liquid refreshments and how you can drink to achieve your weight-loss goals.

The Maker's Diet for Weight Loss Recap: Eat for Your Ideal Weight

1. Change the way you shop for food by purchasing fresh organic foods at a natural food or health food store or local farmer's market, if possible.
2. Understand that processed foods are practically a foolproof guarantee that you'll be consuming genetically modified and refined flour, along with a variety of sweeteners, including bleached white sugar and high-fructose corn syrup.
3. Look for ways to add fiber-rich foods such as nuts, seeds, beans, whole-grain sprouted breads, green peas, carrots, cucumbers, zucchini, tomatoes, and baked or boiled unpeeled potatoes to your diet. Foods high in fiber slow down the digestive process and satiate longer.
4. Take the nutritional type test and determine whether you are a meat or potato type. Eat a diet based on your nutritional type and see how much better you feel.
5. Eat healthy fats such as saturated fats, omega-3 polyunsaturated fats, and monounsaturated (omega-9 or oleic) fatty acids, which are abundant in salmon, lamb, goat's and sheep's milk and cheese, coconut, walnuts, olives, almonds, and avocados.
6. Change the way you eat meat. Choose cuts from grass-fed and pastured cattle, not grain-fed cattle raised conventionally. For fish, purchase only fish that have been caught in oceans and rivers, not raised in concrete-lined "fish farms."
7. Don't eat any more pork, shrimp, lobster, or other shellfish, which contain many more toxins in their flesh than beef and chicken.
8. Double-check the "Dirty Dozen" list and take steps to cross off each of those foods from your shopping list.
9. Realize that the best dairy products come from organic grass-fed cow's milk, goat's milk, and sheep's milk. When consuming dairy products, always choose whole-milk or full-fat varieties.

four

Drink for Your Ideal Weight

Bob DeMoss, an accomplished writer who just turned fifty, has always had to watch his weight since he began tipping the scales in the 225-pound range back in his college years. So he started drinking Diet Coke to save calories without sacrificing his morning caffeine buzz.

Yup, I said *morning*. On a typical weekday around 7:00 a.m., Bob would cruise into Daily's, a gas-'n'-go mini-mart in Franklin, Tennessee, while chauffeuring his daughter to school. Then he'd carry out a Paul Bunyan–sized plastic cup topped off with 44 ounces of sugar-free Diet Coke, or what he called his first "44" of the day. "It had to be Diet Coke," he said. "If Daily's was out of Diet Coke, I'd go somewhere else."

Bob, who works out of his home on collaborative book projects, would nurse his "44" throughout the morning, then return to Daily's at lunchtime for a refill. "Since I always kept the cup, my refill price was considerably cheaper," he said. "A buck-fifty a day, seven days, worked out to ten dollars a week. As liquid treats go, that's not that bad, especially when compared to what you pay at Starbucks for one coffee drink." Because he was such a faithful customer, the friendly clerks at Daily's would occasionally wave him off and not charge him.

After finishing his second "44" in the midafternoon, Bob would mosey over to his private stash of Diet Coke two-liter bottles stacked up in the garage. "Whenever the price dropped from $1.29 to 89 cents, I would buy a stockpile of them," he said. It was time for another refill.

For thirty years, Bob figures that he consumed around 100 ounces of Diet Coke a day, which, according to my math, means he drank the equivalent of 9 12-ounce cans a day, 56 cans a week, 270 a month, 3,285 a year, or at least 98,550 Diet Cokes in his lifetime. But here's where Bob's story takes a twist: his Diet Coke fix came to a sudden halt recently when he walked into his local Publix, strolled over to the soft drink aisle, and, as his hand reached for a two-liter, a voice in his head said, "No, don't do it."

Drink Diet Coke—With Vitamins? by Jordan Rubin and Dr. Bernard Bulwer

Diet Coke has legions of fanatics just like Bob DeMoss. Florida State University football coach Bobby Bowden says that half his diet is drinking Diet Coke and the other half is eating peanuts. Victoria Beckham, married to British soccer celebrity David Beckham, claims to hate the taste of water and drinks nothing but Diet Coke.[1]

Diet Coke is the third-best selling soft drink in America, right behind full-sugar Coke Classic and Pepsi. As sales of diet drinks keep climbing (30 percent of the soda market in 2007, up from 25 percent in 2000[2]), Coke rolled out a new version of Diet Coke in the summer of 2007 with added vitamins and minerals called Diet Coke Plus. The blue-capped bottles contain 10 to 15 percent of the daily requirement of niacin, zinc, magnesium, and vitamins B_6 and B_{12}.

Whoop-de-doo. We fail to see the point, unless it's to fool heavy Diet Coke drinkers to actually think they're drinking something healthy. You're still ingesting aspartame, an artificial sweetener that has sparked debate for decades. H. J. Roberts, MD, an authority on artificial sweeteners, testified at congressional hearings that artificial sweeteners like aspartame, saccharin, and sucralose can be highly addictive and trigger toxic substances to cross the blood-brain barrier, causing neurological problems.[3]

Diet and "lite" beverages featuring industrial nonnutritive chemical sweeteners have been touted as the answer to America's obesity epidemic for decades. Even people with diabetes could supposedly satisfy their sweet tooth. Saccharin—the chemical in Sweet'N Low—was the first artificial sweetener to market, and the compound is up to 700 times sweeter than table sugar. Since its introduction in the 1960s, though, saccharin has created a string of never-ending debates and fights over its safety, especially since laboratory experiments linked it to bladder cancer in rats.

Probably because of its slight metallic aftertaste, saccharin has been supplanted in popularity by aspartame—sold under the brand names NutraSweet or Equal—which has equally evoked controversies over its safety, including a possible link with brain tumors. Aspartame's breakdown products—methanol and formic acid—are known toxins in high concentrations. Aspartame and another popular sweetener, acesulfame K (marketed as Sweet One or Sunett), are up to 200 times sweeter than table sugar.

Sucralose, known commercially as Splenda, came out in 1998 and immediately made a splash by attempting to distance itself from the chemical aftertaste of popular artificial sweeteners. "Made from sugar, so it tastes like sugar" became its slogan. Clearly, this marketing strategy was designed to wrap Splenda in the cloak of being "natural," which is what the manufacturers of artificial sweeteners want you to believe.

"My wife, Leticia, has been after me for ten years to give up Diet Coke," Bob said. "Frankly, she was always lecturing me about it, and, admittedly, I should have listened a long time ago, but Diet Coke was my one little treat. I thought when I squeezed lemon into my Diet Coke that I was adding nutritional value to it."

Bob replaced his addiction for Diet Coke with bottled water. Sure, there were some tough moments while he retrained his taste buds, but eventually his body accepted the "boring" taste of water. During a weak moment or two, however, Bob returned to his Daily's for a "44," but the icky-sweet chemical aftertaste now grossed him out. "It was interesting how quickly I lost desire for my favorite diet soft drink." These days Bob says he's a "water fiend." He now buys a thirty-four pack of bottled water at Sam's Club and keeps them stashed in the garage—where his Diet Cokes used to sit. Whenever he takes a drive, Bob brings two half-liter bottles of water for the road.

What was also interesting was how two other "significant events"—Bob's words—happened after he stopped drinking Diet Coke like it was coming out of a drinking fountain. First, his blood pressure dropped twenty points from a moderately high 149/96 to a nearly normal 130/70. "I wasn't expecting that," Bob said, but the second event surprised him even more. "When I stopped drinking all that Diet Coke, I felt less on edge. What I mean is that when I was drinking 44s and one of my children made the smallest infraction, I'd lose it and overreact. I wouldn't totally blow a gasket, but I'd be quicker to bark. Now I'm a different person. I have a much more even temperament. I don't know if it's caffeine or the artificial sweetener aspartame in Diet Coke, but definitely I seem to have a brighter outlook on life and feel more upbeat."

Bob says he's also moving in the right direction on his weight, and you will too, when you stop drinking colas, diet soft drinks, "energy" drinks like Red Bull, and sports drinks like Gatorade and POWERade. Replacing your old ways of drinking liquid refreshments with water, green tea, certified organic coffee, fresh fruit and veggie juices, and lacto-fermented beverages will do wonders for your health *and* your waistline.

NOTHING LIKE WATER

Let's turn our attention first to plain old water, which is often overlooked as a weight-loss tool because it's so…ordinary. Any fluid replacement that's odorless and colorless seems downright boring compared to the sexier "fitness waters" and candy-colored sports drinks you can buy at a Daily's convenience store, for example. Yet regular ol' water can play a significant role in losing weight because of the way it revs up your metabolism and hydrates cells so that they can process carbohydrates and fat more efficiently. When your body's cells are well hydrated, you accelerate the liver's ability to convert stored fat into usable energy and help your kidneys flush out toxins. If you substitute water for soft drinks—and ignore everything else written in *The Maker's Diet for Weight Loss*—you'll still lose three pounds in short order, according to a study at Children's Hospital and Research Center in Oakland, California.[4]

Water is the ultimate calorie-free and sugar-free substance, the perfect libation. Only water is the perfect fluid replacement to regulate body temperature, carry nutrients and oxygen to the cells, cushion joints, protect organs and tissues, remove toxins, and maintain strength and endurance. Even when bottled, water is still a good deal—unless you're into a natural spring water from Tennessee called Bling H_2O, which comes in wine-sized frosted bottles embedded with Swarovski crystals spelling out its name and going for forty dollars a bottle. Bling, as you would imagine, is big with the Hollywood set, where the entertainment media reports that Paris Hilton fills her dog's water dish with the ultra-expensive couture water.

And I thought San Pellegrino was a treat.

Whenever I leave home for my office, I carry a half-gallon polycarbonate plastic container filled with fresh water that's run through my home filtration system. My goal is to drink the same amount of water daily that Bob DeMoss used to drink in his Diet Coke heyday—at least 100 ounces.

I'm a big water drinker because I know that H_2O hydrates my cardiovascular system, irrigates my digestive tract, keeps my body cool in the stifling Florida heat, and helps eliminate waste products from my body. Regularly sipping on my water bottle means I have to visit the restroom more often, but that's a small inconvenience for participating in one of the healthiest practices available to us. You honestly can't improve on plain water.

If you're looking to slim down, drinking plenty of water is just as important as choosing the right foods to eat. The most rigorous and challenging part of the Weight Loss Eating Plan happens in the first week or two, when the body goes through a "purification" stage. When you suddenly stop eating foods with white sugar, artificial sweeteners, and preservatives, you may experience temporary withdrawal-type symptoms such as headaches, carbohydrate cravings, less energy, mood swings, or even changes in your bowel habits. These "detox" reactions are indications that the body is making adjustments while working to cleanse toxins from the system. Your body needs streams of water during this season of the "blahs." When the body is properly hydrated, the kidneys function normally, effectively removing waste from the body.

You can drink your water cold or lukewarm, as suits your personal taste, but don't drink water with added carbonation, like Perrier. Drinking still or natural sparkling spring water is the best, and consuming water before and during your meals will help you digest your food efficiently and prevent constipation.

How much water should you be drinking? A good rule of thumb is a half-ounce of water for every pound of body weight. As an example, since I weigh between 185 and 190 pounds, that means I should drink 95 ounces of water per day, or around twelve glasses. I know that's a lot of water—considerably more than a half-gallon—but I usually reach my goal of 100 ounces since I carry my 64-ounce plastic container wherever I go. I try to consume around 32 ounces of water before I leave for the office, which is pretty easy for me since I exercise in the morning and guzzle water during my FIT exercise session. (You'll read more on FIT in chapter 9.)

Whenever I travel, I would carry my water jug right onto the plane, but that practice ended when the TSA banned liquids and gels in carry-on baggage a few years ago. These days I either buy a bottle of water before I board, or I ask the flight attendant for two cups (or a bottle) of water each time the beverage cart passes by. Flying is dehydrating due to the extremely dry cabin air, so I try to drink 8 to 16 ounces of water each hour I'm in the air to maintain water levels in my radiator.

What's on Tap?

I mentioned that before I go to work in the morning, I fill a 64-ounce container with filtered water that comes directly from a water dispenser at my kitchen sink. The clear liquid comes from a municipal source responsible for making sure my family's water is safe for public consumption. While dependable and germ-free, municipal water still needs to be filtered before it can become a good source of hydration for you. Most drinking water straight from the tap contains over 700 chemicals, including excessive levels of lead.[5]

Municipal water, be it a major metropolis like New York City to the smallest town in rural outskirts, undergoes a series of filtration steps to remove fine microorganisms and dissolved inorganic and organic materials. Before treated water can be released from a treatment plant, however, it must be disinfected to destroy any pathogens that somehow made it through the filtration process. The most common disinfectant is chlorine or its chemical cousins—chloramines and chlorine dioxide.

Chlorine…yes, I'm talking about the granular white stuff the pool guy dumps into swimming pools so that nobody gets sick when the kiddies urinate in the pool. Chlorine is the disinfectant of choice for municipalities because it's cheap and doesn't seem to harm humans, but it's still a highly toxic substance. If your tap water is treated with chlorine—and it probably is—then I recommend you install water filters at your kitchen sink and between the water line and the refrigerator. A cheaper alternative costing less than thirty dollars would be purchasing a countertop water pitcher with a built-in carbon-based filter.

I went whole hog during the construction of our new home a couple of years ago. I asked the contractor to install a whole-house filtration system using ultra filtration and reverse osmosis that would remove the chlorine and other impurities before the water entered our household pipes. Now, before I leave in the morning, I can fill my half-gallon container with filtered water and confidently know that I'm hydrating my body with the best refreshment resource available to me—right from my home.

You should always have a glass of water nearby as well. Reaching for a sip every now and then may not seem like a big deal, but if you don't keep yourself properly hydrated, reaching your ideal weight becomes that much harder.

WHAT ABOUT OTHER LIQUIDS?

I know that every diet book worth its salt—I hope saying "salt" makes you thirsty—encourages readers to drink at least the proverbial "eight glasses of water each day." I've read, however, that medical experts like the National Academy of Sciences' Institute of Medicine believe that the long-held recommendation to drink eight glasses of water is an old wives' tale. After reviewing more than four hundred studies, the National Academy said the majority of Americans already get enough fluids from the orange juice and coffee they drink, the milk on their breakfast cereal, the juicy orange they eat as a snack, the chicken soup they eat at lunch, and the ice-cold beer they slam down during happy hour.[6] (Just kidding about the last one.)

While I agree that drinking coffee counts some toward your hydration totals—as well as the body producing some water from the foods we eat—I don't think munching on a bowl of cereal topped with milk or slurping chicken soup is the same as drinking pure water. Since many more people are *not* properly hydrated than those who are, my gut says that's because they aren't drinking enough water. Having a bowl of cereal, drinking orange juice, or sipping on soup is not the same as drinking water. Your body tells you there's a difference. When I recommend a half-ounce of water per pound of body weight, I'm talking about pure water. Any other beverages should not count toward that total.

Besides, the state of orange juice and other fruit juices in America is not good. Most juices are full of concentrated sugars with a loss of nutrients from pasteurization and concentration, which makes them as nutritionally void as refined white flour. I recommend that you stay away from OJ and fruit juice while following the Weight Loss Eating Plan unless you buy a fresh-squeezed variety made from organically grown fruit. Fresh-squeezed orange juice should be diluted with purified or naturally carbonated mineral water so that you won't ingest more fruit sugar than you would normally receive when eating a piece of fruit.

In the latter stages of the Weight Loss Eating Plan, it's OK to drink raw vegetable and raw fruit juice, if you use a juicer to make your own. Stay away from canned vegetable juice, especially tomato juice, which tends to be high in sodium and preservatives. Juicing fruits and vegetables yourself gives you all the nutrients nature has provided without anything artificial.

WATER RETENTION

Then there are those who believe that if they drink too much water, they'll gain weight because of water "retention." Unless there is an underlying medical problem, such as liver or kidney failure, just the opposite occurs. Drinking extra water seems to *boost* metabolism, which promotes weight loss, albeit modest. Michael Borschmann, MD, and colleagues from Franz-Volhard Clinical Research Center in Berlin, Germany, tracked energy expenditures from seven men and seven women—healthy and not overweight—who drank 17 ounces of water. This was followed by testing their metabolic rates to see how fast they burned calories.

Within ten minutes of consuming a large glass of water, the test subjects' metabolism increased by 30 percent for both men and women and reached a maximum after thirty to forty minutes. The German researchers estimated that over the course of a year, a person who increased his water consumption by 1.5 liters a day (around 50 ounces) would burn an extra 17,400 calories, which translates into a weight loss of approximately five pounds.[7]

F. Batmanghelidj, MD, and author of *Water: For Health, for Healing, for Life*, contends that sipping on a water bottle will act like a governor on an overheated engine to dampen hunger pangs and prevent you from overeating or cheating. He recommends drinking a glass of water before sitting down for breakfast, lunch, and dinner. "You will feel full and will eat only when food is needed," he said. "The volume of food intake will decrease drastically. The type of craving for food will also change. With sufficient water intake, we tend to crave proteins more than fattening carbohydrates. . . . If you think you are different and your body does not need this amount [eight to ten glasses per day] of water, you are making a major mistake," notes Dr. Batmanghelidj, who believes that many dieters confuse hunger and thirst, thinking they're hungry when actually they're dehydrated.[8]

The sensation of thirst and hunger is generated simultaneously to indicate the brain's needs, but many do not recognize the sensation of thirst and assume both "indicators" to be the urge to eat. Thus, they reach for a bag of chips when they should have been reaching for a glass of water. Dr. Batmanghelidj says that when people reach for water first, they manage to separate the two sensations, which stops them from overeating and taking one step back on their way to reaching their ideal weight.

One way to know if you're properly hydrated is looking at the color of your urine. If your urine is consistently yellow, then you're not drinking enough water. Clear or light yellow urine is the best indicator that you're drinking enough water throughout the day. Cloudy urine, no matter what the color, can indicate dehydration.

When you're at work, keep a water bottle or glass of water nearby. Drinking more water than you're used to will be one of the most important things you can do to lose weight. Filtered water is preferable to "fitness" waters like Propel, which contain sucrose syrup and a bevy of additives. Glacèau Vitamin Water, a trendy "nutrient-enhanced water beverage," is sweetened with crystalline fructose, which, like sucrose syrup, is a variation of high-fructose corn syrup. Depending on what Glacèau Vitamin Water "flavor" you pull from the shelves, a 20-ounce bottle contains 100 to 125 calories and between 20 and 32 grams of sugar, nearly the equivalent of a 12-ounce can of the real thing—Coke. Fresh water has zero calories.

"It is primitive and simplistic thinking that one could easily lace water with all sorts of pleasure-enhancing chemicals and substitute these fluids for the natural and clean water that the human body needs," said Dr. Batmanghelidj. "Some of these chemicals—caffeine, aspartame, saccharin, and alcohol—through their constant lopsided effect on the brain, single-mindedly program the body chemistry with results contrary to the natural design of the body....The intake of wrong fluids will affect the life of anyone who continually consumes them."[9]

Not to mention reaching your ideal weight.

TEA TIME

I have good news to report: drinking tea in moderation—two to three cups a day—certainly contributes to the body's hydration. A published review of tea research conducted at King's College in the United Kingdom—where Dr. Bulwer studied nutrition—showed that tea hydrates the body as effectively as water. "Drinking tea is actually better for you than drinking water," said Dr. Carrie Ruxton, one of the coauthors of the King's College report. "Water is essentially replacing fluid. Tea replaces fluids and contains antioxidants, so it's got two things going for it."[10]

Globally, tea is the most widely consumed beverage, after water. All true varieties of tea come from the leaves of a single evergreen plant, *Camellia sinensis*. (Herbal teas such as chamomile and peppermint should really be called herbal infusions as they are not true teas.) During harvest time, tea leaves are picked, rolled, dried, and heated. The type of tea depends on how the leaves are processed. Green and white teas are nonoxidized and are the freshest. Black or oxidized teas are the most fermented. Oolong or partially oxidized teas are in between.

Green tea accounts for 20 percent of the global tea market, while black tea (or green tea that has been subjected to additional processing that ferments and oxidizes the leaves) accounts for about 78 percent.[11] I recommend green tea because of less processing and its higher levels of antioxidants than black tea.

As far as caffeine is concerned, I believe that tea's benefits are better delivered in teas containing caffeine, which has a mild diuretic effect. Since tea leaves naturally contain caffeine, I believe it's healthiest for us to consume tea in its most natural form. Obviously, if caffeine tends to keep you up at night, you should avoid consuming caffeinated teas in the late afternoon or in the evening.

Even better news is that new evidence is emerging that green tea can help you lose weight. The *American Journal of Clinical Nutrition* published the results of a study at the University of Geneva in Switzerland in which men given a combination of caffeine and green tea extract burned more calories than those given only caffeine or a placebo, meaning that green tea accentuates the stimulant properties of caffeine, which raises the metabolic rate.[12] The clinical trials conducted at the University of Geneva also revealed that the catechins in green tea raised the body's thermogenesis rate (amount of calories burned), which, in turn, increased energy expenditure.

What makes green tea so special? The secret behind green tea lies in its high content of a class of health-promoting agents collectively known as polyphenols or flavonoids—specifically the group known as catechins. Epigallocatechin gallate, or EGCG, comprises up to 40 percent of the dry weight of green teas and has a knack for improving the flow of blood through the vessels, which is good for cardiovascular health. EGCG is a powerful antioxidant ("antirust" agent) that kills many types of cancer cells in vitro without harming healthy tissue; it is also effective in lowering the bad LDL cholesterol levels, which clog our arteries.

Green tea—I also recommend a traditional type of Chinese tea known as oolong tea—should come from organic sources. Some of the best natural, organic teas I've found are imported from the pristine Wuyi Mountains of China, where tea leaves are harvested by hand and not subjected to pesticides and chemical fertilizers. Japan is also a major producer. Unlike conventional produce, you cannot wash herbicide residue off tea leaves, so stick to boxes marked "Organic Tea." Many organic teas are "Fair Trade" certified, which guarantees that workers picking the leaves receive fair wages for their efforts.

There's a different type of tea drink I want to introduce you to, and it's called kombucha, or mushroom tea. Kombucha (pronounced *kom-BOO-cha*) is a fermented beverage made from black or green tea and a fungus culture. Sounds awful, but I have been known to drink several of these exotic beverages a week. They're not cheap, though, at three bucks a bottle, but if you look online, you can find ways to order a kombucha culture and make this sweet-and-sour drink at home.

Many cultures around the world consume lacto-fermented beverages like kombucha for their wonderful health benefits, but it's a beverage unlike anything tasted in this country. One reviewer, Siobhan Roth of the *Pittsburgh Post-Gazette*, compared kombucha to old sweat socks with a lemon twist.[13] I don't think kombucha tastes that bad. Kombucha has a cidery flavor and a definite fizziness, but I like the way the beverage boosts my energy and lightens my mood. My favorite flavor is grape, but you can find flavors like raspberry, mango, and lemon ginger.

Low in calories and sugar—just 8 grams per 8 ounces—you'll find statements like "sparkling Himalayan tonic" or "handmade Chinese tea" on the labels, but kombucha is distinctly Russian in origin. One brand, Kombucha Wonder Drink, started appearing in health food stores several years ago and has developed a cult following. Kombucha is not a drink you guzzle down like a cold bottle of water after playing two sets of tennis. Kathy O'Brien of the Weston A. Price Foundation, which disseminates the research of nutrition pioneer Dr. Weston A. Price, said that you should go slow when drinking this fizzy lacto-fermented beverage—no more than 4 ounces at a time.

Lacto-fermented beverages are very healthy as they're high in lactic and gluconic acids, as well as enzymes and probiotics that are good for digestion. Don't let the pungent aroma or cloudy appearance stop you from trying this healthy drink.

A JAG FOR COFFEE

Although I'm a kombucha fan, I don't see the tart-tasting beverage entering the American consciousness like coffee. This country's obsession with sugared coffee drinks from Starbucks has muddied the waters, so to speak, because any time a barista whips up a coffee confection, you're drinking the equivalent of a liquefied candy bar. Grande sizes of mocha, vanilla, white chocolate, orange mocha, hazelnut, java chip, and caramel-flavored coffees top 400 calories per serving and over 50 grams of sugar.

So, you'll have to put aside your Starbucks fix to reach your weight-loss goals, but that doesn't mean you can't drink coffee. It's fine to consume fresh ground organic coffee flavored with organic cream, honey, or stevia, but exercise moderation, meaning one cup per day or every other day. And just as with tea, I believe coffee is best consumed as it was created—fully loaded. Decaffeinated coffee is highly processed and removes some of the antioxidant benefits contained in the beans.

Personally, I'm not a huge fan of coffee or a coffee drinker myself, but I'm aware that caffeinated coffee, as well as tea, has been consumed for thousands of years by some of the world's healthiest people. As long as your coffee comes from organic sources, you'll be OK. You should buy whole beans, freeze them, and grind them yourself when desired, but you'll be even better off if you put aside coffee until you complete the Weight Loss Eating Plan.

Caution: you should stay away from so-called "slimming" coffees, which are typically a combination of regular ground coffee, herbs, and supplements touted as appetite suppressants, such as hoodia, guarana, hydroxycitric acid, and guar gum, a type of fiber.

The Maker's Diet for Weight Loss Recap: Drink for Your Ideal Weight

1. Make your number-one beverage purified, nonchlorinated water, consuming a half-ounce of water per pound of body weight, or around eight to twelve cups a day, especially if you live in warmer climates.
2. If you drink natural sparkling water, don't choose brands with added carbonation, such as Perrier.
3. Install carbon-based filters at the kitchen faucet and refrigerator, or purchase countertop water pitchers.
4. Brew green tea, or consume presteeped liquid teas (preferably organic), which may be sweetened with a small amount of honey or stevia.
5. Take a step on the wild side and try lacto-fermented beverages like kombucha.
6. If you're a coffee drinker, switch over to certified organic coffee, which can be flavored with organic cream and a small amount of honey or stevia.

five

Snack for Your Ideal Weight

BACK IN THE early 1990s, Melissa Gertz was a missionary in India with Youth With A Mission. After living with and ministering to the Indian people for six years, she returned to the United States and eventually settled in Findlay, Ohio, after marrying her husband, Jeff.

Starting an office job was a bit of a cultural shock for Melissa, who weighed 145 pounds at the time. For one thing, the Ohio diet—heavy on fried foods, light on vegetables, and topped off with sweets—was much different from Indian cuisine, characterized by its extensive use of spices and herbs as well as scintillating vegetarian dishes and flat breads like *roti* and *paratha*. But it didn't take long for Melissa to adapt again to American ways. Monday through Friday, her co-workers would bring boxes of chocolate-glazed doughnuts to work, tempting Melissa until she reached for one or three.

After work, Melissa and Jeff liked to visit Findlay's famous ice cream emporium, Dietsch Brothers, where Melissa would order a sugar cone packed with three scoops of her favorite ice cream—Moose Tracks, heavily ribboned with chocolate. "I became a real chocoholic," she said. "Whenever I wanted a snack, I would hide Dove chocolate in between the seat cushions of my couch and eat them while I watched TV. Within a year or so, my weight ballooned to way over 200 pounds."

I'm pleased to say that Melissa's waistline has greatly improved—she got back down to 180 pounds by following the Maker's Diet for Weight Loss program—but all that harmful noshing nearly did her in. Until she turned her health around, Melissa—and many like her—didn't know what constitutes healthy snacking, nor was she aware that you often *should* eat something between meals. Reason: the body's metabolism resembles a furnace that must be stoked at regular intervals. That's why snacking is an important part of the Weight Loss Eating Plan. Personally, I like to snack, but my in-between treats are healthier—and yummier—than anything Dietsch Brothers' ice cream parlor could serve.

I'm pro-snacking because denying yourself food for long stretches sets you up for three things:

1. Misery

2. Depression

3. Failure

We certainly don't want any of those conditions coloring your experience with the Maker's Diet for Weight Loss. (Melissa said her out-of-control snacking made her feel very depressed, as if she were being controlled.) Snacking wisely can help you satisfy hunger pangs before they become overwhelming. When blood sugar levels fall, you don't want to reach for one of the bad old snacks—honey-roasted peanuts, mesquite-flavored potato chips, crème-filled cookies, vanilla ice cream bars dipped in chocolate, and store-bought snack cakes. These commercially produced snack foods are loaded with refined sugar, chemical preservatives, artificial sweeteners, and processed ingredients that rob your health and set you back two steps after making a stride forward.

To stay one step ahead of hunger, you need to arm yourself with SREs—snacks ready to eat, just as our servicemen and servicewomen carry MREs (meals ready to eat) while on patrol in Iraq. I'm talking about keeping on hand snacks like whole-food nutrition bars or even healthy cacao (chocolate) snacks. (See Appendix C for a list of recommended products.) Drinking a delicious and satisfying high-protein and high-fiber meal supplement will keep you feeling satiated for up to four hours between meals and dampen the munchies an hour or two before lunch or dinner. When you mix a powdered whole-food meal supplement into water, you are receiving two key ingredients to slow the digestion of carbohydrates in your digestive tract: fibertrol and native whey protein.

- *Fibertrol* is a fiber blend that includes glucomannan derived from konjac root, a traditional Japanese food. They help you feel full longer, reducing unnecessary food cravings that can lead to over-eating during meals and overindulging on unhealthy snacks between meals.
- *Native whey* comes from the milk of free-range, grass-fed cattle that graze on pesticide-free pastures. Normally, whey products are by-products of cheese devoid of vital immune and regenerative components that were destroyed during commercial processing. You want a whole-food meal supplement with native whey that's been minimally processed to preserve more of the natural factors, including cysteine, which, Dr. Bulwer says, is an important amino acid with a crucial role in the body's production of glutathione (GSH)— a major antioxidant indispensable for healthy functioning of all body cells, with special protective roles in the liver, the cardiovascular and immune systems, and red blood cells. Laboratory studies have

demonstrated that glutathione has the potential to greatly improve many aspects of our health.

Whole-food meal supplements usually contain probiotics, which are live bacteria cultures shown to enhance the natural flora in the gut. Probiotics increase the number of beneficial or friendly microorganisms present in the digestive tract while improving digestive efficiency. By enhancing the good bacteria, probiotics help drive out bad bacteria, yeasts, viruses, and parasites. Dr. Bulwer says that doctors routinely prescribe probiotics like Lactinex and Florastor to help maintain intestinal balance due to antibiotic use.

As a snack, drinking a whole-food meal replacement will help you maintain healthy blood sugar levels instead of spiking them, like Melissa's Moose Tracks ice cream, for instance. As you would expect, sugary desserts and refined foods have a high glycemic index, which means they are digested very quickly, leaving you hungry in a short time. When you keep nibbling sugary treats to satisfy your sweet tooth, the downward spiral continues. For recommendations on whole-food meal supplements, check out the Maker's Diet for Weight Loss Resource Guide on page 263.

CHECKING OUT THE BAR SCENE

Next on my list of healthy snacks are whole-food nutrition bars, which are commonly known as nutrition or energy bars. If you stroll through a warehouse club these days, you're apt to find a "food demo" for a popular energy bar. Dice-sized squares of various flavors are set on a tray, free for the taking. Energy bars are marketed as a nutritious meal supplement—a candy-bar sized alternative to packing a lunch or purchasing a Snickers from a vending machine. In many ways, energy bars are the perfect snack food for today's grab-and-go lifestyle—portable, nutritious, and tasty.

No longer a niche product for endurance athletes, energy bars have gone mainstream. Energy bars no longer taste like cardboard and sawdust covered with chocolate. Today, you can choose from flavors like chocolate raspberry fudge, cookie dough, dulce de leche, and devil's food cake, to name a few. They really do taste like a candy bar, except for a certain aftertaste. So are they healthy?

I think you already know my answer: most energy bars are not the nutritional powerhouses they are purported to be, nor are they a great meal replacement for those trying to lose weight and stay healthy. These energy bars are a highly processed mix of protein powders (soy or milk), sugars and/or artificial sweeteners, chemicals, preservatives, and synthetic ingredients.

Take soy protein, for example, which is often the first ingredient listed. Most soy protein comes from genetically modified soybeans. Soybeans are high in phytic acid, which can block absorption of essential minerals like calcium, magnesium, copper, iron, and zinc from the intestinal tract. Soy protein must be processed at high temperatures to reduce phytic acid levels, which pretty much destroy the "important proteins" in soy, such as lysine.

The reason why most energy bars taste so sweet is because they're full of high-fructose corn syrup, sucrose, or corn syrup, which are forms of refined sugar and contribute to weight gain and blood sugar imbalances. In my mind, energy bars are nothing more than glorified candy bars. I mean, if it looks like a candy bar, tastes like a candy bar, and has many of the same ingredients as a candy bar...then it's a candy bar and not a nutritious snack for someone trying to lead a healthy lifestyle.

Instead, shop at your local health food store for whole-food nutrition bars that aren't sweetened with high-fructose corn syrup but rather with a natural sweetener like raw honey. The best whole-food bars should contain native whey protein, an organic fiber blend, omega-3 fats, and a superstar ingredient called chia.

I know that when some people hear the word *chia* they think of "chia pets"—those kitschy animal figurines with green chia sprouts growing where their hair should be. The chia I'm talking about come from an edible seed that grows abundantly in desert plants found in southern Mexico and parts of South America. The seeds of the chia plant have long been consumed in Central and South America for use both as food and medicine. The seeds are oil-rich, about one-third of the entire seed, of which 60 percent is alpha-linolenic acid (ALA), thereby giving chia's fiber-rich seeds the highest percentage of omega-3 fatty acids of any plant, including flaxseeds. Because chia seeds have much higher antioxidant levels than flaxseeds, chia seeds don't go rancid as easily as flax.

Best of all for those seeking to lose weight, chia is very filling. Chia seeds swell from seven to nine times inside the stomach, which will pack your tummy in a hurry. You can see why when you mix a small amount of chia in a glass of water, after swirling the water for a few moments, the mixture turns gelatin-like and soon has the consistency of tapioca pudding. We're talking thick, but oh-so-nutritious for you. Again, check the Maker's Diet for Weight Loss Resource Guide on page 263 for recommendations.

I suggest that you eat a food bar or drink a meal-supplement shake as an in-between meal snack once or twice each day, especially during Phase I of the Weight Loss Eating Plan. Each of these two snacks are the answer to a growling stomach in midafternoon.

Other Great Snacks

I'm a constant snacker, one of those who can't go much longer than a couple of hours without eating. I'm not sure why, but when I'm not fasting or on a ten-day "detox" cleanse (as I'll describe in chapter 8), I get hungry quickly and often.

When it comes to whole foods, vegetables and vegetable dips make for fantastic snacks. For instance, you could dip organic baked chips into organically made salsa. A guacamole dip can be made fresh with organic avocados, lemon, cilantro, and sea salt. Carrots and celery can be eaten raw or dipped in hummus.

Fresh fruit and dried fruit are also nutritious snacks. Take a handful of dried raisins, figs, dates, prunes, pineapple, and papaya and combine them with some raw or soaked nuts or seeds. Make sure there is no sugar added or any sulfites. It's very easy to throw some dried fruit, nuts, and seeds into a bag and carry the mixture with you throughout the day for a quick snack.

Also keep in mind that there are many healthy snack and dessert recipes using organic ingredients you can make on your own, like whole-grain blueberry muffins, banana bread, and coconut almond fudge. Popcorn is another popular snack that can be healthy if prepared right. Use this recipe: First, melt some extra-virgin coconut oil in a pan, pour in organic popcorn kernels, and cook them until popped. Pour some melted organic butter over the popped kernels, and sprinkle with your favorite organic seasoning. *Voilà!*

For a list of delicious, healthy recipes and snacks, see the appendices in the back of this book. Some of the most convenient and healthiest snacks are nuts and seeds, which are great sources of fiber, healthy fats, and nutrients. If properly prepared, they are extremely nutritious. "Properly prepared" means raw, soaked, or even dry-roasted nuts and seeds not roasted in vegetable oil. Just make sure they are organic and without added salt. Try almonds, walnuts, cashews, pecans, pumpkin seeds, and sunflower seeds, or make your own healthy trail mix.

Raw nut butters, made from almonds, cashews, and sunflower seeds, are something worth checking out. They're special because they're unheated, not roasted, so their delicate oils haven't been damaged, and they still have their vitamins, minerals, and enzymes intact. Nut butters can be used as a veggie dip or spread onto sprouted bread or fresh fruit. Organic peanut butter is also recommended and can be found in natural-food stores, supermarkets, and even warehouse clubs these days.

THE CASE FOR CHOCOLATE

Back in 1830, British candy makers J. S. Fry and Sons developed the world's first chocolate bar by roasting fermented cacao pods and then grinding them into a fine paste that could be separated into either cacao solids (also known as cocoa powder) or cocoa butter. When they blended the cocoa solids and cocoa butter with refined sugar, the result was chocolate—the "nectar of the gods," as the confection came to be known in Europe.

Americans didn't develop a taste for chocolate until the turn of the twentieth century when Milton Hershey mixed fresh milk with chocolate and created the "nickel" bar, the first American chocolate bar for the masses. As other candy companies chased after a piece of the chocolate business, some chocolatiers discovered they could substitute cocoa butter with cheaper emulsifying agents and gain a price advantage.

These days it's not unusual to see chocolate made with soy lecithin—don't forget that soybeans are a heavily genetically modified crop—or an artificial emulsifier derived from castor oil. This allows manufacturers to reduce the amount of the more expensive cocoa butter while retaining the same melt-in-your-mouth sensation when taking a bite. Chocolate connoisseurs, though, can easily tell the difference between the "real stuff" and heavily processed chocolate in a single bite.

High-quality chocolate creates a taste sensation so intense that people get more excited from eating chocolate than they do when they passionately kiss their lovers, according to recent research carried out by Dr. David Lewis, formerly with the University of Sussex but now with the Mind Lab.[1]

As with anything in the food industry these days, manufacturers can take a perfectly great natural product and completely mess it up. The Chocolate Manufacturers Association, a Washington DC trade organization whose members include Hershey, Nestlè, Guittard, and World's Finest Chocolate, lobbied the Food and Drug Administration (FDA) recently for permission to substitute partially hydrogenated vegetable oils for cocoa butter as well as the right to use artificial sweeteners and milk substitutes. (Can you believe it? Partially hydrogenated vegetable oils are a major source of dangerous trans fats!) Currently, the FDA stipulates that candy makers must call their products "chocolate flavored" or "chocolaty" if the product contains any of these ersatz ingredients. They can't call their confection "chocolate."

Americans, who eat twelve pounds of chocolate each year—that's around a bar of chocolate every other day—don't like the taste of waxy chocolate. They prefer the real stuff: nine of the ten bestselling U.S. chocolate candies, such as Hershey Bars, M&Ms, and Reese's Peanut Butter Cups, use real chocolate.[2]

These days, there's good news for chocolate lovers: there is healthy and organic chocolate available in health food stores and progressive markets. These chocolate products are nutritionally miles ahead of the mass-produced chocolate bars and peanut butter cups found at convenience stores and supermarket checkout stands. The healthiest chocolate comes from dark organic chocolate derived from the seeds of the fruit of cacao trees, which are native to the rainforest regions of South America.

Real chocolate from cacao beans is:

- Super-rich in antioxidant flavonols
- One of nature's best sources of magnesium (a nutrient that supports the heart, increases brainpower, and causes bowel movements)
- High in phenylethylamine (PEA), which is thought to help create feelings of attraction and excitement
- High in fiber, which is great for the heart as well as the gut

Dark chocolate also releases both serotonin and endorphins, which act as antidepressants.[3] Chocolate can lift a dark mood rather quickly, and it diminishes the appetite.

Just be sure to enjoy in moderation. A small handful of cacao chocolate—an ounce—usually contains 100 calories, so this form of organic chocolate remains a treat, not a cheat. (See Appendix C for recommendations on cacao chocolate.)

Naked Chocolate

Slowly roasting the cacao beans and allowing them to ferment brings out the rich chocolate taste, but raw foodists sing the praises of having their chocolate "naked" by peeling and eating raw cacao beans. Raw food enthusiasts David Wolfe and Shazzie (she goes by one name, just like Cher) call the raw cacao bean one of nature's most fantastic superfoods.

"Typical commercial chocolate will contain a mixture of alkalized cacao powder, cacao butter, genetically modified soy lecithin, vanilla extract, and refined sugar," they write in their book, *Naked Chocolate*. "Milk chocolate contains powdered milk with its harmful antioxidant-blocking properties and a vast array of pesticide residues and artificial hormones that have been fed to the animal. After all this, no wonder people want the real thing."[4]

Eating the real thing can be part of a weight-loss program. Wolfe and Shazzie point out that no scientific evidence implicates chocolate consumption with obesity. "In fact," they say, "the reverse seems to be the case. Eating cacao helps one to lose weight. This is why seemingly every weight-loss product on the market contains cocoa powder, which decreases appetite. Diet companies hint they are doing you a favor by providing chocolate weight-loss products, when in fact they use chocolate because it works!"[5]

WHEN A TREAT TURNS INTO A CHEAT

Lifetime habits are hard to change. Many cannot quit eating junk food cold turkey; they often feel like they "deserve" a nutritional indulgence for even trying. Others chafe at restrictions or being told what to do. Indeed, we live in a culture that trumpets the breaking of rules. At one time Burger King told us, "Sometimes you gotta break the rules," while Outback Steakhouses ("No rules. Just right."), Neiman Marcus ("No rules here"), Don Q rum ("Break all the rules"), and even an NFL video game ("No refs, no rules, no mercy") expound the antisocial theme that rules are a drag on life.

So, I'll go with the flow: you have my official permission to cheat.

Why am I giving you my OK to eat a prodigal meal? Because I've learned that allowing people to cheat results in better compliance with the overall Weight Loss Eating Plan. Cheat meals give people a greater feeling of control over their lives. They look forward to their preset cheat meals, when they can feel "normal" again.

I recommend that you cheat on the weekends. That's when most families and couples socialize anyway, so if you want to go for it—just two meals per week, remember—do so sometime between Friday evening and Sunday night. My one request is that you don't eat any of the foods I listed in the Dirty Dozen.

Now, I know this will be a problem for some. You're thinking, "Jordan, everything I ate before I opened this book was one of the Dirty Dozen. Are you telling me that cocktail wienies, Boston Crème Rolls, chocolate-covered pretzels, and Lucky Charms cereal are off limits?"

Yes, if at all possible. You begin by taking steps to remove temptation from your path. You'll find the route to weight loss easier if your pantry isn't stocked with snack cakes, chocolate-covered candy bars, or all your old favorite breakfast cereals. Toss that junk food into the trash. Clean out your cupboards. Scour through the deep recesses of your freezer. Rummage through your refrigerator.

Then, replenish your pantry with organic treats purchased at the health food store: dates rolled in coconut, flaxseed crackers, cashews, and rice chips, to name a few items. Dried fruits such as apricots, peaches, prunes, and raisins are known as "nature's candy" and are ready to eat at any time. These convenient, healthy snacks pack almost as much of a nutritious punch as their fresh counterparts.

What about those occasions when you're invited over to a friend's barbecue or Super Bowl party, and all the old pleasure foods are beckoning from the buffet table? Your resistance melts like a Hershey bar in the warm sun. Within minutes, you're filling a paper plate with hogs in a sleeping blanket, gooey nachos dripping in melted American cheese, and Swedish meatballs drowning in a pool of sweet molasses sauce. You know you're cheating, but you can't stop yourself.

Well, I have good news for you. If you're going to cheat in the scenario I just described, just make sure you do all your cheating in a one-hour time frame.

Why sixty minutes? The husband-and-wife team of Richard and Rachel Heller, PhDs and retired professors from the Mount Sinai School of Medicine in New York, say that when the body has been deprived of insulin-triggering foods high in carbohydrates for two or more consecutive meals—which happens when you're following the Weight Loss Eating Plan—the body makes adjustments. The body learns to release less insulin because it figures that fewer carbohydrates will be coming its way in the future. Since less insulin is released, less fat is stored and more fat is burned up. "The lowered level of insulin also allows the brain chemical serotonin to act as it should—as an appetite regulator," the Hellers write in *The Carbohydrate Addict's Diet*. "You will probably eat far less than you would if you have been eating three consecutive carbohydrate-rich meals."[6]

When you keep eating after halftime of the big football game, the body responds to this onslaught of crummy foods by releasing a second phase of insulin, which produces more fat. Not good. This second insulin phase usually kicks in, say the Hellers, between seventy-five and ninety minutes after you begin eating. If you stop eating those cheesy nachos and Swedish meatballs *before* sixty minutes are up, however, the second phase of insulin release stays much lower. That's why it's important to keep your cheating within a sixty-minute time window.

Summertime barbecues, when the twilight lingers, can be worse than Super Bowl parties. The cheeseburgers might not come off the grill for a couple of hours, leaving your growling stomach plenty of time to graze on sour cream chips and imitation dip while sipping a sugared iced tea. After a leisurely meal with friends, you may wait until you have "more room" for the brownie and ice cream dessert, but eating a rich trifle more than an hour *after* the finger foods and main meal will push your insulin readings over the edge. Result: you've taken *three* steps backward, maybe four. Again, try to keep the cheating within a one-hour time period.

If you are home with your family but absolutely, positively have to cheat at dessert time, munch on cookies made with organic ingredients. In our home, we have tins of Jennies Macaroons available for those times when my sweet tooth wants to be pleased. I like that Jennies Macaroons are made with only three ingredients: coconut, honey, and egg whites. I'm also partial to the aforementioned homemade blueberry muffins and banana bread—both healthy, organic delights. (For more recommended brands, check out the Maker's Diet for Weight Loss Resource Guide on page 263.)

"Jordan, what about ice cream?" you may be asking. *We all scream for ice cream!* OK, if you have a craving for a delicious frozen dessert, you can shop for Julie's Organic Ice Cream in the freezer case of progressive health stores. Another option is to make your own ice cream or frozen yogurt, which I do a couple of times per month. I use a Vita-Mix blender to make the best ice cream and frozen yogurt east of the Mississippi River, using all organic ingredients.

A final thought regarding cheating: nighttime isn't the best time to let yourself have a dessert. You'll be better off cheating in the morning since this will give you extra time to work off those extra calories. No matter what time you cheat, though, you should consume a high-fiber food or beverage to fill up that tummy before the cheat.

Whether you cheat a little or a lot, you can bolster your health by taking nutritional supplements, including an exciting new product made from concentrated fucoxanthin. Our next chapter, "Supplement for Your Ideal Weight," is a primer on the importance and benefits of taking nutritional supplements, especially in relation to weight loss.

The Maker's Diet for Weight Loss Recap: Snack for Your Ideal Weight

1. Drink a whole-food meal supplement to take the edge off between-meal hunger.
2. Look for whole-food nutrition bars with native whey protein and chia, which are extremely high in omega-3 fatty acids and very filling as well.
3. Keep a variety of SREs on hand—snacks ready to eat. Fresh fruit, dried fruit, nuts, seeds, and vegetables like baby carrots can hold you over until dinnertime.
4. Enjoy chocolate produced from cacao beans grown in South American rainforests—the healthiest chocolate and a real tasty treat.
5. Be aware of the difference between a treat and a cheat. You're allowed two cheat meals a week during the sixteen-week Weight Loss Eating Plan, but

don't eat any of the Dirty Dozen foods.

6. Limit your cheating to a sixty-minute time period since eating for a longer period causes the body to raise insulin levels, which makes you gain weight.

six

Supplement for Your Ideal Weight

O NE REASON I like shopping in natural-food stores is the absence of tabloids at the checkout stands. When I do catch some headlines at an airport kiosk, I wonder where they come up with this stuff:

- "Chimp Arrested for Reckless Driving!"
- "Autopsy Proves It! Adolf Hitler Was a Woman!"
- "Guy Calls Phone # on Toilet Wall—& Finds His Missing Mom!"

Listen, we can all enjoy a laugh, but the phoniness stops being funny when you look inside the tabloids, where over-the-top ads promise quick, easy weight loss. These quarter-page ads usually include a blurred photo of a flabby, unhappy woman juxtaposed next to a buff, slimmed-down version who looks vaguely familiar to the Ugly Duckling in the first panel.

"No Diet or Exercise Required!" blares the headline. If you've been looking for a way to finally "take it off and keep it off," then all you have to do is gulp down the $39.95 "all-natural dietary supplements" three times a day and watch the fat melt away.

Weight-loss pills have been advertised since the nation's first tabloid, the *Police Gazette*, was sold a hundred years ago. Back then, weight-loss drugs often contained laxatives (that'll make you lose weight) or synthetic insecticides to purportedly increase human metabolism. These diet potions usually worked for a while—if they didn't cause the runs, blindness, or some other major health catastrophe.

If you're trying to lose weight, I think you should take something *far* different from diet pills. I'm referring to whole-food nutritional supplements, cod liver oil, and supplements made with concentrated fucoxanthin (pronounced *FEW-co-zan-thin*), a carotenoid from brown seaweed that's showing tremendous fat-burning potential. Fucoxanthin can accelerate weight and fat loss when combined with a calorie-conscious diet, according to a clinical study that I'll tell you about shortly.

But first, there's a fascinating backstory to fucoxanthin that I have to share. About seven or eight years ago, I was introduced to a Russian biochemist named

Zakir Ramazanov, PhD, a classically trained biochemist and plant physiologist who graduated from the Soviet Union's North Caucasian State University in 1978 at the top of his class.

While serving with the Soviet army in Afghanistan in the late 1970s, Dr. Ramazanov discovered a tonic that boosted his mental and physical energy—a tea made from the golden yellow roots of a Siberian plant called *Rhodiola rosea*. It seems that a Siberian soldier in Dr. Ramazanov's company received packets of Rhodiola rosea in the care packages sent from home, so Dr. Ramazanov decided to give the special tea a try. Rhodiola rosea, he learned, was a perennial plant that grows in dry, sandy ground at high altitudes in the Siberian arctic, and this herbal tonic would become a research focus after his return to civilian life.

Following his stint as a Soviet soldier, Dr. Ramazanov became the head engineer at the Institute of Solar Energy, where he designed and constructed solar batteries and solar energy stations. It was there that he began experimenting with solar bioreactors and how they affected the cultivation of certain marine vegetables and algae, including spirulina and chlorella.

As his career advanced, Dr. Ramazanov left the Soviet Union in 1989 and eventually made his way to the United States, where he accepted a research fellowship at Louisiana State University at Baton Rouge before he founded a company called National Bioscience Corp., headquartered in Chester, New York.

Dr. Ramazanov's specialty was insolating phytonutrients and antioxidants found in land and ocean plants. For instance, the Russian scientist applied innovative technology to the extraction of lycopene, beta-carotene, and lutein from tomatoes, mushrooms, and algae; the extraction of antioxidants from fruits and vegetables; and the intensive biotechnological cultivation of health-promoting marine plants or seaweed. Dr. Ramazanov helped introduce the healing properties of Rhodiola rosea to an American audience by serving as an essential contributor to *The Rhodiola Revolution: Transform Your Health with the Herbal Breakthrough of the 21st Century* by Richard P. Brown, Patricia L. Gerbarg, and Barbara Graham.

But Dr. Ramazanov's real passion was research into sea vegetables, particularly brown seaweed, because epidemiological data from some of the longest living and healthiest cultures on the planet—most notably the Japanese—showed that the human consumption of brown seaweed portended tremendous health benefits. Dr. Ramazanov informed me early on—this had to be around 2002 or so—that he was having success isolating a carotenoid called fucoxanthin from brown seaweed. Carotenoids are a class of natural pigments found principally in plants and algae. Acting as biological antioxidants, carotenoids protect cells and tissues from the damaging effects of free radicals.

Fucoxanthin, Dr. Ramazanov explained, was the carotenoid—or pigment—that turned brown seaweed "brown." This pigment prevented seaweed floating on the ocean surface from being scorched by the sun. Called *wakame* by the Japanese and a part of Asian diets for centuries, about the only time we're served brown seaweed in this country is when we enjoy a bowl of miso soup or seaweed salad in a Japanese restaurant. Although fucoxanthin was found in abundance in several different types of brown seaweed, the carotenoid was present in far lesser amounts in green and red sea vegetables.

Dr. Ramazanov told me that he believed fucoxanthin could regulate a protein called uncoupling protein 1, or UCP1, which controls the amount of fat stored in the body. UCP1, which regulates the activity of a key gene responsible for maintaining the body's temperature, is found in white adipose tissue, or visceral fat.[1] This type of fat, which usually surrounds the internal organs and sits under our bellies, is one of the major causes of "middle-age spread." White adipose tissue isn't that white; it more resembles a disgusting yellowish glob of tissue. This type of fat gathers toxins, leads to low-level inflammation, and harms people's hormonal health.

Dr. Ramazanov kept me posted on the latest research regarding fucoxanthin after moving his operation to the Canary Islands off the coast of Spain, where he served as director of science for the Institute of Technology and Marine Sciences. In the summer of 2006, he passed along news of a study coming out of Hokkaido University in Sapporo, where Japanese researchers studied the effects of fucoxanthin on more than two hundred laboratory animals. The Japanese study found fucoxanthin effective in fighting flab stimulating the UCP1 protein, which caused stored fat to break down.[2] In tests on the laboratory animals, fucoxanthin resulted in a 5 percent to 10 percent reduction in weight. The Japanese researchers said that since the abdominal area contains abundant white adipose tissue, the compound might be particularly effective at shrinking oversized midsections.

Could fucoxanthin do the same for humans? That became the $64,000 question. Study leader Dr. Kazua Miyashita said his team hoped that fucoxanthin could be developed into a nutritional supplement that targeted harmful fat.[3] Professor Miyashita said that their testing was the first to find that a natural food component had been shown to reduce fat by targeting the UCP1 protein, but dieters shouldn't eat a lot of miso soup or toss strands of brown seaweed in their salad (yuck!) to lose weight. Indeed, Professor Miyashita advised against the consumption of massive amounts of seaweed to lose weight because fucoxanthin was not easily absorbed from whole seaweed.[4]

On the heels of the Japanese study came word from Dr. Ramazanov's Russian sources regarding the results of two double-blind, randomized, placebo-controlled clinical trials involving 150 obese women. These studies (pending publication), a collaboration of multiple organizations including the Center of Modern Medicine and Russian Academy of Natural Sciences in Moscow, involved having overweight women follow a meal plan of 1,800 calories a day while taking fucoxanthin or a placebo. The two key results:

1. Those who received fucoxanthin lost an average of 14.5 pounds in just sixteen weeks, while those who received the placebo pill lost only 3 pounds.

2. Participants taking fucoxanthin raised their metabolic rate an average of 18.2 percent.

In addition, body fat loss was 11.8 pounds in the fucoxanthin group, compared to 2.8 pounds in the placebo group. That's a 383 percent greater weight loss and 321 percent greater fat loss, respectively. The women taking fucoxanthin also received reductions in liver fat, blood pressure, triglycerides, and C-reactive protein (CRP).

What the Russian scientists hypothesized was that fucoxanthin possessed strong thermogenic—or fat-burning—properties. Thermogenesis is defined as a process in which the body generates internal heat and thereby increases its metabolic rate, which in turn requires the utilization of internal stores of energy, such as fat. Translation: thermogenesis raises the temperature of the body's calorie-burning furnace, which burns fat. It's the reason why hibernating animals don't freeze to death during a long, hard winter. Their bodies spend the entire winter burning up stored fat that they accumulated during the feeding season. The same principle could be applied to humans: when stored fat begins burning up, the weight will start coming off.

Another way to explain the thermogenic process is by starting with mitochondria, which are the cells' powerhouses. What the fucoxanthin compound does is increase the UCP1 protein (also known as *thermogenin*) by boosting the metabolic rate within the fat cell so that it burns more fat. In fact, the research showed that users of fucoxanthin increased their metabolic rate by 18.2 percent to 24 percent, depending on the dosage. Participants who consumed the amount of fucoxanthin in three capsules had an average increase in their metabolic rate by 18.2 percent and began to notice results in five to six weeks, while those who took the equivalent of ten capsules increased their metabolic rate by nearly 24 percent and began to see results in two to three weeks. By contrast, green tea—which is known for providing an increase in metabolism—has been shown in clinical studies to raise the metabolic rate by only 4 percent. Taking concentrated fucoxanthin is literally like charging your fat-burning batteries, supporting the metabolism, or breakdown, of fat in white adipose tissue.

The clinical research also indicated that the metabolic boost from taking fucoxanthin did not stimulate the central nervous system, meaning it didn't cause the jitters or lost sleep like caffeine, nicotine, or thyroid hormones. Dr. Ramazanov reported that the fucoxanthin was safe with no side effects, and it even provided other health benefits, including improved cardiovascular health, reduction of inflammation (a major cause of heart disease), healthy cholesterol and triglyceride levels, improvements in blood pressure levels, and healthy liver function. As a carotenoid, fucoxanthin was a powerful antioxidant that protected cells from free-radical damage.

By harvesting the brown seaweed at a young age, Dr. Ramazanov and his team have been able to produce fucoxanthin in a concentration 250 to 500 times greater than by consuming sea vegetables alone. You'd have to drink miso soup by the gallon or use your chopsticks on bowl after bowl of seaweed salad to get a fraction as much of fucoxanthin.

Health food stores and vitamin shops carry nonstimulant weight-management supplements with fucoxanthin, so I urge you to check them out. (You can also find all my recommendations for nutritional supplements in the Maker's Diet for Weight Loss Resource Guide on page 263.) I'm confident these fucoxanthin supplements have shown an ability to break down belly fat by raising the body's metabolic rate without causing jitters, an increase in heart rate, or lost sleep. But don't buy a bottle and think concentrated fucoxanthin is going to work right away. It takes time for your metabolism to shift.

THERE ARE NO MAGIC PILLS

I guarantee that if you toss a basketball into a storefront vitamin store, you'd knock dozens of products marketed as "weight-loss supplements" off the shelves. The Natural Medicines Comprehensive Database lists more than 50 individual supplements and 125 proprietary products being marketed as weight-loss products, although their efficacy and long-term safety are question marks. For example, guar gum, produced from Indian cluster beans, and chitosan, extracted from shellfish, are sold as "fat blockers."

Hoodia, the extract of a South African cactus, is the rage in some weight-loss circles because of the way it purportedly dampens hunger. The supplement "is not thermogenic, so it does not speed up metabolism," explained Fred Pescatore, MD, and author of *The Hamptons Diet*. "It is simply an appetite suppressant. It does work, but it's not a superstar."[5]

Hoodia is mild stuff compared to ephedra, one of the most famous—or infamous—"fat-burner" supplements in the last ten years. Dietary aids containing the herbal supplement ephedra were huge sellers until they were linked to 155 deaths earlier this decade, including that of Baltimore Orioles 6-foot 2-inch, 249-pound pitching prospect Steve Bechler, who died of a heatstroke during a spring-training workout in 2003. Bechler's body temperature rose to 108 degrees, causing his major organs to fail. Toxicology tests on Bechler revealed significant amounts of ephedra in his blood. The Broward County medical examiner in South Florida declared that ephedra was a factor in causing the heatstroke that led to his death.[6]

Following the rash of bad publicity, the U.S. Food and Drug Administration reacted by banning ephedra, but a federal judge threw out the FDA ban in 2005.

The FDA appealed the ruling, and in 2006, the U.S. Court of Appeals for the Tenth Circuit upheld the FDA's ban of ephedra. The sale of ephedra-containing dietary supplements remains illegal in the United States.

Color me a skeptic. Believe me, I know that there are plenty of weight-loss products that tout their ability to burn fat or raise your metabolism. The vast majority don't work, however, or, as in the case of ephedra, are extremely dangerous. But fucoxanthin seems to be the real deal because of the clinical trials with the 150 obese Russian women. I'm confident that fucoxanthin will be one of the greatest fat-loss breakthroughs in the last decade.

What Dr. Bernard Bulwer and Dr. Joseph Brasco Have to Say

I asked my coauthor Bernard Bulwer, MD, and Joseph Brasco, MD, my coauthor on other books I've published, to read Dr. Ramazanov's research on fucoxanthin as well as a pair of double-blind, randomized, placebo-controlled clinical trials authored by Dr. Musa Abidov, professor of medicine at the Russian Academy of Natural Sciences in Moscow, and others on his team. These were the studies involving 150 obese women. Here's what my medical colleagues had to say:

Bernard Bulwer, MD, Cardiology (Noninvasive)/Echocardiography, Harvard Medical School

It appears, from my reading of the research data, that we have a promising weapon to help fight the battle of the bulge. I don't like to use the phrase "the next big thing," but fucoxanthin is a potentially powerful tool in our quest for improved health of Americans.

Many "fat-loss" products have come and gone. A number—both prescription and nonprescription varieties (for example, fen-phen and ephedra)—proved risky, even fatal, and were banned by the FDA. The findings from the Moscow fucoxanthin/pomegranate seed oil study of 150 obese women—which appears to be a carefully crafted study pending publication—indicated that in addition to losing the unhealthiest form of body fat (abdominal and visceral fat), fucoxanthin did not increase heart rate or cause jitters.

I noted with keen interest that fucoxanthin helped to maintain good C-reactive protein (CRP) levels, an indicator of inflammation within our bodies that, when elevated, is a strong and independent predictor of cardiovascular disease. Recent Japanese laboratory experiments in animals showed that fucoxanthin promoted the production of DHA—a healthy omega-3 fat found in fatty fish—that lowers CRP.

Consumption of brown seaweed and pomegranate are age-old practices by some of the world's longest-lived and leanest cultures. Judging from its long history of consumption and safety, and the evidence from published laboratory and animal experiments, and now this first recent clinical trial in humans—and there is even a buzz about fucoxanthin on WebMD.com—I have little doubt that supplements with fucoxanthin will receive a lot more attention in the near future.

Joseph Brasco, MD, Board Certified, Internal Medicine and Gastroenterology

Most weight-loss products offer a multitude of claims with little scientific evidence to back them up, so it was exciting to read a well-designed study that had a reasonable amount of patients and a valid statistical model.

Fucoxanthin doesn't appear to be a cosmetic, shed-a-few-pounds type of supplement. It really seems to have profound health benefits. Not only will I be recommending it to my patients, but I am also planning on conducting a clinical study in my own clinic. When asked who should take fucoxanthin, my answer is: *Who shouldn't?* In fact, as an avid outdoorsman and triathlete, I've been taking fucoxanthin and have lost those last few stubborn pounds. I'm proud to say that I have a six-pack at age forty-eight!

WHOLE-FOOD SUPPLEMENTS

I'm confident that when you consume the right foods, exercise regularly, and take the right supplements, you pose a triple threat against fat. While consuming the right foods is the foundation of overall wellness, you could be missing out on nutrients essential to good health for the following reasons:

- Reducing calories
- Disliking certain foods
- Losing nutrients from cooking
- The variable quality of food supply
- Lack of knowledge, motivation, or time for healthy meals
- Nutrient depletion from farming and processing, stress, lifestyle, pollution, and toxins

If you have been a yo-yo dieter for many years—and eaten nothing but cabbage soup or grapefruit for weeks on end, followed by months of junk food—you have deprived your body of vitamins and minerals that it needs to function at its best. If you found yourself nodding your head as you read those bullet points, then I would like you to consider how a couple of key whole-food nutritional supplements can fill the nutritional gaps in your diet.

I believe supplements are needed more than ever, and it's because of the less nutritious foods we eat. First, a history class: Thousands of years ago, our hunter-gatherer ancestors functioned healthily on the "caveman diet," which was comprised of wild plants, foraged fruits, plant roots, mushrooms, nuts, eggs, fish, local game, and honey for dessert. This "Stone Age diet" ended years ago with the development of agricultural practices—the farming of grains and cereals; domesticating cattle, goats, sheep, and lamb; and the development of fermented foods like cultured dairy, relish, and wine. Life on the farm, so to speak, remained this way until the onset of the Industrial Age in the late 1800s and early 1900s, which led to the introduction of manufactured processes that "refined" foods like grains, cereals, and sugar. The fourth and final trend—the one we're living in today—began in the 1950s with the rise of agribusiness, fast-food restaurants, and convenience foods—fast, nutritionally low, highly processed foods.

I believe we need supplemental vitamins, minerals, and antioxidants because our bodies do not produce these nutrients, so they must come from an outside source. The standard American diet (SAD) contains foods that have been stripped of many of their healthy components and are devoid of many vitamins and minerals. Today's conventionally grown food is usually low in antioxidants and can cause free-radical damage that can compromise cellular health.

Many overweight people are starved of nutrients because their diets contain mostly "empty" calorie foods. If you are among the majority of Americans who begin each day by gulping a multivitamin or two with your orange juice, I have a question for you: Have you checked the label of your multivitamin lately? If you see ingredients such as sucrose, cornstarch, thiamine mononitrate, pyridoxine hydrochloride, or sodium metasilicate listed, your multivitamin is produced from isolated and synthetic materials. When you look on the packaging and see the letters *dl* in front of an ingredient—like "dl-alpha tocopheryl," for example—your multivitamin is using a synthetic version of vitamin E. Again, not all vitamin E is created equal.

Synthetic or isolated multivitamins are never going to be as good or potent as the ones produced from natural sources; studies show that synthetically made vitamins are 50 percent less biologically active than vitamins made from natural sources.[7] So, when you introduce nutritional supplements produced from whole foods and other natural sources into your body, you'll double the nutrients available to the body.

For ensuring proper nutrition while losing weight, I recommend multivitamins fermented with probiotics, which are known in the natural health industry as whole-food or living multivitamins. These vitamins contain important compounds—organic acids, antioxidants, and key nutrients—essential to good health. They are more costly to produce since ingredients like antioxidant-rich fruits and vegetables, sea vegetables, and microalgaes are put through a fermentation process similar to the digestive process of the body. Whole-food multivitamins are well worth the extra money, however.

Whole-food nutritional supplements made with antioxidant-rich fruits and vegetables as well as nutrient-rich cereal grasses are super foods. Cereal grasses are the only foods in the vegetable kingdom that, even if consumed alone, enable animals to continually maintain weight, strength, and optimal health.

Grass is richer in nutrients than spinach, broccoli, eggs, and chicken in virtually all categories, including protein. Grass abounds in unidentified growth factors, powerful antioxidants, immune boosters, and many other health-supporting nutrients. Cereal grasses, including the green leaves of wheat, barley, rye, oat, and kamut, are nutrient-dense foods. Wheat and barley grasses are high in chlorophyll, beta-carotene, vitamins C and E, and are among the best plant sources of protein.

COD LIVER OIL

The benefits of cod liver oil were discovered in the fishing communities dotting the coasts of Norway, Scotland, and Iceland in the nineteenth century. In these remote outposts, taking a spoonful of golden oil pressed from the livers of cod fish carried all sorts of health advantages.

Cod liver oil is a superstar because it contains four nutrients that we hardly get enough of: eicosapentaenoic acid (EPA), docosahexaenoic acid (DHA), vitamin A, and vitamin D. EPA and DHA are long-chain polyunsaturated fats known as omega-3 fatty acids, which are found in cold-water fish and eggs from chickens that run around and eat worms. The omega-3 fatty acids are wonderful not only for maintaining your immune system but also for their ability to promote healthy blood lipids since omega-3 fatty acids can lower blood triglyceride levels. They also support neurological and brain function.

The vitamin A in cod liver oil supports eye health, normal skin and hair structure, and the health and integrity of the mucosal linings of the body, such as the gastrointestinal (GI) tract and lungs.

The vitamin D in cod liver oil builds strong bones, which can prevent bone deterioration in adults. Additionally, vitamin D is suggested to play a pivotal role in supporting muscle tone and strength.

I recommend taking between 1 teaspoon and 1 tablespoon of cod liver oil daily. You can purchase cod liver oils with flavors that mask the "fishy" odor, but for the uninitiated, cod liver oil can be daunting at the outset.

I don't think cod liver oil tastes *that* bad, but then again, I've been either sipping a spoonful or taking easy-to-swallow liquid capsules of cod liver oil for more than a decade. I'm so used to the fishy taste that I could sip the stuff right out of the bottle.

Don't let the fishy taste keep you from introducing this Hall of Fame nutrient into your diet. Cod liver oil helps prevent bone deterioration in adults, improves cardiovascular function, and contributes to long life—great reasons to get cod liver oil off the bench and into the game.

Q&A TIME

I'm going to answer some common questions about the use of nutritional supplements:

1. What if I feel worse after I start taking supplements?

When starting a healthier diet and lifestyle, you should start slowly, and then gradually work up to the recommended amounts. More importantly, check with your health professional to rule out any other reason for these issues. If issues persist and interfere with daily activities, stop supplementation and build up slowly when feeling better.

2. If I'm eating all these healthy foods, why do I need to take so many supplements?

Taking nutritional supplements is a wonderful way to ensure that you're getting all the needed nutrients daily. With whole-food supplements, the dosage amount that satisfies the recommended levels will be higher. They are more like taking concentrated food with your meals than pills. Although they can be taken on an empty stomach with good results, it's better to take them with meals because of the benefits of breaking down foods and carrying nutrients through the bloodstream.

3. After I finish the Maker's Diet for Weight Loss sixteen-week plan, should I still continue to take supplements daily?

After the completion of the Weight Loss Eating Plan, it's entirely up to you whether or not you continue taking the supplements. If possible, though, you should continue taking them since they can help optimize your health.

4. Is there a difference in which supplements I should take based on age? What about children?

No, there isn't a difference, but it's always a good idea to check with your primary care physician before starting a supplement program. Every individual is unique, especially when you consider differences in age and fitness level. As for children, we do not have a suggested usage for those under the age of sixteen. Suggested use is based on a 150-pound individual. Please contact your pediatrician for any recommendations.

5. Can I take supplements with my medication?

As you might anticipate, we are not able to provide medical advice. Please ask your doctor or pharmacist if you can take the recommended supplements with your medication.

The Maker's Diet for Weight Loss Recap: Supplement for Your Ideal Weight

1. Support your body's own breakdown of fat and increase your metabolism with fucoxanthin.
2. Cover your bases with a whole-food multivitamin.
3. Even if you have to hold your nose the first time or two, take 1 teaspoon to 1 tablespoon of cod liver oil. Or, if you're traveling or just can't handle taking oil off the spoon, try cod liver oil capsules.

seven

The Weight Loss Eating Plan

Now THAT WE'VE talked about how you can eat, drink, snack, and supplement for your ideal weight, I'd like to present you with the sixteen-week Weight Loss Eating Plan that's broken down into four phases. Each phase offers approved foods while restricting others. Phase I is the most challenging and requires the most discipline. But, as in life, the more you put in, the more you get in return. If you follow Phase I to the best of your abilities, you should receive excellent results and lose between six and sixteen pounds. The following three phases get progressively easier as certain foods are reintroduced to your diet.

PHASE I
WEEKS 1–4

This sixteen-week program begins with Phase I, the "purification" phase, which is the most rigorous and challenging part of the Maker's Diet for Weight Loss but also the most rewarding. You'll see in the following food list that white sugar, artificial sweeteners, and preservatives are forbidden. Not eating these foods often causes temporary withdrawal-type symptoms such as headaches, carbohydrate cravings, less energy, mood swings, or even changes in your bowel habits. These "detox" reactions are indications that the body is working to cleanse toxins from the system. When you have the "blahs," increase water intake and rest.

Phase I is designed to stabilize blood sugar levels, reduce inflammation, enhance digestion, and balance hormone levels in the body. This phase restricts disaccharide-heavy carbohydrate foods such as pastas and breads but makes up for it in the variety of delicious, high-nutrient, high-fiber foods you can enjoy. You are more likely to see significant weight loss during this phase due to the consumption of higher amounts of protein and healthy fats and less carbohydrates. There is also the added benefit of improved digestion, smoother skin, and increased energy levels.

During Phase I, I recommend that you not drink any alcohol—wine, beer, or mixed drinks—but you are allowed two "cheat" meals per week. The best time to cheat is on the weekend, but do not eat, if possible, any of the "Dirty Dozen" foods listed in chapter 3. Organic treats such as dates rolled in coconut, flaxseed crackers, rice chips, and dried fruits—"nature's candy"—make up "good" cheats.

Try to keep your cheating within a sixty-minute period so the body doesn't release more insulin into the bloodstream.

PHASE I FOODS: WEEKS 1–4
MEAT (GRASS-FED/ORGANIC IS BEST)

Approved	Avoid
Goat	Alligator
Beef or buffalo sausages or hot dogs (no pork casing—natural nitrite/nitrate free is best)	Bacon
Veal	Emu
Elk	Frog
Lamb	Ham
Bone soup/stock	Imitation meat products (soy)
Liver and heart (must be organic or grass fed)	Ostrich
Beef	Pork
Venison	Sausage (pork)
Buffalo	Turtle
	Veggie burgers

FISH (WILD FRESHWATER/OCEAN-CAUGHT FISH IS BEST; MAKE SURE IT HAS FINS AND SCALES)

Approved	Avoid
Salmon	Fried, breaded fish
Tuna	Eel
Scrod	Shark
Halibut	Catfish
Cod	Squid
Grouper	All shellfish (crab, clams, oyster, mussels, lobster, shrimp, scallops, and crawfish)
Haddock	
Pompano	
Trout	
Orange roughy	
Snapper	
Herring	
Whitefish	
Sardines (canned in water or olive oil only)	
Salmon (canned in spring water)	
Tuna (canned in spring water)	
Mahi mahi	
Wahoo	
Tilapia	

Sea bass	
Mackerel	
Sole	
Fish bone soup/stock	

POULTRY (PASTURED/ORGANIC IS BEST)	
Approved	**Avoid**
Chicken	Fried, breaded chicken
Guinea fowl	Processed lunch meats
Duck	
Chicken or turkey bacon (no pork casing—organic and nitrite/nitrate free is best)	
Natural chicken or turkey hot dogs	
Cornish game hen	
Turkey	
Bone soup/stock	
Natural deli meats, including chicken, turkey, and roast beef	
Chicken or turkey sausage (no pork casing—natural and nitrite/nitrate free is best; use sparingly in Phase I)	
Liver and heart (must be organic or grass fed)	

EGGS (HIGH OMEGA-3/DHA OR ORGANIC ARE BEST)	
Approved	**Avoid**
Chicken eggs (whole with yoke)	Imitation eggs (such as Egg Beaters)
Duck eggs (whole with yolk)	

DAIRY (ORGANIC IS BEST)	
Approved	**Avoid**
Whole-milk yogurt (plain)	Soy milk
Sheep's milk yogurt (plain)	Rice milk
Goat's milk yogurt (plain)	Cow's milk and ice cream
Whole-milk cheese	Processed cheese food
Soft goat's, cow's, or sheep's milk cheese	Flavored, low-fat, or fat-free cheese, yogurt, and kefir
Sheep's milk hard cheese	Dry milk (many processed foods contain this ingredient)
Goat's milk hard cheese	
Feta cheese (sheep's milk or goat's milk)	
Full-fat plain kefir	
Full-fat cottage cheese	
Ricotta cheese	
Full-fat sour cream	
Plain almond milk (unsweetened)	
Goat's milk protein powder (for smoothies)	
Cultured buttermilk	

FATS AND OILS (ORGANIC IS BEST)	
Approved	**Avoid**
Flaxseed oil (not for cooking)	Lard
Butter oil (ghee)	Margarine
Hemp seed oil (not for cooking)	Shortening
Avocado	Soy oil
Cow's milk butter	Safflower oil
Goat's milk butter	Sunflower oil
Expeller-pressed sesame oil	Cottonseed oil
Coconut milk/cream (canned or fresh)	Canola oil
Extra-virgin coconut oil (best for cooking)	Corn oil
Extra-virgin olive oil (not best for cooking)	Any partially hydrogenated oil
Peanut oil (cold-pressed and unrefined)	

VEGETABLES (ORGANIC FRESH OR FROZEN ARE BEST)	
Approved	**Avoid**
Squash (winter or summer)	Corn
Asparagus	Sweet potatoes
Cauliflower	White potatoes
Cabbage	
Celery	
Eggplant	
Garlic	
Okra	
Peas	
String beans	
Lettuce (all varieties)	
Artichoke (French, not Jerusalem)	
Leafy greens (kale, collard, broccoli rabe, mustard greens, etc.)	
Sprouts (broccoli, sunflower, pea shoots, radish, etc.)	
Sea vegetables (kelp, dulse, nori, kombu, hijiki, etc.)	
Raw, fermented vegetables (lacto-fermented only, no vinegar)	
Broccoli	
Beets	
Brussels sprouts	
Carrots	
Cucumber	
Pumpkin	
Onion	
Mushrooms	
Peppers	

Tomatoes	
Spinach	

BEANS AND LEGUMES (SOAKED OR FERMENTED ARE BEST)	
Approved	**Avoid**
Small amounts of fermented soybean paste (miso) as a broth	Soy beans
Lentils	Tofu
Black beans	
Navy beans	
Garbanzo beans	
Lima beans	
Tempeh (fermented soybean loaf)	
Kidney beans	
White beans	
Pinto beans	
Split beans	
Black-eyed peas	
Red beans	
Broad beans	

NUTS AND SEEDS (ORGANIC, RAW, OR SOAKED ARE BEST)	
Approved	**Avoid**
Almonds/almond butter	Honey-roasted nuts
Hemp seeds/hemp seed butter	Peanuts/peanut butter
Sunflower seeds/sunflower butter	Cashews
Tahini/sesame butter	
Macadamia nuts	
Hazelnuts	
Pecans	
Walnuts	
Brazil nuts	
Chia seeds	
Pumpkin seeds/pumpkin seed butter	
Flaxseeds	

CONDIMENTS, SPICES, SEASONINGS, COOKING INGREDIENTS, AND SALAD DRESSINGS (ORGANIC IS BEST)	
Approved	**Avoid**
Ketchup (natural or organic)	All spices that contain added sugar
Salsa (fresh or canned, organic)	Commercial ketchup with sugar
Hot sauce (preservative-free)	Commercial barbecue sauce with sugar
Tomato sauce (no added sugar)	White wine vinegar

Soy sauce (wheat free), tamari	
Herbamare seasoning	
Omega-3 mayonnaise	
Homemade salad dressing and marinades using Phase I–allowable ingredients	
Guacamole (fresh)	
Apple cider vinegar	

CONDIMENTS, SPICES, SEASONINGS, COOKING INGREDIENTS, AND SALAD DRESSINGS (ORGANIC IS BEST)	
Approved	**Avoid**
Mustard	
Celtic Sea Salt	
Umeboshi paste	
Bragg salad dressings	
Bragg Liquid Aminos	
Balsamic vinegar	
Red wine vinegar	
Herbs and spices (no added stabilizers)	
Pickled ginger (no preservatives or color)	
Wasabi (no preservatives or color)	
Organic flavoring extracts (alcohol-based, no sugar added, vanilla, almond, etc.)	
Cooking wine (organic red and white)	
Capers	

FRUITS (ORGANIC FRESH OR FROZEN IS BEST)	
Approved	**Avoid**
Blueberries	Bananas
Blackberries	Mangoes
Cherries	Dried fruit
Lemons	Canned fruit
Pomegranates	
Apples (with skin)	
Melons	
Apricots (not dried)	
Peaches	
Grapes	
Oranges	
Pears	
Papayas	
Kiwi	
Nectarines	
Strawberries	
Raspberries	

Grapefruit	
Limes	
Cranberries (not dried)	
Olives	
Pineapple	
Plums	
Fresh figs	
BEVERAGES	
Approved	Avoid
Purified, nonchlorinated water	Alcoholic beverages of any kind
Natural sparkling water, no carbonation added	Preground commercial coffee
Herbal teas (preferably organic)—unsweetened or with a small amount of honey or stevia	Sodas
Raw vegetable juice (beet or carrot juice)	Fruit juices
Lacto-fermented beverages	Chlorinated tap water
Certified organic coffee—buy whole beans, freeze them, and grind them yourself when desired; flavor only with organic cream and a small amount of honey	
SWEETENERS	
Approved	Avoid
Unheated, raw honey in very small amounts (2 tablespoons per day maximum)	Sugar (including organic sugars, all-natural cane sugar, and organic brown sugar)
The herbal supplement stevia in small quantities	Maple syrup
Lo Han Guo in small quantities	Fructose or corn syrup
Xylitol in small quantities or in mints and gum	All artificial sweeteners, including aspartame, sucralose, and acesulfame K
	Sugar alcohol, including sorbitol and malitol
MISCELLANEOUS	
Approved	Avoid
Goat's milk protein powder (for recommendations, see the resource guide)	Milk or whey protein powder from cow's milk
Native whey protein	Soy protein powder
	Rice protein powder
GRAINS AND STARCHY CARBOHYDRATES	
Approved	Avoid
Arrowroot powder (as a substitute for cornstarch)	All grains and starchy foods
	Bread
	Pasta

	Cereal
	Rice
	Oatmeal
	Pastries
	Baked goods
	Corn tortillas

PHASE II
WEEKS 5–8

Phase II allows for a greater variety of foods, but weight loss is not as rapid during this phase. The most important point of Phase II is to maintain blood sugar levels and create and instill healthy eating habits that can last a lifetime. During Phase II, you're cleared to eat all the foods listed in Phase I, plus the foods listed below.

Remember, you should still not drink any alcohol: wine, beer, or mixed drinks. Keep your cheat meals to a minimum; no more than one or two a week.

PHASE II FOODS: WEEKS 5–8	
EGGS	
Approved	Avoid
Fish roe or caviar (fresh, not preserved)	
DAIRY	
Approved	Avoid
Cow's feta cheese	
Blue cheese	
Parmesan cheese	
FATS AND OILS	
Approved	Avoid
Expeller-pressed peanut oil or coconut oil, both good for cooking	
VEGETABLES	
Approved	Avoid
Sweet potatoes	
Yams	
White potatoes	
Corn	
BEANS AND LEGUMES	
Approved	Avoid
Tofu	Garbanzo beans
Soybeans (edamame)	Lima beans

NUTS AND SEEDS	
Approved	**Avoid**
Peanuts	Honey-roasted nuts
Peanut butter	Any nuts or seeds roasted in oil
Cashews	

CONDIMENTS, SPICES, AND SEASONINGS	
Approved	**Avoid**
Healthy salad dressings	Canola oil
	Fat-free dressings
	Dressings with chemicals

FRUITS	
Approved	**Avoid**
Bananas (fresh, not dried)	Canned fruit
Mangoes (fresh, not dried)	Dried fruit, including raisins, prunes, bananas, mango, and papaya
Dates (fresh, not dried)	
Figs (fresh, not dried)	

BEVERAGES	
Approved	**Avoid**
Raw vegetable juice (beet or carrot)	
Coconut water	

SWEETENERS	
Approved	**Avoid**
Unheated, raw honey (no limitation on amount)	Maple syrup
The herbal supplement stevia in small quantities	Heated honey, fructose, or corn syrup
Lo Han Guo in small quantities	Sugars like all-natural cane sugar, organic white sugar, and organic brown sugar
Xylitol in small quantities or in mints and gum	

SNACKS/MISCELLANEOUS	
Approved	**Avoid**
Organic whole food bars (naturally sweetened	

PHASE III
WEEKS 9–12

Phase III allows you to increase the varieties of foods as well as the amount of carbohydrates in your diet. You may be wondering, "Can I maintain weight loss by eating carbohydrates again?"

The answer is yes! Carbohydrates do have a place in our diets and bodies, but the carbs must be in their natural and unrefined state. Fuel your body with simple whole fruits and honey, complex sprouted grains, delightful beans, and healthy vegetables. Supplying your body with these excellent and natural carbohydrates will help you to balance the chemical processes in your body and keep you healthy.

In addition to the approved foods in Phase I and Phase II, you can add the following foods in Phase III:

PHASE III FOODS: WEEKS 9–12	
DAIRY	
Approved	Avoid
Raw cow's and goat's milk	
Organic nonhomogenized cow's and goat's milk	
Parmesan cheese	
FRUIT	
Approved	Avoid
Dried fruit with no sugar or sulfites	
Canned fruit in its own juices	
GRAINS	
Approved	Avoid
Sprouted Ezekiel-type bread	
Sprouted Essene bread	
Fermented whole-grain sourdough bread	
Quinoa	
Amaranth	
Buckwheat	
Millet	
Brown rice	
Sprouted cereal	
Oats	
Kamur	
Spelt	
Barley	
Bulgur wheat	
Whole-grain kamut or spelt pasta in small quantities	

SWEETENERS	
Approved	**Avoid**
Sucanat	Organic sugars like all-natural cane sugar, organic white sugar, and organic brown sugar
Rapadura	
Agave nectar	
SNACKS/MISCELLANEOUS	
Approved	**Avoid**
Healthy trail mixes	
Jennies Macaroons	
Organic chocolate spreads	
Healthy popcorn	

I still recommend that you not drink any alcohol, but if it's a special occasion, organic red wine is preferred. Organic white wine is OK, but it contains less of the antioxidant benefits of organic red wine. As for beer, an unpasteurized organic beer is the best choice. I don't recommend mixed drinks at all.

By now, your desire to "cheat" should have waned considerably.

PHASE IV
WEEKS 13–16

Phase IV is the "lifestyle" phase that will allow you to maintain your ideal weight. As you shed pounds, you should notice significant improvements in your health. If you're feeling great and feeling like you've reached your weight-loss goals, then continue on this lifestyle phase.

Phase IV also provides you the opportunity to step back and ask some questions: Have you reached the goals you've set for yourself? Do you feel and look the way you want? If you are still suffering from symptoms related to insulin resistance or you feel like you've gotten off track, then use this time period to implement Phase I or Phase II again.

You're cleared to resume drinking alcohol, but in moderate amounts. Remember: organic red wine is best, followed by organic white wine and unpasteurized organic beer. Skip the Cosmopolitans and other mixed drinks that use hard spirits. Don't forget that alcohol has twice as many calories per gram as protein or carbohydrates. Cheat meals should be a thing of the past, as well as your cravings for junk food.

Eat meals balanced with whole foods and healthy proteins and fats, watch your portion size, continue to eliminate refined foods, and maintain regular exercise into your week.

I've provided four different health and wellness plans based on your nutritional type, which was determined by your answers to the nutritional-type questionnaire in chapter 3 on page 66. You will find these four plans in chapter 14, "The Maker's

Diet Daily Health Plan." No matter what you eat or what meal plan you follow, it's imperative to think about cleansing your body, which is the topic of our next chapter.

The Maker's Diet for Weight Loss Recap: The Weight Loss Eating Plan

1. Phase I, or the "purification" phase, of the Weight Loss Eating Plan is designed to stabilize blood sugar levels, reduce inflammation, enhance digestion, and balance hormone levels in the body.
2. Phase II allows for a greater variety of food, and although weight loss is not rapid, it does help maintain blood sugar levels and create lifelong healthy eating habits.
3. Natural, unrefined carbohydrates fuel your system and balance the chemical process in your body and keep you healthy. Phase III incorporates a larger, delicious variety of carbohydrates.
4. In Phase IV, or the "lifestyle" phase, you will have the opportunity to step back and ask yourself questions to pinpoint areas where you may have gotten off track.

Section II

MAXIMIZE LIFE AND MINIMIZE LIFE DRAINERS

eight

Cleanse for Your Ideal Weight

WHAT GOES INTO the body must come out.

Alimentary, my dear Watson, but all too often, everything *doesn't* come out, which is why cleansing is an important part of the Maker's Diet for Weight Loss.

The gastrointestinal tract, elementarily known as the alimentary canal, is expertly designed to help the body break down food and absorb its nutrients as well as eliminate unwanted waste products. Not that anyone would want to, but if you stretched your digestive tract from end to end, it would measure 25 to 35 feet—around the width of a singles tennis court.

The digestive tract needs that much length to completely break down the food's nutrients and distribute them throughout the body by way of the bloodstream. Anything that's left over is expelled from the body either through urine or fecal elimination. (The body also eliminates wastes and toxins through exhalation and sweating, but the heavy lifting is performed by the digestive tract.) During your lifetime, sixty tons of food will pass through the gastrointestinal system, making for a lot of...elimination.[1]

When you grab a forkful of pasta or bite into a delicious apple, you begin a physiological process that you have taken for granted since your mother spoon-fed you Gerber's yams in a high chair. Every time you take a bite of food into your mouth, the salivary glands begin their work, filling your mouth with mucouslike saliva that adheres to the food. After you're finished chewing and are ready to swallow, the tongue pushes the soft mass—called the *bolus*—to the back of the mouth and into the pharynx, which is the cavity between the mouth and the windpipe that serves as the body's alimentary passageway to the stomach via the esophagus.

How long your food spends in the esophagus before reaching the stomach depends on how well it was chewed. Food that has been chewed well—properly masticated, as they say in jolly old England—makes the journey in just seven seconds. Food that's dry or not properly chewed can take a full minute to wend its way through the esophagus, which is not good for the delicate tissues lining this 10-inch tube between the throat and the stomach. Improperly chewed food that reaches the stomach takes longer to digest, which creates acute, temporary stress on the entire gastrointestinal process.

Chewing foods properly, however, allows enzymes in your saliva to turn the food into a near liquid form before swallowing, allowing it to shimmy down the esophagus like a fireman sliding down a slick pole to answer an emergency call. The act of working your jaw also sends a neurological message to your stomach and pancreas to increase acid and digestive enzyme production because food's on the way.

Regarding the chewing end of the deal, I'm figuring you've never heard of Horace Fletcher, an American health-food faddist during Victorian times who was known as "The Great Masticator." A raconteur, world traveler, millionaire businessman, amateur painter, speaker, and author, Fletcher tirelessly promoted his theory of good chewing: he recommended that food be chewed thirty-two times—which works the jaw one hundred times per minute—before being swallowed. "Nature will castigate those who don't masticate," he warned. Followers of "Fletcherism," as his doctrine became known, included industrialist John D. Rockefeller and authors Upton Sinclair and Henry James.[2]

I understand that chewing your food many times will seem like an arduous task, but masticating your food thoroughly—especially foods high in carbohydrates—enhances the digestive process and reduces post-meal bloating. More importantly, chewing your food slowly and thoroughly can help you lose weight since the brain will have more time to register the amount of food you are consuming—and perhaps make you eat less. In other words, chewing well will give you time to set your fork down and come to a stop when the stoplight flashes yellow, signaling you're full and it's time to shut down the eating express. Chewing your food thirty-two times before swallowing may be a bit much, but can you chew each bite fifteen or twenty times before gulping and swallowing?

Dr. Fletcher would be proud of me. I've become a much better "chewer" over the years, especially compared to my college days at Florida State, where I wolfed down double cheeseburgers bite-for-humongous-bite with the best of my fraternity buddies. In fact, if you were to dine with me today, you'd be surprised at how long I take to chew my food. It has taken some effort to reprogram the way I eat, but I know that chewing food slowly ensures that plenty of digestive juices are added to each bite before it begins its long, winding journey through the digestive tract.

The reason I'm making a big deal about this mastication business is because properly chewing your food is the first step in cleansing your body as you march toward your ideal weight. Speaking as someone who nearly died from horrible digestive problems, I can assure you that the health of the gastrointestinal tract is imperative for overall wellness. Unfortunately for many of us, the typical American diet never allows the body to cleanse itself properly. Eating the wrong foods—I'm thinking greasy chicken and sticky sweets—is like filling your car's fuel tank with crude oil rather than 93-octane fuel.

Furthermore, a diet heavy in processed foods does not provide the deep-seated nutrition the body needs to build and repair muscles, grow strong bones, or keep things moving where it counts. Processed foods strain the gut, causing the digestive system to work harder to extract nutrients. This explains why many Americans feel "down in the dumps" after they eat; they feel stuffed, bloated, or constipated. When an overloaded gastrointestinal system gets backed up, fecal matter can ferment in the colon and cause painful bowel problems. The colon wall absorbs the remaining water in the feces, turning the stool hard as stone pebbles. The harder the feces, the more difficult it is to eliminate.

The goal is for the digestive tract to run like a Swiss train: everything leaving the station on time. Under ideal conditions—and the consumption of whole foods—twelve to twenty-four hours should pass between the moment the meal is finished until the moment waste is eliminated at the other end. The amount of time that foods stay in the digestive tract before you have to go to the bathroom is called "bowel transit time." Food that leaves the body in less than twelve hours—which happens when you have diarrhea—cannot be adequately absorbed. The body cannot extract the nutrients it needs in such a short time, which is one reason why you feel weak and uneasy after a bout of diarrhea.

On the other hand, those who munch throughout the day on glazed doughnuts, french fries, pretzels, and snack cakes present the body with *too many* carbohydrates to digest. Leftover undigested carbs camp in the gut longer than twenty-four hours and impair digestion. Instead of everything being eliminated on time, the substances linger inside the intestines, causing an overgrowth of harmful bacteria and yeasts, which can lead to abdominal discomfort and mischief.

In addition, those who consume too many desserts with refined sugars unwittingly feed the "bad" microorganisms in the intestines. Sugary foods feed harmful bacteria that irritate and unbalance the delicate flora lining of the gastrointestinal or GI tract. Sugary foods also encourage specific kinds of intestinal bacteria to flourish at the expense of others. More than four hundred different types of bacteria or "gut flora" live inside our intestines, and what we eat influences the ratio of "good" versus "bad" gut flora by allowing some kinds to out-compete others.

Habitual intake of a diet high in refined and highly processed foods leads to accumulation of toxins, increased contact time, and damage to the lining of the gut due to constipation and higher pressures developing inside the bowel. In plain language, such foods gunk up the digestive tract like a mass of cookie dough in a garbage disposal.

Enough already! That's what the body is saying after years, if not decades, of abuse. If the digestive system isn't given a chance to restore itself—through body therapies known as cleansing and fasting—then digestive-related disorders and diseases can and will occur.

Reaping What We Sow by Dr. Bernard Bulwer

The famous British surgeon Sir Dennis Burkitt, who worked in Africa during World War II and for decades afterward, remarked that he rarely saw the "diseases of civilization"—constipation, hemorrhoids, diarrhea, etc.—among the African people. As for the British and Americans he treated, he concluded that the West's highly refined diet resulted in hard, dry stools that passed sluggishly through the intestine and required a large increase in luminal pressure for their evacuation.

The longer toxins hang around your body, including inside your gut—the greater their potential for discomfort and problems. From where do these toxins arise? Toxins are literally everywhere in our environment. No food is guaranteed 100 percent safe. We live on a fallen planet. We drink, eat, inhale, and produce toxins. This is not an alarmist statement.

Don't believe me; check out the facts yourself. The foods we eat contain untold numbers of agents that are *not* food: pesticides, additives, colorants, extraneous hormones, chemicals, and heavy metals, not to mention prescription and nonprescription drugs—which our bodies, especially the liver, are forced to detoxify, which is why we have elimination systems, especially in our urine and stool.

This is why I strongly recommend that you embark on the Maker's Diet Cleanse, a ten-day detoxification and cleansing system that I recommend be done four times a year. Toward the end of this chapter, I give a complete hour-by-hour road map of the Maker's Diet Cleanse, broken down by the seasons, that you can follow.

WHAT THE MAKER'S DIET CLEANSE IS ALL ABOUT

The Maker's Diet Cleanse is a ten-day detoxification cleanse that should be done quarterly in January, April, July, and October. During your ten-day Maker's Diet Cleanse, you will eat five times a day, every two to three hours. Most people eat breakfast around 7:30 a.m., followed by a second meal at 10:30 a.m., lunch at 1:00 p.m., a midafternoon meal at 3:30 p.m., and dinner at 6:00 p.m. The first day of each seasonal detox cleanse is crucial.

Winter Cleanse

For the Winter Cleanse, you should consume only homemade chicken soup (or a broth from a vegetable soup) for all five meals on the first day. My wife, Nicki, who's a wonderful cook, and I have come up with an excellent recipe that we call, tongue in cheek, "Cleansing Chicken Soup." This recipe was inspired by my late Grandmother Rose.

Cleansing Chicken Soup

1 chicken, whole or cut (free range, pastured, or organic)

3–4 quarts filtered water

1 Tbsp. raw apple-cider vinegar

4 medium-sized onions, coarsely chopped

8 carrots, peeled and coarsely chopped

6 celery stalks, coarsely chopped

2–4 zucchinis chopped

1 pound green beans

½ cup fresh or frozen green peas

4 inches grated ginger

4 Tbsp. extra-virgin coconut oil

1 bunch parsley

5 garlic cloves

2–4 Tbsp. sea salt

¼–½ tsp. cayenne pepper

If you are using a whole chicken, remove fat glands and gizzards from the cavity. Place chicken or chicken pieces in a large stainless steel pot with the water, vinegar, garlic, ginger, salt, cayenne pepper, extra-virgin coconut oil, and all vegetables except parsley. Let stand for 10 minutes before heating. Bring to a boil, removing the scum that rises to the top. Cover and cook for 8–12 hours. The longer you cook the stock, the more cleansing it will be. About 15 minutes before finishing the stock, add parsley. This will impart additional mineral ions to the broth.

Remove from heat and take out the chicken. After it cools, remove chicken meat from the carcass, discarding the bones. Drop the meat back to the soup. You may purèe for even easier digestion.

On days 2–4, consume Cleansing Chicken Soup during the four daytime meals, followed by a healthy salad for dinner containing all the colored vegetables you can think of. Greens and sprouts are wonderful high-fiber foods, but be sure to add slices of cucumbers, carrots, red onion, cabbage, tomatoes, and celery. Garnish with half an avocado, and add 2 tablespoons of a healthy raw salad dressing. (Please see Appendix C for recommended brands.) You can also make your own dressing from the following ingredients:

- Extra-virgin olive oil
- Apple-cider vinegar or lemon juice
- Some of your favorite herbs, spices, and seasonings
- A dash of sea salt, liquid aminos, or soy sauce

You can eat as much salad as you want, limiting the avocado to one-half and the dressing to 2 tablespoons, but make sure you finish eating by 7:00 p.m. After that, I'm afraid, you're done eating for the day, and that's the toughest part, especially for those used to a bowl of Ben & Jerry's or a handful of chocolate chip cookies before going to bed.

On days 5–7, you can add raw nuts and seeds to your salad after eating Cleansing Chicken Soup throughout the day.

On days 8–10, eat Cleansing Chicken Soup for the first four meals, but you may add 4 ounces of plain whole-milk yogurt or kefir and 1 tablespoon of raw honey for your third and fourth meal.

For your fifth meal, it's advisable to add some fatty fish (salmon, mackerel, herring, sardines, or tuna) and raw cheese to your salad, which will help you transition into the Weight Loss Eating Plan once the Maker's Diet Cleanse is over. In addition to the five meals, it is important to drink ¾ of an ounce of water per pound of body weight per day.

Spring and Fall Cleanses

For the Spring and Fall Cleanses, the first two meals of the day are fruit. Be sure to eat only one type of fruit—1 or 2 cups—at each meal. Try to eat high-sugar fruit like mangoes, pineapple, and papaya early in the day rather than late. Lower-sugar fruits are apples, cantaloupe, watermelon, berries, grapefruit, oranges, peaches, plums, and tangerines.

The lunch and midafternoon meals are Cleansing Chicken Soup, and your fifth meal is a salad. As with the Winter Cleanse, you can make your salad with your favorite greens and vegetables. Garnish with half an avocado, and add 2 tablespoons of a healthy raw salad dressing or make your own. Follow this regimen for the first four days.

On days 5–7, you can add raw nuts and seeds to your salad after eating fruit for the first two meals and Cleansing Chicken Soup for the third and fourth meal.

On days 8–10, during your fruit meals (meals one and two), add 4 ounces of whole-milk plain yogurt or kefir and 1 tablespoon raw honey. Consume Cleansing Chicken Soup for meals three and four. At your last (fifth) meal, add cheese and fatty fish (like wild-caught salmon) to your salad, which will help you transition into the Weight Loss Eating Plan once the Maker's Diet Cleanse is over.

As mentioned earlier, you can eat as much salad as you want, but make sure you finish eating by 7:00 p.m.

Summer Cleanse

For the Summer Cleanse, the first day is a mono diet where you will eat the same fruit at each meal for the entire day, marked by five fruit servings (1 or 2 cups of fruit for each serving). The best fruits for cleansing have a lot of water: watermelon, grapes, apples, and oranges. Bananas don't have nearly as much water.

On days 2–4, eat four servings of fruit during the day, separated by two to three hours, followed by a healthy salad for dinner containing all the vegetables you can think of. Greens and sprouts are wonderful high-fiber foods, but be sure to add slices of cucumbers, carrots, red onion, cabbage, tomatoes, and celery. Garnish with half an avocado, and add 2 tablespoons of a healthy raw salad dressing or make your own.

On days 5–7, follow the same regimen, but now you can add raw nuts and seeds to your salad.

On days 8–10, eat one serving of fruit during the first two meals of the day. For your third and fourth meal, eat one type of fruit, 4 ounces of whole-milk plain yogurt or kefir, and 1 tablespoon of honey. Add raw cheese and fatty fish (like wild-caught salmon) to your salad meal, which will help you transition into the Weight Loss Eating Plan once the Maker's Diet Cleanse is over.

During each of these seasonal cleanses, you should increase your water consumption to ¾ ounce per pound of body weight, compared to the ½ ounce I recommended earlier. That means, for a 160-pound person, drinking 120 ounces of filtered water. I know, that's almost a gallon of water, but if you start sipping in the morning, you can make it. You need these liquids to really flush the system.

Going Ape in Great Britain

OK, it was a publicity stunt, but nine Brits pitched a tent at Paignton Zoo in Devon, right next to the monkey exhibit. Their goal: cast aside processed foods in favor of a twelve-day "Evo Diet," consuming up to 5 kilos (12 pounds) of raw fruits and vegetables a day. TV cameras were on hand twenty-four hours a day to film their exploits for a reality show.

Dieticians from King's College Hospital devised a three-day rotating menu of fruit, vegetables, nuts, and honey. In the second week, standard portions of cooked oily fish were added to their diet. Water was the only liquid refreshment allowed.

The cleansing diet provoked significant weight loss (4.4 kilos or 9.7 pounds), dramatic drops in cholesterol (23 percent) and blood pressure levels (an average of 140/83 to 122/76), and odorous flatulence inside the tent (no comment). One volunteer, Jon Thornton, a thirty-six-year-old driving instructor, explained that he hadn't eaten vegetables since he was a very young child. Following his "release" from the zoo, Mr. Thornton said he had vegetables with his Christmas dinner for the first time in thirty-six years.[3]

Although the Maker's Diet Cleanse may seem similar to the Evo Diet, I won't ask you to camp out next to the ape house.

I've been asked why I don't recommend drinking vegetable and fruit juice during a cleanse. While vegetable and fruit juices are great sources of nutrients, they are quickly absorbed and are often times higher in sugar, which leaves you feeling hungrier than when you started. When you eat whole fruits and their fiber, however, you shouldn't get as hungry, especially if you're eating every two to three hours or so. Don't drink any whole-food meal supplement shakes, however, because the first seven days of the cleanse should be dairy-free to help your body get rid of any allergens.

While cleansing, you should take the recommended supplements, which you learned about in chapter 6. The supplements recommended for the Winter, Spring,

Fall, and Summer Cleanses are a whole-food multivitamin, a fucoxanthin supplement, and omega-3 cod liver oil.

I realize that doing a Maker's Diet Cleanse four times a year is asking a great deal and that not every reader will attempt this (some of you are wimps). But how about giving it a try? Even if you don't make it past the fourth day of a ten-day cleanse, you'll still be better off for having made the attempt. I did two of these cleanses while writing *The Maker's Diet for Weight Loss* and keeping up with my other responsibilities. I wasn't able to go the full ten days on each occasion because I was traveling, but the results were super.

After my second cleanse, I began an intense exercise program I call Functional Interval Training (FIT) (which you'll hear about in chapter 9) and gained several pounds of muscle.

When you're ready to do the Maker's Diet Cleanse, you can follow the hour-by-hour road map I've included toward the end of this chapter.

TAKE YOUR MAKER'S DIET CLEANSE TO THE NEXT LEVEL

If you think it's normal to have a bowel movement every two or three days, then it's no wonder you feel lousy! You should eliminate every day—and better yet, two or three times a day—just as infants do. If you don't go potty, you have constipation, and the retention of waste inside the colon presents all kinds of health problems: harmful bacteria, intestinal parasites, yeasts, and hemorrhoids.

My bowel consciousness was raised by nutritionist Bernard Jensen, PhD, who owned a health sanitarium in Escondido, California, called the Hidden Valley Health Ranch. Dr. Jensen had become kind of a hero of mine for his pioneering work in digestive cleansing and his book *Tissue Cleansing Through Bowel Management*. Back in 2001, when Dr. Jensen was ninety-two years old and in failing health, a friend and I visited him at his ranch outside of San Diego. I knew he was dying (in fact, Dr. Jensen would pass away three weeks later), but I had always wanted to meet him. He was confined to his bed but willing to see me. After his wife, Marie, made the introduction, Dr. Jensen told me to get my notepad out. I eagerly agreed, feeling like a freshman student sitting at the foot of his professor. Dr. Jensen reminded me that cleansing doesn't affect just your gut but everything in your body.

"What goes in doesn't always come out," he declared. The bowel holds on to waste materials longer than anyone realizes, he said, and the toxic material decaying in the large colon is a good place for health issues to get started. He called chronic constipation a "modern plague" and the greatest present-day danger to health. He blamed America's love for fast foods and being clueless about the importance of colonic cleanses. Dr. Jensen urged me—as someone just starting to speak and write books—to carry on the message of good health. I felt humbled that afternoon.

That meeting with Dr. Jensen is one of the major reasons why I believe that a gentle digestive cleanse can contribute to overall health and wellness. You'll find many digestive cleanse products available in health food stores and vitamin shops, or you can turn to the Maker's Diet Resource Guide on page 263 to learn what I recommend. I know that when some people hear the phrase "digestive cleanse," they picture themselves taking a harsh laxative that will keep them chained to a porcelain throne for the next week. Or maybe your idea of a cleanse is being hooked up to a colonic machine, where a tube is inserted into the rectum and your bowel is flooded with several gallons of water in a matter of seconds. But there are internal cleanse programs available that don't disrupt everyday activities. Thy are not expensive, time consuming, or challenging to perform.

You may think that embarking on a digestive cleanse is one of the wackiest things you could ever do, but I urge you to put away that thinking. If you've never tried this type of cleanse, I urge you to view this like a spring cleaning, a chance to complete an—ahem—top-to-bottom scrubbing of every nook and cranny of your digestive tract. You need to reduce the toxic load that has built up over the years from exposure to toxins in the air, water, and food. Excess toxins can make you feel lethargic and impact your health in many ways.

A digestive cleansing reduces the toxic load on your body via the lungs, kidneys, and particularly the liver. Every minute, around the clock, a properly functioning liver eliminates small amounts of toxins, heavy metals, bacteria, and other impurities from the blood before returning the life-sustaining substance to the rest of the body.

Another liver function is the secretion of about one to two quarts of bile each day to carry processed, nonfunctional, nonnutrient environmental compounds—this is a polite, scientific way of saying "junk food"—to the large intestine, where they are expelled from the body. The liver also carries toxins, metals, microbes, and other metabolic by-products that must be eliminated through the gastrointestinal tract.

Capturing and binding toxins secreted through the bile for transport out of the body is crucial for effective support of the body's normal internal detox and cleansing functions. Normally, eating foods high in fiber—such as green vegetables—helps the body capture toxins in the gastrointestinal tract, binding them for transport out of the body. While dietary fibers from edible fruits, vegetables, and grains are capable of absorbing environmental pollutants and other impurities, some types of fibers are easily broken down by intestinal flora.

What is intestinal flora? The normal human gastrointestinal tract contains hundreds of different species of harmless bacteria, otherwise known as intestinal flora. When the normal balance of bacteria is impacted by a poor diet heavy in processed foods, imbalances can occur and may result in occasional constipation or diarrhea.

You can expect some changes in your bowel movements when undergoing a digestive cleanse. Your stools are likely to become more frequent, softer, and change color. You may require more sleep, and you may feel tired during certain parts of the day. All of these changes are a result of the body's efforts to eliminate toxins.

So take a load off your digestive tract and cleanse. A digestive cleanse will leave you feeling lighter on your feet and with a brighter outlook, working in harmony with your body to release and remove toxins naturally so that you will feel like a better you. Again, without getting into too many bathroom details, you will be impressed with the results.

What a Digestive Cleanse Did for Me by Duong Sheahan

I'm a busy mom and live with my three school-age children and loving husband in the Chicago area. Last New Year's, following my sweet tooth marathon over the holidays, I knew it was time to clean house. Perhaps it was the sugar overload I felt in my system. At any rate, I began doing a digestive cleanse.

I had incredible results the first day. By the third day, I felt like a revived person because the toxic buildup in my system was leaving my body. My energy level increased immensely as well as my mental alertness. Trust me, I need to be alert and full of energy every day.

I've recommended a digestive cleanse to a few of my friends, and they loved the results as well. I love the way I even lost my cravings for sweet things, like chocolate, and that's not easy!

(Note from Jordan: I met Duong at one of my Weekend of Wellness conferences while writing this book. At the tender age of six, she was one of the fortunate "boat people" who escaped to the United States after the fall of Vietnam back in 1975. I loved her servant heart.)

THE SEASONAL CLEANSE PROTOCOLS

As promised, here's a complete protocol that you can follow during a ten-day seasonal Maker's Diet Cleanse.

WINTER CLEANSE

The mealtimes are approximate; obviously, feel free to adjust the times to eat based upon your schedule. Keep in mind that a single serving of fruit is either one cup (berries, grapes, and cut-up pineapple, for example) or one or two pieces (for example, grapefruit, peaches, plums, apples, or oranges).

	Winter Cleanse			
Upon waking	**Days 1–10:** Drink 16–24 ounces of water.			
	Days 1–10: Perform the Healing Codes exercise. (You can learn about the Healing Codes exercise on pages 184–185. I recommend that you perform the Healing Codes exercise twice a day—once in the morning and once in the evening—but feel free to try this two-minute exercise three, four, or five times a day.)			
7:30 a.m.	**Days 1–10:** Eat one serving (1 or 2 cups) of homemade Cleansing Chicken Soup.			
	Days 1–10: Drink 12–16 ounces of water.			
	Days 1–10: Take two or three whole-food multivitamin caplets and one to four capsules of concentrated fucoxanthin.			
10:30 a.m.	**Days 1–10:** Eat one serving of homemade Cleansing Chicken Soup.			
	Days 1–10: Drink 12–16 ounces of water.			
1:00 p.m.	**Days 1–7:** Eat one serving of homemade Cleansing Chicken Soup.	**Days 8–10:** Eat one serving of homemade Cleansing Chicken Soup, 4 ounces of plain whole-milk yogurt or kefir (cow's, goat's, or sheep's milk), and 1 tablespoon of raw honey.		
	Days 1–10: Drink 12–16 ounces of water.			
	Days 1–10: Take two or three whole-food multivitamin caplets and one to three capsules of concentrated fucoxanthin.			
3:30 p.m.	**Days 1–7:** Eat one serving of homemade Cleansing Chicken Soup.	**Days 8–10:** Eat one serving of homemade Cleansing Chicken Soup, 4 ounces of plain whole-milk yogurt or kefir (cow's, goat's, or sheep's milk), and 1 tablespoon of raw honey.		
	Days 1–10: Drink 12–16 ounces of water.			
6:00 p.m.	**Day 1:** Eat one serving of homemade Cleansing Chicken Soup.	**Days 2–4:** Mix a large green salad with any of the following: mixed greens; carrots; cucumbers; celery; tomatoes; red cabbage; red onions; red, yellow, and orange peppers; radishes; sprouts; and half an avocado.	**Days 5–7:** Mix a large green salad with any of the following: mixed greens; carrots; cucumbers; celery; tomatoes; red cabbage; red onions; red, yellow, or orange peppers; radishes; sprouts; half an avocado; and raw or soaked and dried nuts or seeds.	**Days 8–10:** Mix a large green salad with any of the following: mixed greens; carrots; cucumbers; celery; tomatoes; red cabbage; red onions; red, yellow, or orange peppers; radishes; sprouts; half an avocado; and raw or soaked and dried nuts or seeds. Add 4 ounces of cold-water fatty fish (salmon, mackerel, herring, tuna, sardines) and 2 ounces of raw cheese (cow's, sheep's, goat's).
		Salad dressing: use 2 tablespoons of one of the following: Homemade dressing: extra-virgin olive oil, apple-cider vinegar or lemon juice, sea salt, herbs, liquid aminos, and soy sauce A healthy store-bought salad dressing (please see Appendix C for recommended brands)		
	Days 1–10: Drink 8–12 ounces of water.			
	Days 1–10: Take two or three whole-food multivitamin caplets, one to three capsules of concentrated fucoxanthin, and 1 to 3 teaspoons (or three to nine capsules) of a high omega-3 cod liver oil complex. (See Appendix C for recommended products.)			
Before Bed	**Days 1–10:** Perform the Healing Codes exercise on pages 184–185.			
	Days 1–10: Go to bed by 10:30 p.m.			

THE SPRING/FALL CLEANSE

The mealtimes are approximate; obviously, feel free to adjust the times to eat based upon your schedule.

Spring/Fall Cleanse			
Upon waking	Days 1–10: Drink 16–24 ounces of water.		
	Days 1–10: Perform the Healing Codes exercise. (You can learn about the Healing Codes exercise on pages 184–185. I recommend that you perform the Healing Codes exercise twice a day—once in the morning and once in the evening—but feel free to try this two-minute exercise three, four, or five times a day.)		
7:30 a.m.	**Days 1–4:** Eat one serving of grapefruit.	**Days 5–7:** Eat one serving of apples.	**Days 8–10:** Eat one serving of plums, 4 ounces of plain whole-milk yogurt or kefir (cow's, goat's, or sheep's milk), and 1 tablespoon of raw honey.
	Days 1–10: Drink 12–16 ounces of water.		
	Days 1–10: Take two or three whole-food multivitamin caplets and one to four capsules of concentrated fucoxanthin.		
10:30 a.m.	**Days 1–4:** Eat one serving of oranges.	**Days 5–7:** Eat one serving of strawberries.	**Days 8–10:** Eat one serving of grapes, 4 ounces of plain whole-milk yogurt or kefir (cow's, goat's, or sheep's milk), and 1 tablespoon of raw honey.
	Days 1–10: Drink 12–16 ounces of water.		
1:00 p.m.	Days 1–10: Eat one serving (1 or 2 cups) of homemade Cleansing Chicken Soup.		
	Days 1–10: Drink 12–16 ounces of water.		
	Days 1–10: Take two or three whole-food multivitamin caplets and one to three capsules of concentrated fucoxanthin.		
3:30 p.m.	Days 1–10: Eat one serving of homemade Cleansing Chicken Soup.		
	Days 1–10: Drink 12–16 ounces of water.		
6:00 p.m.	**Days 1–4:** Eat one serving of homemade Cleansing Chicken Soup.	**Days 5–7:** Mix a large green salad with any of the following: mixed greens; carrots; cucumbers; celery; tomatoes; red cabbage; red onions; red, yellow, or orange peppers; radishes; sprouts; half an avocado; and raw or soaked and dried nuts or seeds.	**Days 8–10:** Mix a large green salad with any of the following: mixed greens; carrots; cucumbers; celery; tomatoes; red cabbage; red onions; red, yellow, or orange peppers; radishes; sprouts; half an avocado; and raw or soaked and dried nuts or seeds. Add 4 ounces of cold-water fatty fish (salmon, mackerel, herring, tuna, sardines) and 2 ounces of raw cheese (cow's, sheep's, goat's).
		Salad dressing: use 2 tablespoons of one of the following: Homemade dressing: extra-virgin olive oil, apple-cider vinegar or lemon juice, sea salt, herbs, liquid aminos, and soy sauce A healthy store-bought salad dressing (please see Appendix C for recommended brands)	
	Days 1–10: Drink 8–12 ounces of water.		
	Days 1–10: Take two or three whole-food multivitamin caplets, one to three capsules of concentrated fucoxanthin, and 1 to 3 teaspoons (or three to nine capsules) of a high omega-3 cod liver oil complex. (See Appendix C for recommended products.)		
Before Bed	Days 1–10: Perform the Healing Codes exercise on pages 184–185.		
	Days 1–10: Go to bed by 10:30 p.m.		

THE SUMMER CLEANSE

The mealtimes are approximate; obviously, feel free to adjust the times to eat based upon your schedule.

Summer Cleanse				
Upon waking	Days 1–10: Drink 16–24 ounces of water.			
	Days 1–10: Perform the Healing Codes exercise. (You can learn about the Healing Codes exercise on pages 184–185. I recommend that you perform the Healing Codes exercise twice a day—once in the morning and once in the evening—but feel free to try this two-minute exercise three, four, or five times a day.)			
7:30 a.m.	**Day 1:** Eat one serving of grapes—any variety.	**Days 2–4:** Eat one serving of mango.	**Days 5–7:** Eat one serving of papaya.	**Days 8–10:** Eat one serving of kiwi.
	Days 1–10: Drink 12–16 ounces of water.			
	Days 1–10: Take two or three whole-food multivitamin caplets and one to four capsules of concentrated fucoxanthin.			
10:30 a.m.	**Day 1:** Eat one serving of grapes—any variety.	**Days 2–4:** Eat one serving of watermelon.	**Days 5–7:** Eat one serving of peaches.	**Days 8–10:** Eat one serving of pears.
	Days 1–10: Drink 12–16 ounces of water.			
1:00 p.m.	**Day 1:** Eat one serving of grapes—any variety.	**Days 2–4:** Eat one serving of pineapple.	**Days 5–7:** Eat one serving of raspberries.	**Days 8–10:** Eat one serving of blueberries, 4 ounces of plain whole-milk yogurt or kefir (cow's, goat's, or sheep's milk), and 1 tablespoon of raw honey.
	Days 1–10: Drink 12–16 ounces of water.			
	Days 1–10: Take two or three whole-food multivitamin caplets and one to three capsules of concentrated fucoxanthin.			
3:30 p.m.	**Day 1:** Eat one serving of grapes—any variety.	**Days 2–4:** Eat one serving of cherries.	**Days 5–7:** Eat one serving of apples.	**Days 8–10:** Eat one serving of strawberries, 4 ounces of plain whole-milk yogurt or kefir (cow's, goat's, or sheep's milk), and 1 tablespoon of raw honey.
	Days 1–10: Drink 12–16 ounces of water.			

		Summer Cleanse		
6:00 p.m.	**Day 1:** Eat one serving of grapes—any variety.	**Days 2–4:** Mix a large green salad with any of the following: mixed greens; carrots; cucumbers; celery; tomatoes; red cabbage; red onions; red, yellow, and orange peppers; radishes; sprouts; and half an avocado.	**Days 5–7:** Mix a large green salad with any of the following: mixed greens; carrots; cucumbers; celery; tomatoes; red cabbage; red onions; red, yellow, or orange peppers; radishes; sprouts; half an avocado; and raw or soaked and dried nuts or seeds.	**Days 8–10:** Mix a large green salad with any of the following: mixed greens; carrots; cucumbers; celery; tomatoes; red cabbage; red onions; red, yellow, or orange peppers; radishes; sprouts; half an avocado; and raw or soaked and dried nuts or seeds. Add 4 ounces of cold-water fatty fish (salmon, mackerel, herring, tuna, sardines) and 2 ounces of raw cheese (cow's, sheep's, goat's).
		Salad dressing: use 2 tablespoons of one of the following: Homemade dressing: extra-virgin olive oil, apple-cider vinegar or lemon juice, sea salt, herbs, liquid aminos, and soy sauce A healthy store-bought salad dressing (please see Appendix C for recommended brands)		
	Days 1–10: Drink 8–12 ounces of water.			
	Days 1–10: Take two or three whole-food multivitamin caplets, one to three capsules of concentrated fucoxanthin, and 1 to 3 teaspoons (or three to nine capsules) of a high omega-3 cod liver oil complex. (See Appendix C for recommended products.)			
Before Bed	**Days 1–10:** Perform the Healing Codes exercise on pages 184–185.			
	Days 1–10: Go to bed by 10:30 p.m.			

ON DECK

We've just addressed the inside of the body and how we can to make it function at its best. In our next chapter, we'll focus on making the outside match how good you feel inside by discussing the importance of getting fit for your ideal weight.

The Maker's Diet for Weight Loss Recap: Cleanse for Your Ideal Weight

1. The next time you're eating alone, count the number of times you chew your food before swallowing. Try to chew your food fifteen to thirty times before swallowing.
2. When starting the sixteen-week Maker's Diet for Weight Loss program, consider going on the Maker's Diet Cleanse, a ten-day detoxification program. Make this a quarterly routine.
3. Concurrent with the Maker's Diet Cleanse, consider using a digestive cleanse product. (See Appendix C for recommendations.)

nine

Get FIT for Your Ideal Weight

I SWIVELED MY HIPS to maintain my balance on the stability ball and then gave the 7-kilo medicine ball (15½ pounds) a two-handed chest pass toward my workout partner, Mike Yorkey.

Mike, seated on a stability ball about six feet away, caught the heavy ball and immediately thrust it back into the air in my direction. I deftly caught it and glanced at my watch. "Another minute to go," I huffed.

"You're killing me," a red-faced Mike exerted. "I won't be able to comb my hair tomorrow morning if we keep going."

"Last series," I said. "Not too much longer."

For the last half hour Mike and I had squatted on stability balls and tossed medicine balls back and forth to each other. We started with the lightest ball—a 2-kilo ball about the size of a volleyball—and played toss-and-catch for two timed minutes before taking a break. During each "rest" interval, Mike held the medicine ball with outstretched arms while I reached the next ball—a bit heavier—and cradled it. After one minute of ball holding, it was back to playing catch with the next heavier medicine ball for two minutes.

Mike, who's been my research and writing partner on my last fifteen books, is twenty years my senior. For a member of the baby-boom generation, he's in good shape. Mike does meaningful exercise five or six days a week, either working out in the gym, playing doubles with his tennis buddies, or bike riding with his wife, Nicole. On this occasion, Mike had flown to Florida from his San Diego home to work on *The Maker's Diet for Weight Loss* with me. When I suggested we take a break from brainstorming and work out together in my home gym, Mike was gung-ho to raise his heart rate with me. "I want to show you some exercises I'm working on for the book," I said.

I told Mike that the exercise chapter in *The Maker's Diet for Weight Loss* would be absolutely crucial to the program, but to issue the standard health-and-fitness book advice—"Start exercising in a gym"—wouldn't cut it. My preference is that you adopt an exercise system that I call FIT—Functional Interval Training—into your daily schedule, or at least four times a week.

Interval training involves alternating short, intense bouts of exercise with brief recovery times. That's why Mike and I "rested" between sessions of tossing the medicine ball back and forth, although holding a 3-kilo medicine ball demanded its own effort. By sharply increasing and decreasing our heart rates, we burned more calories than if we had spent the same amount of time striding on side-by-side treadmills. Interval workout training will improve your resting metabolic rate (RMR) as well as your VO_2 max rate, which is the maximum amount of oxygen that can be used by an individual, in milliliters, in one minute per kilogram of body weight.

In addition, FIT exercises that work the body's "core" muscles with dumbbells, resistance bands, stability balls, medicine balls, or even Russian kettlebells are examples of "functional" exercises long on exertion and short on duration. If you will give me twenty minutes of concentrated, huff-and-puff exercise, you will benefit from huge caloric expenditures and continue to burn fat long after I've kicked you out of the gym and told you to take a shower.

You see, you can't lose weight—or at least sustain any weight loss—without stoking the body's furnace to burn up reserves of fat. When you complete a series of FIT exercises, you increase your oxygen intake as well as your heart and lung capacity so that your body turns into a fat-burning engine that incinerates fat cells long after you've stopped working out. You do this by building muscle—or restoring muscle that's been lost over the years—through functional, anaerobic, or, as I like to call them, anabolic (building) exercises. Even if you add a pound or two from gaining muscle, you'll be better off because one pound of muscle burns thirty to fifty calories a day while one pound of fat burns only three calories a day. It goes without saying, but be sure to check with your doctor before starting any fitness program, especially if it's been awhile since you've exercised.

My experience in fitness—I received my certification in fitness training in my early twenties—augurs my belief that engaging in intense workouts designed to deplete oxygen stores will cause the body to switch on the fat-burning cells. In other words, the standard "cardio" exercises—that is, walking on a treadmill like a mind-numbed robot for forty-five minutes—are somewhat helpful; however, intense oxygen-depriving anaerobic exercise does two important things to help you lose weight:

1. Anaerobic exercise increases the percentage of calories and fat burned as compared to the percentage of carbohydrates burned.

2. Anaerobic exercise raises your metabolic rate, which helps you burn off even more calories when you're at rest.

You may be wondering what "anaerobic exercise" is all about. When the body exercises, it works in two basic ways: aerobically and anaerobically. The body is said to be working aerobically when it operates at a pace that allows the cardiorespiratory system—the lungs, heart, and bloodstream—to replenish energy as you exercise. Put another way, aerobic exercise causes the body to utilize oxygen to create energy. This is basically anything that gets the heart going, like walking on treadmills, cycling on stationary bikes, or stepping on stair-stepper machines.

Aerobic exercise is generally associated with nonresistance exercises such as:

- Aerobics classes
- Basketball
- Bicycling
- Calisthenics
- Dancing
- Gardening
- Golfing
- Hiking on level terrain
- Ice-skating
- Inline skating
- Racquetball
- Scuba diving
- Snowboarding
- Snow skiing
- Soccer
- Softball
- Squash
- Table tennis
- Tennis
- Volleyball
- Walking
- Water skiing

In general, aerobic exercise is performed at a low to moderate intensity level. You're said to be exercising aerobically if you can pass the "talk test," meaning you can hold a conversation and exercise at the same time. The fitness bar is raised when you're very proficient at one of the aforementioned sports and can expertly compete against top-flight competition that demands your very best effort. An energetic set of singles between a pair of advanced tennis players can be more anaerobic than aerobic exercise, for example. Ditto for high-intensity "step" aerobics classes.

Long-Duration Exercise: Not That Good for Your Health

Low-intensity exercise—like walking on a treadmill or jogging around the neighborhood—is long on making repetitive steps but short on cardiovascular variation. While we could all afford to walk more each day (the average American accumulates only three thousand to five thousand steps per day, according to researcher David R. Bassett Jr., professor of exercise science at the University of Tennessee[1]), stepping on a treadmill to make up the shortfall is a shortsighted answer.

"Routinely forcing your body to perform the same continuous cardiovascular challenge, by repeating the same movement, at the same rate, thousands of times over, without variation, and without rest, is unnatural," declared Alan Sears, MD, and author of *PACE: Rediscover Your Native Fitness*.[2] Long-duration exercise "downsizes" the heart's capacity to rapidly provide you with big bursts of energy when you need them, increases LDL cholesterol and triglycerides, elevates clotting and inflammation factors, and creates loss of bone density.

We need to look no further than the Amish for an example on how to meld low-intensity exercise with quick bursts of energy and the great health that results. During his research, Professor Bassett placed pedometers on ninety-eight Amish adults and learned that men averaged an astounding eighteen thousand steps a day, but they also performed ten hours of vigorous physical activity a week—anaerobic activities like heavy lifting, shoveling trenches, and tossing hay bales. Women averaged fourteen thousand steps a day and three and a half hours of vigorous physical activity on the family farm each week.[3] This level of exertion goes a long way toward explaining why obesity in the Amish community ranks at a paltry 4 percent, as compared to 31 percent of American adults.[4]

On the other hand, anaerobic exercise is any form of nonsustained physical activity that typically involves a limited number of specific muscles over a short time, such as strength training or lifting free weights. You're said to be working the body anaerobically when the cardiovascular capacity cannot replenish the muscles with energy—and you're so out of breath that you can't pass the "talk test." In fact, a good test to see if you're in the anaerobic zone during your workout—where you're strengthening your heart and lungs—is the fact that you're panting and sweating between each set. I know during my FIT sessions that I'm certainly doing both.

Anaerobic exercise causes the body to make energy without oxygen because the demand for energy is so fast and huge that the body must create it from numerous body chemicals.

Examples of anaerobic exercise are:

- Lifting weights
- Using strength-training machines such as Nautilus and Hoist
- Jumping rope or jumping on a rebounder
- Sprinting
- Working the body's core muscles through the use of functional exercises with rubber bands, stability balls, medicine balls, and kettlebells

I can explain the differences between aerobic and anaerobic exercise further by using a word picture. Let's say you've been exercising on a stationary bike all winter long at your fitness club. Your usual routine is to pedal two or three times a week for thirty-minute stints. Spring is in the air, so you decide to take advantage of the warm sun by going on an outdoor bike ride. The temperature is just right on this Saturday morning—around 70 degrees. It feels good to pedal briskly in the fresh air on a level bike path. You are performing classic aerobic exercise.

In the distance, you spot a series of hills. You pedal over the first one with little exertion, but you can feel it in your legs on the second hill. The final climb, however, is a killer: to keep up your cadence and speed, you stand on your pedals and give that little extra *oomph* to clear the rise.

Practice Deep Breathing Too

I've seen many people forget to breathe when they're exercising—or breathe shallowly and use only the top half of their lungs. When performing FIT exercises, it's imperative that you inhale deeply as you begin the exercise movement and exhale completely, removing the air from your lungs during the eccentric portion where the exertion of the exercise kicks in. When the lungs are fully oxygenated, two things occur:

1. The body receives enough oxygen to nourish the cells.
2. The body expels waste products like carbon dioxide.

When you're tossing the medicine ball to a friend, concentrate on filling the lungs completely as you hold the ball up. Exhale with each toss. When the ball is tossed back to you, hold your breath for several seconds before exhaling again on the toss back. Visualize the diaphragm moving up and down to provide more room for your lungs to expand.

One of my personal trainers, Ron Kardashian, said it takes practice to voluntarily exchange the oxygen within the respiratory system through deep-breathing exercises. "The beauty of FIT anaerobic, high-intensity bursts of exercise is that they increase this voluntary exchange," he said. "This creates a utilization of oxygen from the top of your head to the toes of your feet."

Failing to inhale and exhale deep breaths when you exercise can be responsible for restricting the intensity and duration of a workout. Many people stop exercising when they experience an overwhelming feeling of shortness of breath, but doing proper breathing exercises can help you exercise longer and more intensely. I know I get more out of my workouts when I concentrate on my breathing.

What you've just done on that third hill is switch over from aerobic to anaerobic exercise. You handled the first two hills aerobically, but to maintain speed on the final rise, you needed extra help. When you stood on the pedals and pumped those tired leg muscles, you crossed a threshold and began exercising the body *anaerobically*. Chances are you couldn't sustain that type of energy exertion very long since only elite athletes can do *any* form of anaerobic exercise beyond a few moments. Yet anaerobic exercise is the best way to build muscle and lose weight. Many studies have shown that anaerobic exercise burns more calories and thus more fat than aerobic exercise—up to *five* times more, according to this Colorado State University study:[5]

CALORIES BURNED IN SIXTY MINUTES OF EXERCISE			
Exercise	During exercise	Two hours after exercise	Three to fifteen hours after exercise
Aerobic	210	25	0
Anaerobic	650	150	260

As you can see, we're talking about a huge difference in caloric expenditures. What happens is that aerobic exercise typically burns 25 percent muscle and 75 percent fat for body energy, but anaerobic exercise burns 100 percent body fat for body energy.

The dirty little secret in the weight-loss world is that the first thing you lose when you diet—and casually exercise—is muscle tissue. Your body cannibalizes muscle tissue to support your energy needs, but the fat stays on your tummy and hips. Trying to lose weight without exercising anaerobically would be like running a 10K race with ankle weights: it's going to take you a lot longer to reach the finish line. It's extremely difficult to lose fat permanently without exercising anaerobically.

You can achieve your fitness goals as well as drop gobs of weight by incorporating functional interval training exercises into your lifestyle. But first I interrupt this chapter to issue a health advisory: functional interval training is not recommended for those new to exercise or out of shape. You may have to spend the first week or two, maybe your first month, getting your body reacquainted with physical exertion. You should walk on a treadmill, pedal a stationary bike, or jump on a rebounder before tackling intense interval training.

The sooner you transition into FIT, however, the better, because the benefits become evident almost immediately. You can see results as soon as two weeks, according to a 2005 study published in the *Journal of Applied Physiology*. Six of the eight college-age men and women who were asked to ride a stationary bicycle until they were exhausted doubled their endurance after two weeks of interval training. All eight volunteers in a control group, who skipped interval training but followed their normal "aerobic" training, didn't improve their endurance rates at all. Researchers at McMaster University in Hamilton, Ontario, expressed surprise with the results because the volunteers were already reasonably fit before the study, having jogged, biked, or performed aerobic exercise two or three times a week.[6]

In a similar study at the University of Guelph in Ontario—why are the Canadians taking a lead in this area of study?—researchers had the test subjects alternate short bursts of high-intensity exercise with easy-does-it recovery times. Eight women in their early twenties pedaled a stationary bike for four minutes of hard riding, then rested for two minutes on their way to completing ten sets. After this interval training, the amount of fat burned increased by 36 percent. Jason L. Talanian, the lead author of the University of Guelph study, said it didn't matter how fit the subjects were before because sedentary adults and college athletes both showed similar increases in fitness and fat burning: "Even when interval training was added on top of other exercise they were doing, they still saw a significant improvement."[7]

Get Thee to a Doctor by Bernard Bulwer, MD

What kind of shape are you in? If the last time you exercised was when comedian Jerry Seinfeld was still taping original episodes of *Seinfeld*, then it's incumbent upon you to see a medical physician before embarking on a fitness program. Skipping a medical checkup before attempting to lose a solid amount of weight is foolhardy at best and death-defying at worst, especially if you're over forty.

You can expect your doctor to register some concern if:

1. You've been smoking cigarettes or puffing on cigars.
2. You're overweight by forty or more pounds.
3. You have a history of heart disease or sudden death in the family.
4. You have received an abnormal stress electrocardiogram (EKG) test.
5. You complain about arthritis in your joints or bones.
6. You have suffered a debilitating illness in the last five years.
7. You're on medications for diabetes or hypertension.

During a routine physical, your physician will check your eyes, ears, nose, throat, heart, height, weight, blood pressure, abdomen, lungs, neurological and skeletal systems, and urinary tract. Ask your doctor how your medications may affect your exercise plan. Drugs for diabetes, high blood pressure, and heart disease, as well as sedatives, antihistamines, and cold medications, can cause hypoglycemia (low blood sugar), dehydration, weakness, impaired balance, and blurred vision; in addition, some medications can affect the way your body reacts to exercise.[8]

Scheduling a physical examination is one of those prevention ideas that's high in common sense, so don't hesitate to see your family physician before engaging in any vigorous physical activity.

GRAB A TOWEL

Every person is different, every person is in different shape, and you know yourself best, but I'd love to get you started with FIT as soon as possible since intense exercise, followed by periods of rest, enhances the body's ability to metabolize both carbohydrates and fat. If you visited me at my home gym, the first thing I'd tell you is that we will be targeting the body's core—the area around your trunk and pelvis—because this is where fat lives, either as subcutaneous fat (which the whole world can see) or visceral fat (which is hidden but is even more unhealthy since it latches onto your vital organs). Working your core muscles also works more muscles at the same time. Toning up your muscles makes them less flabby, which improves your shape and posture.

If you perform these exercises consistently and with determined effort, there's no reason why you shouldn't finish a FIT workout in twenty minutes or so. Feel free to mix and match, but the goal is to exert yourself and raise your target heart rate into the anaerobic zone, which is 80 to 90 percent of maximum heart rate.

Your maximum heart rate is about 220 minus your age, so if your target heart rate is 85 percent, you want to see your heart rate reach the following number sometime during your workout:

Age	Target Heart Rate Zone (85 percent)	Average Maximum Heart Rate (100 percent)
20	170	200
25	166	195
30	162	190
35	157	185
40	153	180
45	149	175
50	145	170
55	140	165
60	136	160
65	132	155
70	128	150

Be advised that you will find it difficult to reach the 85th percentile if you're not in good shape. And I don't want you to die trying. This is just a goal to work toward. What I would like you to do is push yourself for as long as you can, then rest for a few minutes before exerting yourself again. That is one of the fundamental ideas behind FIT.

START OFF EASY

Before starting any moderate to intense physical activity, it's a good idea to warm up your muscles. If you're in a gym, the most obvious method of warming up is stepping on a treadmill. Others prefer to pedal an upright exercise bicycle or a recumbent exercise bike, which is easier on the back than traditional upright bikes. If you're working out at home, a series of stretching exercises will get you limber.

A more anaerobic way to warm up is by using a rebounder (mini-trampoline) or an elliptical machine, which is a cross between an exercise bike and a cross-country ski trainer, with a bit of stair climber thrown in for good measure. Your feet loop forward while your hands grasp the handlebars, which are also known as the pedal arms. You can dial up the pedaling resistance to deplete oxygen in a hurry, which will raise your heart rate quickly into the "target zone." Nearly all elliptical trainers, as well as stair steppers, exercise bikes, and treadmills, have metallic sensors that you can grasp, which allows a heart rate monitor to measure your pulse.

If you have five minutes to warm up, great, but if you're pressed for time, even two minutes will suffice. Beginning on page 159 is a list of my favorite exercises that you can pick and choose from to get FIT. Commitment and effort will be the keys to success.

What Personal Trainers Can Do for You

Every club has them—personal trainers who guide, show, exhort, motivate, educate, encourage, and stimulate you to physical levels you never thought possible. I'm a great believer in PTs, or personal trainers, and it's not because I used to be one. A good personal trainer knows dozens of ways to exercise those core muscles by using stability balls, medicine balls, and other toys that you will never think of. A good personal trainer will also be up to speed on the latest fitness innovations to keep your workout fresh and exciting.

The biggest drawback to trainers is cost: most charge between forty and seventy-five dollars an hour, which means if you employ the services of a personal trainer twice weekly, eight times a month at fifty dollars per workout, you'll receive a four hundred dollar add-on to your health club bill. That's more than a nice car payment.

If your budget can handle the extra expense, however, I highly recommend personal trainers, especially if you're walking the fitness comeback trail. Trainers can help you lose weight, reduce chances of injuring yourself, and motivate you in a million different ways. Most personal trainers I know "get it" when it comes to the importance of functional anaerobic training and pushing you with short but intense exercise that helps you burn body fat.

Personal trainers not only will show you how to exercise anaerobically, but they also hold you accountable. You *have* to show up at the appointed time (unless you're willing to forfeit a fifty-dollar cancellation fee for standing up your PT). They won't let you slack off. They put you through a vigorous workout, track your progress, correct your form, come up with new and exciting ways to exercise, and help you accomplish your fitness goals. You get a better workout and end up making more progress than if you were on your own. Personal trainers help prevent injuries since the most common training mistakes are related to technique. Many people have a tendency to use too much weight, resulting in poor form. Incorrect technique decreases the effectiveness of anaerobic training and greatly increases the risk of injury.

A good personal trainer will work muscles you never thought you had, but the soreness will feel good! Personal trainers are knowledgeable about different exercises, how to properly use strength-training equipment, and how to work past your fitness plateaus and avoid boredom.

Please know, however, that all you need to call yourself a personal trainer is a business card. No regulatory or licensing agency governs the industry, and no law demands trainers to be certified, although many gyms require it. If you are a woman, then I understand why you may feel more comfortable having another woman at your side. This is a hands-on profession, so a good personal trainer will be touching and pushing you. On the other hand, some women prefer having a gung-ho guy barking out, "Give me four more reps!"

Finding a personal trainer should be easy. Ask friends for recommendations, and when you get a name, watch that person put someone else through the paces. You should interview your potential personal trainer, asking questions that can reveal why he (or she) got into the field and how he plans to help you reach your ideal weight. Consider the personal trainer's attitude, interpersonal skills, and appearance. Does he practice what he preaches? What are his credentials and educational background? Was he certified by the National Strength and Conditioning Association (NSCA) and American Council of Sports Medicine (ACSM), the gold standards of certification? The American Council on Exercise (ACE), Aerobic and Fitness Association of America (AFAA), and National Academy of Sports Medicine (NASM) are acceptable.

I think you would be well served to solicit the expertise of a trainer, especially during the early stages of trying to lose weight. Over the last ten years, I have apprenticed and trained with some of the best personal trainers and strength coaches in the world, including renowned trainers, fitness innovators, and authors Charles Poliquin and Juan Carlos Santana.

I was still putting together my favorite FIT exercises when I put Mike Yorkey through the paces. A couple of months later, a good friend and one of the top trainers in the country, Ron Kardashian, was in town, and I invited him over to the house to see what he thought. Ron was one of three persons nominated for Personal Trainer of the Year by the National Strength and Conditioning Association (out of 26,000 NSCA members!) in 2003 and 2004, and although he didn't receive this prestigious award, he's called the "Fitness Evangelist" in his industry because he is a minister as well as a strength and conditioning coach.

Over the years, Ron has served me as a personal fitness coach, but on this occasion, it was my turn to put this popular trainer—Ron estimated that he's given twelve thousand hour-long sessions since the late 1990s—through the paces. Here's what Ron had to say.

"I had a great time hanging with Jordan in his home gym, but I was critiquing him as he went. As usual, he had an answer for everything. We went through what Jordan called 'The Big 5,' where he introduced me to Russian kettlebells. Believe me; we did a full kettlebell workout. We had such a good time that we did two workouts that day, one in the late morning, the other three hours later. Believe me, these workouts were tough, but afterward I felt phenomenal.

"I would recommend the FIT program to anyone, from the forty-five-year-old female who wants to lose some fat to those muscle heads in the gym who spend all of their time doing bench presses and curls. It's quick, it's easy, and it's highly beneficial."

Ron has trained NFL football players, NBA players, and Hollywood celebrities, so he had to bust my chops a few times, but we had a great workout that day.

STABILITY BALLS

You've probably seen them—giant, soft rubber exercise balls used for strength exercises, improving balance and coordination, and really giving the core muscles a workout. These exercise balls are known as stability balls or Swiss balls, but they aren't made of cheese or chocolate. These jumbo exercise balls have been used for many years in physical therapy and for good reason. Just sitting on the ball places the spine in neutral alignment and targets your core muscles—abdominals, obliques, and back.

Most people should use a 55-cm stability ball. If you've never sat on a stability ball, it may take you a few minutes to find the right balance. Keep your feet wide on the floor and move your hips slightly side to side. This provides you with a "feel" for the ball and the balance needed to stay upright.

Chest exercises

1. Position yourself with your stomach resting on the ball, which is called the plank position. Put your hands on the floor. Roll your body forward until the ball reaches the feet. Then perform a push-up.

2. Start in the plank position and roll your legs until your knees are on top of the ball. Press your knees into the ball, using your abdominal muscles to bring your knees into your chest.

Abdominal muscles

1. Lie on the floor and place your legs on the ball. Put your hands behind your head, and perform crunches.

2. Position yourself with your back lying on the ball. Raise your arms and interlock your fingers. After finding the right balance, perform abdominal crunches as your arms reach for the sky.

3. Sit tall on your ball with your feet resting on the floor. Fold your arms across your chest so that your hands are resting on the front of your opposite shoulders. Slowly lean backward until you feel your abdominal muscles kick in. Hold this position for several seconds before returning to the start position.

4. Lie on your back on the floor and rest your legs on top of the ball. Your legs should be hip-distance apart. Squeeze your legs together and raise the ball off the floor. Hold for three deep breaths before returning to the start position.

Leg and calf exercises

1. Trap the ball between the small of your back and a wall. With your arms outstretched for balance, perform deep knee bends.

2. To perfect hamstring stretches, lie on the ball on your stomach. Then raise your right leg and the left arm at the same time, followed by left leg and right arm raises.

Prone back extensions

1. Kneel on the ground behind the stability ball. Slowly lower yourself so that you are lying on your stomach on top of the ball while your knees and feet stay on the ground. Begin by curling your upper body around the ball and placing your hands underneath your chin for support. Lift your upper body backward off the ball in a reverse crunch motion.

MEDICINE BALLS

1. When sitting on the stability ball, hold a medicine ball in front of you. Swing the ball and your body from one side to another, almost like you're a quarterback making a handoff.

2. If you have a training partner, toss a medicine ball back and forth to each other for one minute; then rest for one minute. If you feel up to it, go for two minutes before resting for one minute. Use heavier medicine balls if they're available.

3. Stand with your feet hip-width apart. While holding a medicine ball in your hands, make a backward lunge with your right foot. Lower your body by bending at the hip while keeping your chest upright. Return to start position, but don't let the right foot touch the ground. Bounce the medicine ball off your knee and then make another backward lunge.

4. Lie on your back with your arms at your side with palms down on the floor. Raise your legs with your knees bent. Place the medicine ball between your knees and rotate your legs from one side to the next.

5. With the medicine ball still between your knees, bring your knees toward your abdominal area, raising your glutes (butt) off the floor.

Russian Kettlebells

Ron Kardashian's eyes popped out when I introduced him to Russian kettlebells. Hefting these kettlebells—which look like oversized cannon balls with handles—is one of those old-school workouts that's been around so long that it's new again.

The Pied Piper for kettlebells is Pavel Tsatsouline, a Red Army Special Forces trainer back in the USSR days, who immigrated to the United States with a half-dozen kettlebells in his suitcase (that's a joke). He opened his first gym in an abandoned bank vault (that's not a joke), which was perfect, he said, because you could drop the kettlebells without problems and "nobody could hear my victims' screams."[9] No wonder he was given the nickname "The Evil Russian." Tsatsouline began advising elite units of the U.S. Marine Corps and various law enforcement agencies on how to develop overall strength and fighting capability as well as writing books like *Enter the Kettlebell!* and *From Russia With Tough Love* for the comrade ladies. CNN and *FOX News* gave him airtime because he was different: a muscular, well-cut fitness instructor with a Russian accent swinging kettlebells every which way.

All the publicity has helped put Russian kettlebells on the map, and more fitness gyms are stocking cast iron kettlebells, starting at 4 kilos (or around 9 pounds) for the women and 12 kilos (around 26 pounds) for the men. I have a heavy kettlebell that resembles a basketball with a handle in my home gym; it weighs in at 48 kilos or 106 pounds.

Technique is important when you swing a kettlebell around, unless hernias are unimportant to you. A beginning exercise is holding a kettlebell by the horns, chest-height, and making proper squats, keeping your weight on your heels. You can make like a Harlem Globetrotter by making under leg passes to yourself. Swing the kettlebell around the front of your right leg and through your legs by passing the kettlebell to your left hand behind your left leg.

Need a Demo?

If you're wondering what a Russian kettlebell workout looks like, Russian kettlebell maestro Pavel Tsatsouline has a Web site at www.dragondoor.com, which will give you ideas for how to exercise with kettlebells.

Sprinting

I realize that sprinting will be outside the realm of possibility for many, but alternating brisk walking with ten or fifteen seconds of running as fast as you can is a great high-intensity exercise you can do. Periods of walking in between will allow you to recover.

After having not sprinted much since my high school days, I was pleased to add wind sprints to my training regimen. I wear a special athletic shoe (one with a raised heel) and complete a half-dozen 40-yard sprints behind my house. That pushes my heart rate into the 85 percent zone—and higher—rather quickly!

RESISTANCE BANDS

If you travel a great deal, as I do, and find it hard to work out, then pack resistance bands in your suitcase. Resistance bands are basically giant surgical-like rubber tubing that stretch to provide resistance. Just about any muscle group can be worked using these bands, but they're great for upper- and lower-body strength training.

When I'm in my hotel room, I wrap them around my door handle, turn around, and perform a series of chest presses. Placing the resistance bands under both feet and bringing my hands just over my shoulders are called overhead presses. I press the arms up over my head and then lower.

All you need is a good imagination or a good exercise guidebook to use resistance bands for an excellent workout.

JUMPING ROPE OR JUMPING ON A REBOUNDER

Jumping rope or bouncing up and down on a rebounder (or mini-trampoline) are two of the best lung-bursting exercises out there. A mini-trampoline is typically three feet in diameter and about nine inches off the ground. Jumping up and down is one of the best and most complete anaerobic exercises you can do since jumping strengthens muscles, tendons, and ligaments—and demands great energy. The acceleration, deceleration, and gravity pull positively stress your bones, which results in higher bone density. Rebounding affects the efficiency of the lymphatic system, which helps to shuttle nutrients to the cells and remove waste from the body.

Many people are not aware that the lymphatic system, unlike the body's cardio-vascular system that uses the heart to pump blood and oxygen cells through the veins and arteries, has no pump. The lymphatic system relies on body movement to open and close the one-way valves that transport lymphatic cells throughout the body, as well as release toxins. The up and down rhythmic bouncing from jumping rope or jumping on a rebounder promotes increased lymph flow by as much as fifteen times. Instead of toxic by-products like germs, viruses, and bacteria remaining locked within the lymphatic system, jumping around on a rebounder breaks up the inertia and sends the germs and toxins on their way to elimination by the body.

If the last time you jumped rope was back in elementary school, bring your jump rope out of mothballs. You'll be surprised how winded you get, but that's a good thing. The same goes for mini-trampolines, which are available at large merchandise and sporting-goods stores. You can find good ones for less than fifty dollars, and many come with videos that you can follow.

EXTRA CREDIT

It's a triple FIT day when I can have time to do three of my favorite body therapies:

1. A twenty-minute FIT workout in my home gym
2. A twenty-minute session in my far infrared sauna
3. A twenty-minute FIT swim session in my saltwater pool

You know all about the workout with a stability ball and my medicine balls, but let me tell you more about the sauna. When we constructed our new home, we installed a Sunlight Saunas three-person far infrared sauna in the master bathroom area. After a good workout, I like to relax in the sauna and crank up the heat to 150 degrees. Within a few minutes, I can feel the tension and sweat pour out of my body through my skin.

You may be wondering if you can lose weight sitting in a sauna. Yes, a sauna will gently raise the heart rate and increase the number of calories you burn, but any weight loss is likely to be a form of water loss from perspiration. You'll gain weight right back as soon you replace those lost fluids, but you will rid your body of harmful environmental chemicals, fat-soluble toxins, and heavy metals. I have owned and used a far infrared sauna for over eight years and highly recommend it.

After working out and taking a sauna, I'm pretty wiped, so it's nice to jump into our backyard pool for a refreshing dip. The cool water stimulates the body and boosts oxygen use in the cells.

I understand that few folks have a home gym, sauna, and pool on the premises, but fitness clubs do. If you work out hard for twenty minutes, retreat to the club's sauna to open those skin pores. Finish with a few laps in the pool, and you'll have a triple FIT workout in sixty minutes—and feel like a million bucks.

Let the Sun Shine In

You may not see much correlation between sunning yourself and losing weight, but let me explain. When your face or your arms and legs are exposed to sunlight, the skin synthesizes vitamin D from the ultraviolet rays of sunlight. The body needs vitamin D to produce adequate blood levels of insulin. I recommend intentionally exposing yourself to at least fifteen minutes of sunlight every other day to increase vitamin D levels in the body. That is often not possible because we're indoors during the day, or it's winter and the sun refuses to break through the gray cloud cover. That's why I recommend taking omega-3 cod liver oil, an important source of vitamin D. A teaspoon or three capsules a day are all you need.

LOOKING FOR MORE TO DO?

Here are some of my favorite exercises you can perform during an exercise session. If possible, perform eight to twelve reps for four times, resting one minute in between reps. Don't overdo it, though, especially at the beginning.

V-leg crunches

Begin by lying down comfortably on the floor, preferably on carpet or a foam pad. Lie so that your knees are bent and your legs up so that your thighs are perpendicular to your body and your calves parallel to the floor. Open your legs so that they form a V shape. Place your fingertips behind your head with your elbows pointing out to the sides.

Exhale as you slowly raise your head, shoulders, and upper back off the floor in a slow, controlled motion. Keep your abs tight and your lower back pressed to the floor. Hold for a count of two. Inhale as you lower your legs. Rest for a few seconds and then restart.

Diagonal curl-ups

Begin once again by lying comfortably on your back with your feet flat on the floor and your back flat. Place your fingertips behind your head with your elbows out to the sides. Slowly raise your head, shoulders, and upper back, rotating so that your left shoulder comes toward your right knee. Exhale as you lift. Many beginners of this exercise have a tendency to pull their left elbows across their bodies. Instead, you want to keep the left elbow pointing out to the side. Hold for a count of two. Slowly lower and inhale. Repeat the exercise in the opposite direction.

Single-knee lifts

Start in the same position as you did for the diagonal curl-ups. Simultaneously raise your left knee and torso, bringing your forehead and both elbows toward the knee. Don't pull on your neck and head with your arms. Exhale as you lift. Hold for a count of two. As you inhale, slowly lower your upper body and leg. Repeat with the opposite leg.

Bent-knee crossovers

This exercise starts differently. You begin by getting down on all fours, paying attention to keeping your back flat. With your left knee bent and at a 90-degree angle, lift up your left leg and back, then cross it over the calf of your right leg. Keep your buttocks tight at all times. Return to the starting position. Do one set, then repeat with the other leg. For those who want an advanced workout, you can add 1-pound ankle weights to make this exercise more difficult.

Lunges

This is an exercise that looks easy to do but leaves you feeling sore afterward. Start by standing with your feet about six inches apart and your toes pointed straight ahead. For balance, rest your hands on your hips. Step forward as far as possible with your left foot. Bending your knees, slowly lower your right knee toward the floor. Don't let your left knee extend beyond your toes. Hold for a count of two. Pressing off with your left foot, stand back up. Do one set of eight to twelve reps, and then repeat with the right leg. For an even more complete workout, try bending down and touching your foot as you extend it out for the lunge. This will make your lunge a two-part exercise as you will be bending your back after you lunge. You can also do this with a pair dumbbells or a medicine ball. This advanced version of the exercise is called a reaching lunge and provides added functionality to an already great exercise.

The Cobra

Equally important are exercises that strengthen your back. The Cobra is a great exercise. Start by lying flat on your stomach. Rest your elbows on the ground and hold your head up. Stretch the stomach and muscles while contracting the back. To deepen the stretch, you can lift up onto your hands. You will feel a greater stretch in your stomach and greater contractions in your back.

Opposite leg-arm lift

Lying flat on your back, lift your left arm off the ground twelve inches while you lift the right leg twelve inches. This exercise strengthens flabby stomach muscles and can also be done on a stability ball, as previously mentioned.

Gluteal tightener

Lie flat on your back. Lift one leg off the ground, keeping the leg as straight as possible, and hold for five seconds. Rest. Lift the opposite leg off the ground and hold for five seconds. This exercise tightens the *gluteus maximus*—the butt muscles—by contracting the glute muscles and extending the hip flexors. Make sure you keep your hips on the ground so that you can gain the maximized stretch.

Hamstring curl

Get on all fours on your knees. Bend your right leg and then lift until you feel mild tension. Hold for five seconds. Never lift to the point of pain. You can feel the contraction in the hamstring and the stretch in your hip. After doing a half-dozen sets, do the other leg. Be sure to breathe out each time you perform the hamstring curl.

Back flexion

Lie flat on your stomach with arms straight ahead of you. Lift your arms, head, and legs off the ground simultaneously. The only thing on the ground is your chest and your belly. This will strengthen the back muscles while stretching the front of your body. All of us very rarely stretch the front side of our torso since we constantly bend over all day long.

MOVING ON

Exercising with stability balls, medicine balls, and Russian kettlebells are all great examples of intense, strength-resistance movements that push the body to make great gains in strength, balance, and flexibility. Just like making the choice to eat junk food, going through the rest of your days on Earth without intentional exercising is tantamount to choosing a shortened life span and lower quality of living. A Finnish study of nearly eight thousand men and women, for instance, found that those who did not exercise increased their risk of dying by 400 percent compared to individuals in the high-activity group.[10]

Next to an excellent diet, exercise is the second essential for achieving and maintaining optimal physical health. When you exercise, you reduce your risk of developing high blood pressure. You reduce your feelings of depression and anxiety. You build and maintain healthy bones, muscles, and joints. You become stronger and better able to perform tasks.

Exercise is essential to losing body weight and visceral or "killer fat." In fact, regular physical activity is one of the simplest, least expensive, and most rewarding ways to maintain a healthy body. For example, when you lose 10 pounds of body weight, it will feel more like a 30-pound weight loss on your knees—and when you walk upstairs, those 10 pounds will feel like 70 pounds less of weight to your knee joints. Losing an excess 10 pounds can have a dramatic impact.

Your knees are not the only beneficiaries of exercise. You can also live "younger." Men who exercise right live eight years younger, and women who do so live nine years younger.[11] Exercise helps restore the metabolism by increasing insulin sensitivity. Overall, people who exercise look younger and have more vitality and fewer health problems than those who do not exercise.

When you exercise, you are actually helping the body remove toxins through breathing more deeply, which releases toxins from the lungs, and from perspiration and muscle activity. If you do not take advantage of the toxic elimination properties of exercise, these toxins may remain in your body, disrupt immune function, and make you more susceptible to infection and illness.

I think—and this is coming from a former personal trainer—that the toughest thing about exercise is not the exertion it demands but finding time to do it. You will have to set your mind to getting the body moving again. You will have to discipline yourself. The good news is that you don't have to spend many hours exercising with the FIT program. I'm talking about twenty to thirty minutes a day, but it'll take four times a week.

When is the best time to exercise? You're probably expecting me to say in the morning, and the morning is the best time, if for no other reason than you can't cancel a workout that you've already finished. But the best time to exercise is when it works for you.

Now, I know what you're thinking: "But Jordan, I don't have time to exercise. You don't know how hectic my life is."

Although I can't walk a mile in your Nikes, we all manage to find time for the things that are important to us, whether it's volunteering to host the Girl Scout troop, pace the sidelines while your son or daughter runs up and down the soccer field, attend an important civic or charity dinner, or view the latest must-see Hollywood release. We are given 168 hours each week, and from that amount, you must find 4, 5, or 6 half hours to exercise most days of the week.

You don't have to belong to a gym to get your workout done. I understand that fitness club memberships are expensive and that there are a host of reasons why they don't work for you: too far away, no babysitting, no time in the day. If that's the case, you will have to work out at home. All you need is to get started.

You can do deep knee bends, push-ups, lunges, wall squats, and a number of other exercises with no equipment at all. This can be accomplished while cooking dinner or even during the commercials of your favorite TV show. Even better, spend a few bucks to buy a stability ball. While perched on the exercise ball, you can use a bag of potatoes to provide resistance for various exercises. A 16-ounce can of tomato sauce can be a poor man's Russian kettlebell. A jump rope and rebounder are inexpensive additions.

What about used exercise equipment? You often pay a fraction when buying a used elliptical trainer, for example. Check www.craigslist.com for classified advertisements in your hometown. Another idea is to gather a couple of friends in the neighborhood and hire a personal trainer to come to your house and put everyone through their paces, making it more affordable for everyone.

Whether you're at home or on the road, in the gym or in your living room, whatever you do, just get started. Use your desire to lose weight to give you a dose of determination to carry out your goals. You can promise yourself that tomorrow is the day you'll *finally* work out, but that's just paving another road with good intentions. You won't get FIT for your ideal weight until you get up and do something *today*.

Are You a Sleepy Head?

Sleep seems to be in short supply these days. A nationwide sleep deficit means that we're packing in as much as we can from the moment we wake up until we crawl into bed sixteen, seventeen, or eighteen exhausting hours later. American adults are down to a little less than seven hours of sleep each night, a good two hours less than our great-great-grandparents slept a hundred years ago.[12]

If you're looking to control your weight, sleep can help out. University of Chicago researchers found a link between the lack of sleep and the risk of weight gain. They were able to identify how a lack of sleep boosts the appetite, especially for high-calorie, high-carbohydrate foods. What happens is that sleep lowers leptin, a hormone that tells the brain that it doesn't need more food, and elevates ghrelin, a different hormone that triggers hunger. When test subjects slept only four hours nightly, leptin levels decreased by 18 percent and ghrelin levels increased 28 percent.[13]

How many hours of sleep are you getting nightly? The magic number is eight hours, say the sleep experts. That's because when people are allowed to sleep as much as they would like in a controlled setting, like in a sleep laboratory, they naturally sleep eight hours in a twenty-four-hour time period.

The Maker's Diet for Weight Loss Recap: Get FIT for Your Ideal Weight

1. Realize that aerobic exercises—walking on the treadmill and enrolling in low-intensity aerobics classes—burns calories but not body fat. Look for ways to exercise that improve your heart and lung capacity by performing FIT exercises that rev up the body's furnace to burn up fat reserves.
2. When you exercise, can you pass the "talk test"? In other words, can you exercise and carry on a conversation at the same time? If so, you're not working yourself anaerobically, which requires intense, oxygen-depriving exercises.
3. Start working out harder for shorter amounts of time. Lift weights, use strength-training equipment like Nautilus or jump rope, or work out with stability balls, medicine balls, and Russian kettlebells.
4. When you perform functional interval exercises, you'll witness near-immediate results and burn fat long after you've finished your workout.
5. If it's been years since you've lifted a dumbbell or participated in any meaningful exercise, seek out a medical physical with your primary care doctor.
6. If you're looking for motivation and/or deeper instruction when you exercise, look into hiring a personal trainer.
7. Make a date in your day planner to exercise at least four times a week, although five or six times weekly will be much better for you.
8. If you're getting less than seven hours of sleep each night, you're operating with a sleep deficit. The body needs adequate rest, so turn off the TV and go to bed earlier.

ten

Reduce Toxins for Your Ideal Weight

WITH APOLOGIES TO King David, I now offer you the Dieter's Psalm, based on Psalm 23:

Strict is my diet. I must not want.
It maketh me to lie down at night hungry.
It leadeth me past the confectioners.
It trieth my willpower.
It leadeth me in the paths of alteration for my figure's sake.
Yea, though I walk through the aisles of the pastry department,
I will buy no sweet rolls, for they are fattening.
The cakes and the pies, they tempt me.
Before me is a table set with green beans and lettuce.
I filleth my stomach with liquids,
My day's quota runneth over.
Surely calorie and weight charts will follow me all the days of my life,
And I will dwell in the fear of scales forever.[1]

Humor is often a welcome salve to the emotional pain that comes from being overweight. Perhaps that's why we see cute bumper stickers warning other drivers: "Caution: Hungry Dieter on Board."

I'm one of those fortunate souls who have never had to lose weight. Wait a minute—before you grab the nearest brick and toss it in my direction, hear me out. As President Bill Clinton once famously said, "I feel your pain," and I can commiserate with you because I've put my body through periodic fasts and Maker's Diet Cleanses. I know what it's like to experience light-headedness, dizzy spells, and an inability to concentrate on anything more than my next plate of food.

If you've struggled with your weight, then you've surely experienced the same sense of deprivation. It doesn't matter what diet you've tried, be it Atkins, cabbage soup, or grapefruit halves. By midafternoon you wish someone would stuff you into a wooden barrel and push you over Niagara Falls.

Physiologically speaking, there's a reason you feel horrible. The more fat cells that take up residence in your torso, the more toxins you've potentially stored in your body. When you lose fat cells, you release toxins into your bloodstream, which is why you feel atrocious and search for the nearest couch on which to lie down.

We have toxins inside our bodies because they are present everywhere in our environment—the air we breathe, the water we drink, the lotions and cosmetics we rub on our skin, the products we use to clean our home, and even the toothpaste we dab on our toothbrushes. If your blood and urine were tested, lab technicians would uncover dozens if not hundreds of chemical toxins in your bloodstream, including PCBs (polychlorinated biphenyls), dioxins, furans, trace metals, phthalates, VOCs (volatile organic compounds), and chlorine.

The main toxic hit comes through the foods we eat and the beverages we drink. Liz Lipski, PhD, author of *Digestive Wellness*, points out that the average American consumes fourteen pounds of additives a year.[2] The supermarket shelves are crammed with packaged foods containing food colorings, preservatives, flavorings, emulsifiers, humectants, and antimicrobials.

I've already had something to say about what I believe to be some of the worst—and most widely consumed—additives out there, and they are the no-calorie and low-calorie artificial sweeteners such as aspartame, saccharine, and sucralose. As many as 180 million Americans regularly eat and drink sugar-free products, according to recent statistics by the Calorie Control Council.[3]

Besides the long-alleged health risks, sugar alcohols and polyols such as sorbitol, malitol, isomalt, and a whole lot of other scientific-sounding names found in popular sweeteners can create significant digestive problems. Our bodies have a hard time breaking down sugar alcohols. In large amounts, they can cause diarrhea, gas, and bloating.

The digestive system has enough work to do without having to deal with an overload of toxins. Fortunately, some toxins are water soluble, meaning they are rapidly passed out of the body and present little harm. Unfortunately, many more toxins are fat soluble, meaning that it can take months or years before they are completely eliminated—if ever—from your system. Some of the more well-known fat-soluble toxins are dioxins, phthalates, DDT, and chlorine, and when they are not eliminated from the body, they become stored in your fatty tissues. "Consider those love handles as a hiding place for stored toxins and poisons," says Don Colbert, MD, and author of *Toxic Relief*. "In other words, fat is usually toxic, too."[4]

The best way to flush fat-soluble toxins out of your bloodstream is to increase your intake of drinking water, which helps eliminate toxins through the kidneys (which I'll get into shortly). Increasing the fiber in your diet eliminates toxins through the bowel, exercise and sweat eliminate toxins through the lymphatic system, and practicing deep breathing eliminates toxins through the lungs.

Another way to reduce your toxin load is to consume organic or grass-fed meat and dairy. Remember: most commercially produced beef, chicken, and pork act as chemical magnets for toxins in the environment, so they will not be as healthy as eating grass-fed, organic meats. In addition, consuming organic produce purchased at health food stores, roadside stands, and farmers' markets (only if produce is grown locally and unsprayed) will expose you to less pesticide residues as compared to conventionally grown fruits and vegetables.

Canned tuna is another food to eat minimally, although many popular diets include tuna and salad as a lunchtime or dinner staple. Heavy metal compounds, like those of mercury, lead, and aluminum, continue to be found in the fatty tissues of tuna, swordfish, and king mackerel. Shrimp and lobster, which are shellfish that scavenge the ocean floor, are loaded with toxins and should be exorcised from your diet. I recommend you limit the consumption of canned tuna to two cans per week (try low-mercury, high-omega-3 tuna) and avoid shellfish completely.

WHAT TO DRINK

I've already touted the health benefits of drinking pure water in chapter 4, but when it comes to reducing toxins in your environment, water is especially important because of its ability to flush out toxins and other metabolic wastes from the body. Overweight people tend to have larger amounts of stored toxins.

Our bodies are between 60 percent and 70 percent water. Increasing your intake of water will enhance your metabolism—which can lead to weight loss—and allow your body to assimilate nutrients from the foods you eat and the nutritional supplements you take. Since water is the primary resource for carrying nutrients throughout the body, a lack of adequate hydration results in metabolic wastes assaulting your body—a form of self-poisoning. That's why the importance of drinking enough water cannot be overstated: water is a life force involved in nearly every bodily process, from digestion to blood circulation.

Nothing beats plain old water—a liquid totally compatible with your body—especially when you're trying to lose weight. When the body is properly hydrated, the kidneys function optimally, and the liver can convert stored fat into usable energy. In other words, the liver—acting like a traffic cop—will direct the body to tap into its fat reserves when you are eating leaner, healthier foods and consuming fewer calories, and when you are exercising more.

Since bodies with excess weight tend to have sluggish (fattier) livers, the liver's ability to convert stored fat into usable energy can be greatly increased by the consumption of an abundance of clean, healthy water. Cold or lukewarm, it doesn't matter. Water helps you digest your meals more efficiently, reduces fluid retention, and prevents constipation. You will also notice a difference in your skin as water plumps up the skin, thereby reducing the appearance of fine lines and wrinkles while giving the skin a healthy, well-hydrated glow.

Watch out, though, when water soaks your skin during a shower. Standing underneath a nozzle blast of steaming warm or hot water for ten or fifteen minutes is the toxic equivalent of ingesting six to eight glasses of chlorinated water. Since chlorine is a gas, not only does it penetrate the skin, but it is also inhaled during a shower. Municipalities routinely treat public water supplies with chlorine or chloramine, chemical compounds used as disinfectants to kill, destroy, or control bacteria and algae. These potent chemicals are hard on your skin and give your body one more dangerous toxin to deal with.

You can install a whole-house filtration system that removes the chlorine and other impurities out of the water *before* it enters your household pipes, as we did, but a far less expensive option would be installing an inexpensive carbon-block shower filter. Once installed, these shower filters remove toxic chlorine for six months to a year until the filter needs to be changed.

To Microwave or Not to Microwave?

You won't find a microwave in the Rubin household, which puts us into a diminutive minority. Ninety percent of American kitchens come equipped with a microwave oven to heat up leftovers or frozen meals, but I nixed microwave ovens the day Nicki and I set up house after the honeymoon. I told Nicki that I had done my homework: microwave ovens emit radiation in the form of radio frequencies, and when those waves of energy bombarded food, the agitation caused molecular friction to occur, which heated up the food but also destroyed the fragile structure of vitamins, minerals, and enzymes in food.

The Food and Drug Administration (FDA) regulates microwave ovens and believes they are safe for use, but the jury is still out on the possibility of a link between microwave exposure and diseases such as cancer. My feelings could be summed in three words: *Why risk it?* Nicki, though skeptical at first, went along with the program, and we haven't had a microwave in any home we've lived in.

I realize some readers think that we must live like the Flintstones since we don't have a microwave in the home. What I've noticed about microwaves, though, is that they're never used to heat up "normal" foods—fruits, vegetables, and meats. Instead, I would wager that microwaves in this country are used 90 percent of the time to heat up frozen, heavily processed meals like Hot Pockets sandwiches, Swanson's chicken pot pies, and Lean Cuisine Chicken Florentine Lasagna. These are definitely not meals you should be eating when you follow the Maker's Diet for Weight Loss program.

But what about heating up infant formula? We've survived just fine with the addition of two infants recently. It only takes a couple of minutes to heat a pot of water and warm up their bottles. When Joshua started eating solid food, we never fed him commercial baby food out of a jar anyway, so heating up those jars was never an issue.

What Nicki and I found was that the old-fashioned toaster oven is more than adequate when it comes to heating up something quickly. Our favorite toaster-oven meal on the go is homemade pizzas from sprouted English muffins, which not only are a healthy source of fiber and other nutrients, but also they heat up in a jiffy and don't have a soggy aftertaste as some microwaved foods do. On occasion, we've cooked lamb chops, baked potatoes, and just about any leftover in the fridge with our handy toaster oven. Toaster ovens heat up faster than regular ovens, use less energy, and are easier to clean.

TOXINS ELSEWHERE IN YOUR ENVIRONMENT

There are other toxins lurking in our environment that aren't directly related to losing weight but are important enough to mention:

Plastics. There's a reason I carry a 64-ounce polycarbonate water bottle with me: the presence of dioxins and phthalates added in the manufacturing process of plastic. Phthalates are used to increase the flexibility and resilience of plastic. The problem with phthalates is that this petroleum-derived product has been linked to cancer in lab tests.[5]

Polycarbonate water bottles are safer in regard to the leaching problems associated with plastic. It's impossible to get away from plastic in our modern lives, but Nicki and I make it a point to store leftovers in glass containers and not wrap food in plastic wrap, just to be safe. And you won't find Styrofoam cups in our house either.

Household cleaners. Many of today's commercial household cleaners contain potentially harmful chemicals and solvents that expose people to VOCs—volatile organic compounds—which can cause eye, nose, and throat irritation. There's a reason why companies recommend that you keep these household cleaners out of the hands of children.

All-purpose cleaners contain chlorinated phosphates, complex phosphates, dry bleach, kerosene, petroleum-based surfactants, sodium bromide, glycol ether, and naphtha. These compounds are stored in human fat cells, adding to the toxic load on the liver, and they are not absolutely necessary to keep countertops, sinks, and floors clean. Nicki and I have found that natural ingredients like vinegar, lemon juice, citrus oils, and baking soda are excellent substances that make our home spic and span. Natural cleaning products from companies like Seventh Generation and Ecover aren't harsh, abrasive, or potentially dangerous to your family, and they are becoming more and more available in natural-food stores and progressive grocery stores.

Toothpaste. By reading the fine print, you will find that your tube of toothpaste contains a warning: "In case of accidental swallowing, you should contact the local Poison Control Center." What's that all about? Most commercially available toothpastes contain artificial sweeteners, potassium nitrate, sodium fluoride, and a whole bunch of long, unpronounceable words. Those red, white, and blue swirls in some of the leading brands don't come from fresh strawberries, coconut, and blueberries.

You can search out a healthy, natural, fluoride-free toothpaste in health food stores. On occasion, we've used natural peppermint oil-based tooth drops to clean Joshua's teeth. We think our three children will have a great shot at going through life cavity-free since we won't be feeding them candy or any treat with refined sugar.

Skin care and body care products. Toxic chemicals such as chemical solvents and phthalates are found in lipstick, lip gloss, lip conditioner, hair coloring, hair spray, shampoo, and soap. Ladies, when you rub a tube of lipstick across your lips, your skin readily absorbs these toxins, and that's unhealthy. Lipstick deserves an award for being the most toxic cosmetic. When you spread lipstick across your lips, you're applying a substance that contains several carcinogens, including polyvinyl-pyrrolidone plastic (say that three times), saccharin, mineral oil, and artificial colors. It's human nature to lick your lips, but when that happens, you're merely delivering its toxic ingredients sooner into the body's bloodstream. Mascara, eye shadow, powdered blush, and face powder fall into the same category.

Scented products such as perfumes and colognes are a soup of chemicals, solvents, alcohol, and chemical fragrances and a substitute for something that would actually be good for you—natural essential oils. It's a pity that approximately 95 percent of the ingredients in perfumes are derived from petrochemicals.[6] More research needs to be done on the health effects of scented products, but we have all known friends or family who have experienced skin irritation, headaches, and even nausea when they are around certain perfumes and aftershaves. Others are highly allergenic or environmentally sensitive to the overwhelming smell.

It's tough, though, making cosmetic changes. I have this favorite eye shadow... that's a joke, but in our master bathroom, Nicki prefers her tried-and-true, nonorganic mascara, lipstick, and lip liner, along with a certain hairspray that I'm sure contains every carcinogen known to man. She tried an "organic" hairspray one time, but that left her hair feeling like sticky wax. "I don't go for the crunchy look," she said.

Listen, I've learned something in eight years of marriage: women want to look their best, so when Nicki reaches for the hairspray bottle, I excuse myself from the bathroom. At least I don't have to inhale all those toxins.

Organic cosmetics and skin care products are improving as consumer demand escalates, however. A company called Aubrey Organics, also listed in Appendix C, is producing superb natural and organic hair and skin care products free of synthetics and petrochemicals. You should find brands like Aubrey Organics in natural-food stores and progressive grocery stores, although they are becoming more widely available in drug stores and beauty stores.

Air quality. We spend 90 percent of our time indoors, according to the American Lung Association, usually in well-insulated and energy-efficient homes and offices with central air conditioning in the summer and forced-air heating during the winter.[7] Double-pane windows, when tamped down shut, don't allow any fresh air into the home and trap "used" air filled with harmful particles such as carbon dioxide, nitrogen dioxide, and pet dander.

Perhaps you've noticed all the attention given to mold-related illnesses and how homes have been torn up to rid walls and studs of spores of green and black mold. Those living in mold-infested environments have been diagnosed with impaired thyroid and adrenal problems, chronic fatigue, and memory impairment. It's tough to stick with a lifestyle change—or remember to do so—if poor indoor air quality drains your energy.

I recommend opening your doors and windows periodically to freshen the air you breathe, even if the temperatures are blazing hot or downright freezing. Just a few minutes of fresh air will do wonders, far better for you and the family than spraying the house with synthetic room fresheners and fragranced cleaning products, which provoke skin, eye, and respiratory reactions. In homes where aerosol sprays and air fresheners are used frequently, mothers suffered 25 percent more headaches and 19 percent more depression, and infants under six months of age had 30 percent more ear infections and 22 percent higher incidence of diarrhea, according to a study done at Bristol University in England.[8]

Don't buy air fresheners, deodorizers, and odor removers. Instead, purchase a quality air filter, which will remove and neutralize tiny airborne particles of dust, soot, pollen, mold, and dander. I have set up four high-quality air purifiers in our home that scrub harmful impurities from the air. Indoor houseplants scrub the air as well, but you could also place flower sachets in strategic areas around the house. Health food stores also sell fragrance jars and dried botanicals.

The Maker's Diet for Weight Loss Recap: Reduce Toxins for Your Ideal Weight

1. Drinking plenty of water—at least a half-ounce for each pound of body weight—will give the body the fluids it needs to pull those toxins out of the bloodstream.
2. Install shower filters to remove chlorine and toxins from your water.
3. Use glass or polycarbonate containers instead of plastic containers whenever possible.
4. Improve indoor air quality by opening windows, strategically placing natural houseplants, or buying an air filtration system.
5. Use natural cleaning products for your home.
6. Try out organic cosmetics and personal care products, which are good for the body and for the environment.

eleven

Think for Your Ideal Weight

I F YOU'RE AMONG those who've watched *Extraordinary Health*, my half-hour TV program that airs on the Trinity Broadcasting Network and other networks nationwide, then you've probably enjoyed the cooking segments I've done with Carol Green, a bubbly and talented executive chef from South Africa.

Carol has a lilting accent—not quite British, not quite Australian—that's pleasing to American ears. More importantly, she very much enjoys eating to live and teaching others how to cook for their ideal weight. You wouldn't know it by looking at her while she whips up wonderful flans and creamy sauces on our kitchen set, but Carol was an "emotional" eater for many years, someone whose weight yo-yoed whenever black moods or unsettling stress happened in her life. If you have battled emotional ups and downs regarding your weight, then you'll appreciate Carol's story:

> I grew up in a picturesque province called the Eastern Cape on my parents' wheat farm. I have three brothers: Robert is older, and Michael and Gavin are younger. All my brothers were very athletic—Robert was a national rugby star—but their athletic abilities didn't rub off on me. I was really short, and if truth be told, rather chubby as a child. My sporty brothers could eat a ton of food, so I ate big boy portions as well. I guess I never learned what a normal-sized portion of food really was.
>
> Unlike me, my mum is tall, but she is a lovely lady who was always on and off a diet. She was always searching for the next miracle regimen. When she was on a diet, she starved herself and was miserable; when she was off a diet, she ate all the things she had been deprived of. This behavior impacted me deeply, especially as I grew older. I was a fat kid and teased unmercifully at school. "Carol the Barrel," they called me. I also heard lots of comments like, "How can you possibly be Robert's sister?" Even back then, I didn't measure up.
>
> So I began to go for long runs—and go on crazy diets. I joined the cross-country running squad in high school and became obsessed with running.

The weight melted off, down to a point where I weighed 92 pounds. At 5 feet 3 inches tall, I was really skinny, and I liked that.

My final year at high school, though, I got injured and had to stop running, so I concentrated on studies. The pounds came back, not many, mind you, but enough to capture my attention. I really thought I was headed to the fat farm, although when I look back at photos from that time, I was actually thin. That just goes to show you how completely distorted my body image was becoming.

I went into the fashion industry after finishing school, becoming a buyer for one of the leading department stores in South Africa, working in Cape Town. Looks became super important to me; they were paramount since I worked in the fashion industry, where image was everything. So I had to keep any pounds from creeping on, which exacerbated the on-a-diet and off-a-diet cycle that had engulfed Mum. I felt great mental anguish and wondered why I kept failing on diets.

I kept putting on the same 20 to 25 pounds two or three times a year. I had fat clothes and thin clothes in my wardrobe, things I could fit into and things I couldn't fit into. At times, I got up to 150 pounds. When the fat clothes came out of the closet, I'd follow the cabbage soup diet for a week (*blech!*) or eat nothing but grapes.

Whenever I came off a diet, I would eat everything in sight—just like Mum. And the weight would come rushing back, which mentally weighed on me again.

I tried on diets like the models tried on clothes before setting off for the runways. If eating grapefruit for a week straight didn't reap results, I followed Weight Watchers for a while. If the latest miracle cure didn't pan out, I tried Jenny Craig. Over a ten-year period I did 'em all: no fat, low fat, low carb, high protein, high carb—I just mixed and matched the regimens, figuring something had to work.

I thought that leaving the fashion industry might help. Ten years ago, out of the blue, I got an opportunity to sail in the Caribbean on a small yacht as the cook, and being the adventurous sort that I am, I took it, even though I had no formal experience as a chef. I had always loved to cook growing up and even thought of going to cooking school, but back in the mid-1980s, there weren't many opportunities for chefs.

I must tell you that I really enjoyed working in the galley as the private yacht glided across the light blue waters of the Caribbean. I found that cooking for others agreed with me. After my first winter in the Caribbean, I found a better job—this time cooking on a beautiful and swift 130-foot yacht owned by an American couple. I didn't do very well being surrounded by all this fancy food; I constantly snacked and overate, gaining 20 to 25 pounds and two clothing sizes. I hated putting on a bikini to take a refreshing dip in the tropical water and trying to "be good" when I was cooking all the time.

During this time I either cooked or followed the latest diet out there, as the rich, thin ladies I cooked for were always obsessing about their weight too. I became resigned to the idea that I would always be overweight. "If I'm going to be fat, by golly, I'm going to enjoy it," was my attitude. I was tired of the mental anguish of always being on a diet.

After a couple of years onboard a luxury yacht, I wanted to take my cooking skills to the next level, so I asked for a sabbatical and traveled to Lyon, France, where I enrolled in a four-month intensive cooking school. I learned the basics of traditional French cooking and *boulangerie*. Several things stood out to me. One, I never cooked with so much butter and eggs and cream in my life—but even with all that butter and cream, the French people weren't fat. They cooked and ate real food, a contrast to the directive to prepare low-fat and fat-free dishes and desserts onboard Caribbean yachts.

I noticed several other things about the French. Inside Carrefours—the big supermarket chain in France—potato chips and other snack foods comprised just one-half of one aisle. But in America, where I spent some time during my Caribbean travels, the potato chips and snack chips were stacked up in *two* aisles. (You could also buy a half-dozen different flavored versions of Doritos.) And what was the story with fat-free sour cream and chive chips?

In addition, French people ate their meals sitting down. They weren't in a hurry to eat, preferring stimulating discussion and a leisurely pace with their knife and fork along with a glass of Bordeaux, even in the middle of the afternoon. No matter what they had pressing on their schedules, the French took their time whenever a meal was served. The Americans I cooked for on the yachts often wolfed down their meals and didn't appreciate the food or the time I took to prepare it. Some would fill up a paper plate from the buffet line and eat standing up.

After receiving my culinary training in France, I returned to the Caribbean and cooked on private yachts for a couple more years. Waking up in the Grand Cayman Islands one morning or shopping for provisions in Castries, St. Lucia, was a lifestyle very much removed from reality, so I decided to return to land when I accepted a personal chef position with a prominent Houston family. During this time, I developed a serious heart condition called atrial fibrillation, which meant the heart wasn't beating properly. I was prescribed strong drugs to control the heartbeat, all of which had terrible side effects. Seeking a different path to getting well, I began researching nutritional supplements that could help me. I took various vitamins and minerals by the handful each day, but nothing seemed to help. This all happened in my late thirties.

I found a doctor who put me on a detox program to cleanse my body. "You know, when your body is clean, it can function much better," he said as he wrote me a "prescription" to go purchase some Garden of Life products at a health food store. I felt dramatically better within days, which prompted more curiosity on my part.

I learned that the person behind Garden of Life was a fellow named Jordan Rubin. He had a new book out called *The Maker's Diet*. I read the book in nearly one sitting; everything made absolute sense to me. When I graduated from the detox program, I ate the food in *The Maker's Diet*, focusing on nutritional healing, and the weight loss followed. I realized the damage I had done to my body for years with yo-yo dieting and artificial "fat-free" diet foods. Over a period of three months I lost 23 pounds and attained my ideal weight.

Maintaining your weight and your health is really the same thing. You begin by focusing on eating real food. If I want cake or ice cream, I want to know if they are made from the best quality ingredients I can find without hydrogenated oils and preservatives in them. I love every bite of a cake or ice cream, when it's made the healthy way. I eat calmly, enjoying every last bite.

If you are dealing with emotional issues that are keeping you from your weight-loss goals, you need to do three things:

1. **You need to understand the real reason why you overeat.** Deal with emotional issues, and you'll understand why you overeat. Stop self-medicating with food. I had to deal with the reasons why I overate and stop blaming it on a diet that didn't work. No diet is ever going to work unless you make it a lifestyle program.

2. **Focus on only eating real food.** When you supercharge your body with nutrition, cravings are way less, and this will help you stay on the program. That's the message in the "Eat for Your Ideal Weight" chapter, but it's amazing how many folks will purchase factory foods and eat pure junk.

3. **Don't eat on the fly.** How you receive your food is important. Make every meal an occasion. Pray over your food. Eat calmly. Eat with joy every bite.

I've been at my ideal weight for two years. Occasionally when I allow myself too many treats, I do gain a pound or two, but I make sure I follow the Maker's Diet program, exercise, and, most importantly, don't stress about it. I don't tell myself, "You're going to weigh 150 pounds again." Instead, I get back to basics, and within a week, I'm in good shape again.

For me, cooking is a joy. I have not only turned my health around, but I have also found my life's purpose, which is helping others lose weight and achieve God's purpose for their lives. If you are struggling with your weight today, I urge you to give up all the other fad diets you've ever tried and follow the Weight Loss Eating Plan. Eat whole and natural foods that have been around for thousands of years. You will look and feel better than you ever have, you will age well, and you will enjoy your life as God intended.

THE MIND-BODY CONNECTION

I love Carol's story, and it's illustrative of how our active minds have a considerable impact on our weight and our health in ways that we never thought imaginable. The mind-body connection has always fascinated me, but I wanted to bring in an expert who's become a dear friend to me. His name is Alex Loyd, PhD, and he and Ben Johnson, MD, are the creators of an emotional health system called "Healing Codes."

I asked Alex to read Carol's story and then comment on how readers of *The Maker's Diet for Weight Loss* can "think" for their ideal weight. Alex believes this area of emotional health could be the missing link for those trying to shed pounds. He'll be providing you with a Healing Codes exercise at the end of this chapter that I recommend you perform two to five times per day. But first, here's what Alex had to say:

My partner, Dr. Ben Johnson, and I have been lecturing around the world talking about the Healing Codes for over five years now, trying to help people heal the source of their problems. It seems that at every event we are inundated with people who tell us they want to lose weight. "Will the Healing Codes help me lose weight?" they ask. "I've been trying for years. Is this going to be the thing that finally does it for me?"

And our answer every single time is this: "No, because your problem is not what you think your problem is."

Many overweight people think something has gone haywire in their bodies, that something's not working the way it is supposed to work, or they are reacting to foods in ways that they shouldn't react. They are looking for the one magical diet that is going to turn everything around, which was Carol Green's story growing up in South Africa.

I greatly identified with what Carol had to say because when I was growing up, the junior high years were the absolute worst time of my life—period, end of discussion. One of the big reasons why is because I was overweight. I wasn't obese, however, or anything like that. I was just kind of soft and squishy.

I can vividly remember going to David Lipscomb Junior High School in Nashville, Tennessee, and hearing kids yell across the school yard: "Hey, chunky!" And I would laugh. And then I would go home and cry. Of course, while I was crying, I would snack on a whole bag of Lay's potato chips and maybe a couple of white sugary doughnuts. I learned that one of the things that made me feel good after feeling so *bad* was eating something fattening and good tasting.

Sometime late in junior high, I made up my mind that my classmates were never going to make fun of me again because of my weight. I started jogging eight or ten miles every day—just like Carol—and knocking off hundreds of sit-ups and push-ups before I went to bed. I laid off high-fat foods, or if I did indulge, I ate them early in the day so I could burn them off.

Sure enough, I lost weight, and people never made fun of me again. I went from being teased all the time to dating cheerleaders and homecoming queens. Wow, I must have lived happily ever after, after that, right? No, absolutely not. Why? Because I solved my weight issues for all the wrong reasons. My single-handed purpose to lose weight was so that people would look at me and think good things instead of thinking how fat I looked. My problem wasn't on the outside; it was what was on the inside, and that's illustrated by the fact that we have one hundred million sensory receptors for things that are outside, but we have ten thousand billion sensory receptors for things happening inside our bodies.[1] When things happen on the inside, it's always an emotional or spiritual issue.

Let me share with you how this all came together for me. More than three thousand years ago, wise old King Solomon in the Book of Proverbs said this: "Above all else, guard your heart, for it affects everything you do" (Proverbs 4:23, NLT). I'm told that if you read that original passage in Hebrew—which I can't because I don't know Hebrew—then what Solomon is saying is that heart issues are the source of 100 percent of our problems.

This observation makes sense to me. If you ask anybody who has a weight problem, "Is this an issue for you?" every one of them will reply, "Absolutely." A vast majority will confide that it's the *biggest* issue of their lives. Well, according to Solomon, your issue with being overweight does not originate with your body's thyroid or the health of your endocrine system or how fast your body metabolizes fat. They originate with issues of the heart.

A story in the *Dallas Morning News* on September 13, 2004, really drove this point home. The gist of the news article was that researchers at the University of Texas Southwestern Medical Center were finding that cells record their experiences—called cellular memory—all without the benefit of a brain. Scientists believe these cellular memories might mean the difference between a healthy and unhealthy life, even death.[2]

For instance, cancer can be the result of bad cellular memories replacing good ones. Psychological trauma, addiction, and depression may all be furthered by abnormal memories inside cells. Health issues that crop up later in life may be due to errant memories programmed into cells as people age. Dr. Eric Nestler, the University of Texas chairman of the psychiatry department, said that for many ailments, medical treatments aren't much better than Band-Aids since they treat the symptoms, not the source.[3]

That source is from the heart. If you read the more than eleven hundred passages in the Bible that talk about the heart, including what Solomon said about the heart affecting everything you do, and then consider what the Southwestern Medical Center research says about cellular memory—which really is about what lies inside our hearts—it's the same thing! Modern medical science is finally catching up with what Solomon said thirty centuries ago: that the issues of the heart are the source of just about any problem that we can have in our lives. Said another way, if we can fix the issues of the heart, we can fix just about any problem we have.

Now, is this principle applicable to weight loss? You bet your boots it is, and here's why: Whenever we are experiencing—a lot of times this is unconscious and not conscious—anger or fear or anxiety or low self-worth, we are experiencing issues of the heart. They are the spiritual issues that manifest themselves in a thousand different ways: irritation, being overwhelmed by life's circumstances, being afraid of the future, worries about money, relationship difficulties. We can go on for days just naming them. Those are all issues of the heart.

When we have an issue of the heart like one of the things I just mentioned, there is a mechanism in the brain called the hypothalamus. The hypothalamus is responsible for turning the stress switch in the body on or off. When the stress switch is turned on, the first thing it does is suppress the immune system. The second thing it does is start to suppress or shut down normal bodily functioning, such as food digestion, metabolizing of fat, cleansing the blood of toxins, and movement of the bowels.

Dr. Bruce Lipton of the Stanford University Medical School, in his bestselling book *The Biology of Belief*, says that every cell in your body is in one of two modes: it's either in stress mode, or it's in a growth mode.[4] A cell that is in stress mode does not do the job it's supposed to do, so if it's a cell responsible for metabolism, or the proper digestion of food, or pulling nutrients out of food, or dealing with fat so that it's burned or stored appropriately, it's not going to do the job it's supposed to do. Furthermore, the "stressed" cell does not cooperate with other cells around it. It doesn't grow or reproduce but chooses to do its own thing. These cells cannot absorb nutrients the way they're supposed to or release toxins as they need to. Many bodily functions are put on hold or stopped.

Regarding the stress mode, did you know that you're only supposed to go into stress when you're put into a severe, dangerous situation—like being chased by a bear or confronted by an armed intruder in the house? The problem is—and many studies show this—the average person encounters lower levels of stress many, many times a day. We get stressed out by the MasterCard bill, making the house payment, getting into a fender bender, keeping up with the Joneses, wearing the right dress, driving the right car, and a thousand other things. The cumulative effect makes us feel like we are running as fast as we can on a hamster treadmill but getting nowhere quickly.

Dr. Ben and I talk to people all the time, and invariably we ask them to describe their diets to us. "You know, I eat organic, I eat fruits and vegetables, and if I eat meat, it is very lean and in limited amounts. And I still can't lose any weight and keep it off."

Well, OK, tell me about the rest of your life. Are you stressed?

"Oh, man, to the max, over the top. I am under water. I feel like I am going crazy half the time."

When they are in that situation, their immune system is being suppressed, and the physiological systems that control their weight issues are not functioning the way they're supposed to work. Very often, when you heal the underlying issues of the heart, not only do you feel better emotionally, but your physical systems also start to work the way they should. The Healing Codes can help you deal with the issues of the heart, and when that happens, the hypothalamus will turn off the stress switch. The immune system will come back up, the systems of the body will start doing what they were designed to do, and the cells will start functioning properly the way nutrition and metabolism are concerned.

The following Healing Codes exercise will help you work on and improve the issues of the heart. Normally, I recommend that you go through this exercise early in the morning before you start your day, but Jordan believes that performing the Healing Codes exercise before meals will reduce stress and make for better digestion. In fact, if you are upset, nervous, fearful, angry, or stressed out before *any* meal, you won't digest your food as well, and you're more likely to emotionally overeat, so that's when it would be a good time to perform the Healing Codes exercise.

THE HEALING CODES EXERCISE

1. Focus on your overall stress level related to your weight, and rate it from 0 to 10, with 10 being the highest. Your first thought should be: "How much does this [the issue in your life] bother me?" When you think about this stressful situation, what feelings, emotions,

or thoughts do you feel? Are they anger, frustration, irritation, or a feeling that life is never going to change? When you think about this issue, where do you feel it in your body? What do you feel—pain, heaviness, flutter, or pressure?

2. Place your hands one on top of the other, with your right palm over your belly button and your left palm over the back of your right hand.

3. Focus on the stress you want to leave your body—physical, emotional, or spiritual.

4. Do power breathing for ten seconds. Breathe rapid and powerful "belly breaths" in and out. Forcefully blow out and suck in through your mouth, using your diaphragm so your belly moves out as you breathe in and moves in as you breathe out. If you feel a little lightheaded, breathe the same way, but reduce the intensity.

5. Leave your right hand over your belly button and move your left hand over your heart as you relax for fifty seconds. Think or say "stress out" while you focus on the stress leaving your body. If you like, you can also visualize stress leaving your body as you relax and think or say "stress out."

6. Move your left hand back on top of your right hand over your belly button.

7. Focus on physical, emotional, or spiritual peace.

8. Do power breathing for ten seconds. Breathe rapid and powerful "belly breaths" in and out. Forcefully blow out and suck in through your mouth, using your diaphragm so your belly moves out as you breathe in and moves in as you breathe out. If you feel a little lightheaded, breathe the same way, but reduce the intensity.

9. Leave your right hand over your belly button and move your left hand over your heart as you relax for fifty seconds. Think or say "peace" while you focus on peace entering your body. If you like, while you say "peace," imagine peace flowing into your body from God or visualize a peaceful scene that calms and strengthens you.

10. Rerate your overall stress level from 0 to 10, as you did in step 1.

11. Rerate your overall stress level ten minutes later.

12. Do another Healing Codes exercise if your stress level is still at 4 or above.

WRAP-UP FROM JORDAN

This Healing Codes exercise has greatly helped me deal with the stresses in my life—running an international health and wellness organization with more than one hundred employees, writing books, taping TV shows, speaking around the world, being interviewed by the media, and formulating nutritional supplements. Then there are my personal responsibilities that—wonderful as they are—can still be stressful: spending quality time with my wife, Nicki, and being a great father to our three children. At the same time, I understand my stresses are unique to me, and the daily stresses in your life are unique to you as well. We must all cope with the busyness of life.

The Healing Codes exercise can help you deal with any lingering "issues of the heart." One issue that is often overlooked is unforgiveness, which is common for those who grew up being overweight. Perhaps you were teased unmercifully in the school yard, like Carol and Alex. When you reached adulthood, the digs were delivered in a more subtle form: "Are you really going to eat that?" or "Have you thought about trying this diet?"

If you are harboring resentment in your heart, nursing a grudge into overtime, or plotting revenge against those who hurt you, these issues of the heart will produce toxins similar to bingeing on a dozen glazed doughnuts. The efficiency of your immune system decreases noticeably for up to six hours, and staying angry and bitter about those who have teased you in the past can alter the chemistry of your body—and even prompt you to fall off the healthy food wagon again. An old proverb states it well: "What you are eating is not nearly as important as what's eating you."

This is not the time to revert to old habits: consuming a deep-dish large pizza in one sitting, scarfing a package of Oreo cookies, or plying yourself with "comfort" foods filled with fat and sugar as Alex did back in his junior high days. If you're still annoyed by those who teased you about your body shape, made snide comments about your plus-size clothes, or told you that you'll never lose weight, you have to let it go. The Healing Codes exercise will help you do that.

No matter how badly you've been hurt, put your past in the rearview mirror and move forward. It's still possible to forgive.

The Maker's Diet for Weight Loss Recap: Think for Your Ideal Weight

1. Realize that your issue with weight may be related to something happening on the inside—an issue of the heart.
2. Perform the Healing Codes exercise, which focuses on letting go of stresses in your life.
3. Practice forgiveness every day, and forgive those who hurt you.

Section III

MAXIMIZE CARE AND MINIMIZE CARELESSNESS

twelve

Take Weight Off the World

URING ONE OF my seasonal cleanses in the midst of writing *The Maker's Diet for Weight Loss*, I conceived a lofty goal: eat only locally grown fruit, salad, and vegetables.

I knew I needed some help, so I enlisted the aid of Paul Nison, one of the world's leading experts on eating raw foods and author of a half-dozen books, including *The Raw Life*. Paul lives in West Palm Beach, and our paths had crossed several times since we're both speakers and health authors.

In addition, Paul also faced a major health crisis when he was twenty years old—the same age I was—when sudden stomach pains grew so intense that he had to be hospitalized. Doctors diagnosed him with Crohn's disease, just like me, and told him to deal with it because they had no cure. His physicians also declared that he would be on medications for the rest of his life.

Such bleak news prompted Paul to chuck his life as a Wall Street trader and move to West Palm Beach, where he settled into an apartment right next door—as fate would have it—to the Hippocrates Health Institute. He had no idea what the institute did, but he soon learned that they taught people how to live with debilitating diseases with a raw-food diet and lifestyle.

Within months Paul's chubby body was transformed, which set him down a new career path to tell others about the health benefits of eating raw foods. Even though I'm not a raw foodist—someone who primarily consumes raw, uncooked, and unprocessed foods—I certainly agree that many health benefits can be derived from eating raw, especially for short periods of time. After all, the Summer Cleanse means eating raw fruits during the day and a raw salad for dinner, which was my goal when I contacted Paul about my idea of eating local. We made arrangements to meet one morning.

I hadn't seen Paul in a year or two, so I had forgotten that he was a whirling dervish of energy. Midthirties, a bushy beard, hair slicked back, and wearing khaki clothes and leather sandals, Paul looked like an extra from Cecil B. DeMille's *The Ten Commandments* movie set. He stands 5 feet 7 inches and weighs 145 pounds.

Paul brandished a pair of perilous tools in his hands—a mean-looking machete that looked to be razor-sharp and an extension pole pruner to pry away coconuts lodged high in the tall palms of South Florida. The plan that morning, as he outlined it, was to visit a nearby organic farm that cultivated exotic fruits not normally found in supermarkets *or* health foods stores, as well as cherry-pick coconuts from coconut trees growing in the midst of suburbia.

Our first stop was Josan Growers, a mom-and-pop fruit farm located in the rural outskirts of West Palm. With Paul as my personal shopper, we filled the back of my car with eggfruit, durian, mangoes, and a 14-pound jackfruit, which, at $3 per pound, cost $42. My total bill was $91. "You'll like that durian," Paul said. "It tastes like vanilla custard with a hint of garlic and onion."

That's an interesting taste combination...

Meanwhile, Paul kept up a steady chatter, telling me about his life as a "minimalist," even though he rued the fact that he was picking up more "stuff" now that he was in his second year of marriage.

"Really?" I said, cocking an eyebrow.

"Yes," he replied. "Except for the furniture in our apartment, everything I own fits in one suitcase."

By now, nothing that Paul could say would surprise me. There was the time he returned to Central Park in New York City and picked leaves off the trees for a snack—and got arrested. Prior to his marriage, he lived out of a van for a year and foraged empty fields for wild food to keep body and soul together. "There are all sorts of wild foods in South Florida that are quite edible," he instructed. I decided I would take his word for it.

After we filled up my trunk with exotic fruit, we drove around Forest Hill—a tidy bedroom community about seven miles southeast of West Palm Beach—hunting for coconuts in front yard trees. Paul guided us to a neighborhood where he had knocked on doors before to ask the occupants if it would be OK to snag a few of their coconuts.

"Stop here," he directed. I watched as Paul—with a long, flowing beard that threatened to touch his sternum—approached the front door of a well-kept, mustard-hued single-family home with a menacing machete gripped in his right hand. Whoever answered the door would be more likely to call the cops than give him permission to chop down their coconuts.

After several rejections, we found an owner who said it would be OK to prune the coconut tree in her front yard. Up went the extension pole, and with a jerk of the blade, coconuts rained down. We probably packed fifteen or twenty coconuts for the trip home.

I drove Paul back to his car and thanked him for his time. Over the next several days, I split open the fresh coconuts, gulped the mineral-charged coconut water, and feasted on young coconut spoon meat. My "local" salad came from lettuce grown in a hydroponic tower situated in my backyard patio—but more on that later. One crucial ingredient was missing from my salad, though. Florida's famous avocados, so mouth-watering that I call them "butter pears," were out of season, so I had to purchase organic California avocados at my local health food store.

So much for eating 100 percent local, but I came close. In a small and local way, though, I was participating in a burgeoning movement called "sustainable food," which means the establishment of a shorter food chain by consumers and restaurant chefs eager to buy meat, fruits, and vegetables produced locally. Currently, only 1 to 2 percent of American's food is locally grown, and the produce you eat is shipped an average of fifteen hundred miles to your local supermarket, according to a study by the Leopold Center for Sustainable Agriculture at Iowa State University.[1]

The transportation of lettuce or any type of food—or just about anything we do in life—leaves a "carbon footprint," a term referring to the impact that human activity has on the environment in terms of the amount of greenhouse gases produced. Eating foods shipped from another state, driving a car, taking an airline flight, and heating and air conditioning our homes are some of the everyday examples of leaving a "carbon footprint" on the planet.

The leaders of the sustainable food movement urge consumers to leave a smaller carbon footprint by seeking out local organic alternatives to mainstream food from co-ops, natural-food stores, farmer's markets, roadside stands, and backyard gardens and fruit-bearing trees. Every time you shop locally for food, your buying decision has ramifications for the health of your body as well as the planet.

While purchasing organic apples from Washington State, organic strawberries from California's Salinas Valley, and organic avocados from San Diego County sends an important message to agribusiness—namely, you're choosing organic over conventionally grown produce—shopping for organic fruits and vegetables grown locally (or growing your own lettuce, tomatoes, fruit, and vegetables in your backyard) sends an even better message: you're trying to live a more sustainable life that places less environmental demands on the planet. You're attempting to meet the physical needs of the present without compromising the ability of future generations to provide for their own needs.

Sustainable Fisheries

The term *sustainable* also applies to our fish habitats.

Scientists at Dalhousie University in Halifax, Canada, are worried that stocks of commercial fishing species will collapse by 2048 due to overfishing. They say that 90 percent of the big fish—tuna, cod, and swordfish—are gone from the oceans and that only 6 percent of the global fish catch can be certified as "sustainable," meaning that fish are not being pulled from the ocean any faster than they can reproduce.[2]

We can do our part for the environment—and help ensure that there will be a nutritious protein source for our children and children's children—by looking for the blue-and-white label from the Marine Stewardship Council that the fish are certified as sustainably caught.

Living sustainably is an important part of "living green," which is the idea that we should use our natural resources wisely to restore and maintain a balanced world. The choices we make every day regarding the food we eat, how much water and energy we consume, the type of cleaning products we use in the home, and the kind of car (and how often) we drive have a positive or negative impact on the earth.

It's important to take weight off the world too.

TAKING WEIGHT OFF THE PLANET

Living a sustainable lifestyle is part of my DNA, and I have my Grandpa Joshua Rubin to thank. My father, Herb Rubin, tells me that his family grew up in Floral Park, New York—a suburb of Long Island—without any grass in their backyard. Grandpa ripped out the lawn to cultivate a vegetable garden, using every available square inch to plant cucumbers, tomatoes, and lettuce. Peach and pear trees delivered scrumptious fruit by the bushel. The soil was incredibly fertile because of a compost pile that took up a good corner of the yard. Dad says he can remember approaching his father as a four- or five-year-old boy—this had to be in the mid-1950s—and asking, "Daddy, how do you know the soil is so rich and wonderful to grow plants in?"

Grandpa replied, "Just put your hands in the soil, son, and let it slide over your hands. Don't you feel the richness and life in that soil? It's a feeling! The deep, dark, almost black color means the soil is rich in nutrients."

Dad was too young to comprehend what nutrients were in those days, but he knew he could kill twenty worms every time he jammed a spade into the black earth. My grandpa was such a conservationist that he had their family of four share the same bathwater! "That was his way to save water," my father remembers. "Disgusting!"

Grandpa couldn't let all that gray water run down the drain, either. No, they got a bucket brigade going and dumped the dirty bathwater on their compost pile. "We had the largest tomatoes in the neighborhood," my dad said with a tinge of pride.

When Dad was entering high school, Grandpa had him read Rachel Carson's *Silent Spring*, a book widely credited with launching the environmental movement and inspiring widespread public concerns over pesticides and pollution. "He told me that what Rachel Carson wrote would come to pass if we didn't do something and make a difference."

My father, as I mentioned in the introduction, walked to the beat of a different drum as he came of age and married. He and Mom were among the first of their generation to pursue a hippielike "natural" lifestyle, as it was called in the 1970s. Unfortunately, even though my grandfather cared about the environment, he lacked discipline in the area of his personal health. Nearly 60 pounds overweight at the age of sixty-three, my grandfather died of a sudden and massive heart attack when I was nine years old. In the eyes of this youngster, he was my favorite person in the whole wide world. I can still remember seeing the cherry-red, plump tomatoes and hefty cucumbers in his backyard garden.

Although I haven't torn up my backyard to plant a garden, I am growing my own cucumbers as well as four varieties of lettuce in a pair of hydroponic towers situated in my backyard patio.

I can hear the question being asked: *What is a hydroponic tower?*

A hydroponic tower is a way of cultivating plants with water and nutrients without soil. I have two towers, each standing around five feet tall. The bottom of the tower holds a water reserve tank with nutrients. A small low-voltage electric water pump transports the water to the top of the tower and descends by gravity, irrigating the plants and returning to the bottom tank. The plants grow out of small holes in the tower. One can plant lettuce, herbs, leek, broccoli, cauliflower, Swiss chard, cucumbers, strawberries, tomatoes, and medicinal herbs—just about anything you want.

A company called Future Growing produced my hydroponic towers. The owner and president of Future Growing is Tim Blank, who worked for Disney's Epcot theme park in Orlando until 2005. At Epcot, which is an acronym for Experimental Prototype Community of Tomorrow, Blank used his training in hydroponic agriculture to manage Epcot's agricultural showcase of food crops from around the world. "I was responsible for Epcot's futuristic, cutting-edge agricultural display, open 365 days a year, utilizing hydroponics and sustainable growing practices from around the world," Blank explained. "I believe one of the greatest futurists who ever lived was a man named Walt Disney."

Walt Disney's pioneering vision of a better tomorrow is one of the reasons why Tim Blank founded Future Growing with the dream that someday every human on the planet would have access to healthy, pesticide-free food right in their own home and local community. (Check out their Web site at www.futuregrowing.com.) The company installs residential glasshouses and glass rooms that attach to homes like sunrooms so that people can grow their own organic fruits and vegetables year round. Those seeking a smaller investment can purchase hydroponic towers, which cost around $500 apiece, as a way to get into organic and hydroponic gardening.

"With our Future Growing Tower Gardens, people tend to grow a lot of lettuce, herbs, tomatoes, peppers, and cucumbers, but it's the gourmet lettuce that seems to be making the biggest impact," Blank said. "People are used to spending good money in the store for healthy, clean lettuce, but with our tower systems, they can grow lettuce in half the time at very little cost with no pesticide on the leaves."

Nicki, Joshua, and I can barely keep up with the escarole, endive, and lamb's lettuce sprouting from our tower. Tower 2 is our cucumber tower, which fascinates my son Joshua. As I'm writing these words, he's constantly interrupting me with this preschooler plea: "Daddy, can we go see the cucumbers?" They're huge—in fact, I just ate part of an 18-inch long cucumber in my dinner salad this evening.

"With our growing systems, you have real quality control of the food going into your body," Blank said. "Our company, Future Growing, is introducing this technology to the green and eco-friendly community. What I tell people is that lettuce is one of the easiest crops in the world to grow. Commercial lettuce production, however, is one of those terrible examples of leaving a huge carbon footprint on the world when you consider the environmental costs to grow, harvest, and deliver that one head of lettuce from the fields to a grocery store near you. Think about it: Farmers of conventional lettuce use lots of water and petroleum-based chemicals to maintain it and grow it. After harvesting, the lettuce is packaged and then refrigerated to keep chilled. All that takes gobs of energy, plus the fuel costs to ship the lettuce across the country. Supermarket lettuce sits on a chilled store shelf for several more days, where it has a very short shelf life."

Blank says the new growing technologies make sustainability fun because the food is exploding with flavor and nutrition. "Children want to eat healthy when the food tastes great, and they can actually help and watch it grow," he said. "My wife, Jessica, and I often enjoy having our friends and family over for dinner, and they literally cannot believe the robust flavors in the lettuces, herbs, and vegetables they are eating. No matter how many times someone has enjoyed a meal in our home, we are always asked why the food in the store doesn't taste nearly as good as our home-grown dinner.

"Although Jessica and I are fairly handy in the kitchen, the real secret is Future Growing's proprietary blend of pH-balanced water-soluble nutrients and minerals that provide the plants with great nutrition and abundant growth. We produce such an abundance of almost labor-free food that our friends usually leave our home with a bag of produce."

The technology behind Future Growing recycles 100 percent of the nutrients and water and uses only 5 to 10 percent of the water that conventional or organic farmers use in the field. "Obviously, we have to use a tiny bit of electricity to run a recirculation pump," Blank said, "but you don't have to store your lettuce in the fridge to keep it cool or chilled. Just pick it when you're ready to make a salad. I see this as being a key component to the future sustainability of our planet."

I do too. Just as I have a burden to help people take weight off their bodies, I have a burden to do my part to take weight off the planet. Everyone has become aware of the environmental challenges lying ahead of us because of global warming. While there's scientific disagreement behind the root causes of global warming—and this book is not taking sides on this contentious issue—the fact remains that climate changes are happening right before our eyes. I haven't forgotten how hot the summer of 2005 was—the hottest year on record—or the buffeting our home took when Hurricane Wilma roared through South Florida. We are all responsible for climate change when we turn on the air conditioning in our homes; drive our cars to work, school, and on errands; take an airline flight; and consume goods and services.

In a few moments, I'll share some ideas that we can all implement at home that will collectively make a big difference, but for now, let me tell you about some of the things we're doing at the Garden of Life headquarters in West Palm Beach to be more "green." Our office building is a fairly typical two-story concrete affair situated in a business park. A couple of years ago, our team developed a program to start producing our products in the "greenest" way possible as well as taking steps to consume less energy to run our business.

We've taken some important steps to get there. We purchase renewable energy certificates equal to 100 percent of the company's energy expenditures from our offices and distribution center, and the light switches in our employee restrooms and several of our common areas automatically go off when the motion sensor doesn't detect anyone inside. Our warehouse ships hundreds of boxes each day, but whenever practical and possible, we use recycled or biodegradable packaging in our shipping boxes, marketing materials, product containers, and wrapping. Our catalogs and product boxes are printed with soy-based inks void of toxins. Of course, we like to think that the natural and organic products we produce are part of lightening the weight of the planet.

What pleases me most is how some of our employees are buying in. Some have traded in their gasoline-powered cars for hybrids. Some started carpooling. The lunchroom recycling is going great guns. Many of our suppliers had the same reaction and have made the move to using organic or recycled products.

We feel, corporately speaking, that Garden of Life has a chance to expand its mission from "Empowering Extraordinary Health" to being part of the solution to improve our air, water, food sources, homes, and workplaces. We have even donated, on behalf of our top 250 retailers, wind power certificates to offset their electricity usage in their stores.

The Farm of the Future

A couple of years ago, I spoke at a conference in Grantham, Pennsylvania, where I had the opportunity to visit what I call the farm of the future. Their grass-fed raw-milk ice cream was otherworldly. That afternoon I tried scoops of vanilla, maple, strawberry, and peanut butter and couldn't decide which I liked best.

I'm talking about Hendricks Farm and Dairy in Telford, Pennsylvania (their Web site is www.hendricksfarmsanddairy.com). The owner, Trent Hendricks, has a passion to raise food sustainably and locally. In fact, his award-winning raw-milk cheese, eggs from pastured chickens, and meats like lamb sausage aren't available outside of Pennsylvania, which is why health-minded people drive hundreds of miles to buy their superior grass-fed meats and dairy products.

Hendricks Farms and Dairy is licensed to provide Grade A, certified humane, grass-fed raw, unpasteurized dairy from cow's, goat's, and sheep's milk—over twenty varieties of cheese, cottage cheese, yogurt, cream, ice cream, and, of course, raw milk. On the meat side, they provide organic beef, chicken, eggs, and lamb and beef sausage. If I lived within two hundred miles of Hendricks Farms, I would be there every other week to pick all the necessary protein foods for my family.

I've come to respect Trent as a leader in the sustainable food movement. We had this question-and-answer exchange, and I thought you would be interested in what he had to say.

Jordan: I know that you urge consumers to seek out local, sustainable alternatives to mainstream food. Why is it important to consume local and sustainable meat and dairy products?

Trent Hendricks: This question can be answered on several levels. First, there is an argument that believes food produced in the same environment as the consumer lives in will lead to the greater health of that consumer, based on the foods' ability to survive that environment. Second, there is the aspect of community building, supporting businesses on a local level, and returning dollars to the region in order to build strength and longevity in our communities, maintaining open spaces, and environmental balance. Third, and perhaps most importantly, local agriculture has the potential to reduce our carbon footprints, thereby protecting and healing the environment. As greater demands are placed on our resources, it behooves us to consider the ramifications not only for ourselves but for future generations as well. Earth can most certainly support our growing population and feed us organically, but it will require stewardship and vision.

Jordan: Why do you think customers drive hundreds of miles, across state lines, to buy your meat and dairy products?

Trent Hendricks: We practice what we preach! We are actively researching a complete package for our energy needs, but in the meantime, we have implemented many conservation, sustainable practices, such as heating our water for the dairy and our buildings with wood that would have otherwise ended up in a landfill. Our buildings are located to take advantage of a natural breeze, eliminating the need for fans for the cattle. We compost our animal manure with leaves and ground wood chips from the community and provide an excellent soil enhancer for gardens, lawns, and fields. We recycle our wastewater and use it to irrigate our pastures. We employ animal traction to supply much of our power needs, such as spreading manure, hauling, and trimming pastures.

Also, we absolutely will not sacrifice quality for quantity. The most valuable way to get folks to "eat better" is to make healthy food "taste better," and our farm produces grass-fed, all-natural, humane, and award-winning food. Make it easy for people to eat well, and they will support a viable, sustainable local business.

Jordan: Is it getting easier to find local and sustainable meat and dairy products, or are operations like yours getting scarcer? Is there good news to report?

Trent Hendricks: There is good news, but too many folks entering the industry are looking to make a buck, or simply "live the dream," and are far less focused on the above-mentioned aspects that we feel are very important. This industry is screaming for strong leadership, which is something we hope to assist in providing.

Jordan: Do you consider Hendricks Farm and Dairy a "farm of the future"? If so, why?

Trent Hendricks: Absolutely! We have embraced the best of the old along with the best of the new. We use mules to spread manure to reduce our usage of fossil fuels, yet we have one of the nation's first fully robotic cow milkers, allowing true free-range options to our cows. We are certified humane, certified freedom milk, and we have a fully integrated product line, taking healthy, local, sustainable grass-fed products into universities, hospitals, schools, and outlying communities, educating and feeding folks along the way. Our commitment to social stewardship is unrivaled, and we most definitely have put our money where our mouths are.

A Dozen Ideas for a Greener Home

Simple changes around the house can also make a big difference for the environment. With inspiration from my friend Stephen Hennessey's *In Pink* magazine,[3] here are some suggested changes that we all could afford to do:

1. Change your incandescent light bulbs to compact fluorescent.

Here's an idea that's really caught on, but it's a no-brainer since fluorescent light bulbs burn twelve times as long as regular light bulbs and consume 50 to 80 percent less energy. When we built a new home a year ago, we asked the contractor to install full-spectrum fluorescent light bulbs, which is even better for the environment than compact fluorescent. Full-spectrum lights effectively emit the same kind of light that streams from the sun, as well as ultraviolet rays, which makes this type of lighting extremely healthy since UV light causes the body to produce vitamin D. Full-spectrum lights are more yellowish, which makes reading bedtime books to our children easier with less eyestrain.

2. Bring your own shopping bags or reusable canvas bags to the health food or grocery store.

Whenever I travel to Europe, I notice that the supermarkets don't provide plastic bags for their customers. Instead, paper bags can be purchased for around 25 cents each, so the locals bring leather satchels or recycle paper bags from previous trips. What a simple yet effective "green" habit to get behind.

I think supermarket chains on this side of the Atlantic should adopt the same "bring your own bag" policy. One warehouse club already has: Costco stopped providing plastic bags for their customers, and I predict other retailers will follow in their footsteps. Plastic bags, made from toxic polyethylene, are not biodegradable and litter the landscape whenever the wind kicks up.

3. Use rechargeable batteries.

Did you know that you're not supposed to throw your old batteries in the trash? In most parts of the country, used batteries are considered "e-waste," just like computers and old TV sets. Batteries contain a high concentration of metals that seep into the ground when the casing erodes. The technology behind rechargeable batteries is improving all the time.

4. Recycle your newspapers, junk mail, and plastic bottles.

You want to know what I dislike about my neighborhood? We don't have separate bins to recycle our newspapers and paper trash. Recycling just the fat Sunday papers alone would save more than a half million trees every week. I can always tell when I have California visitors to my home: they ask where the recycling bin is when they have some paper or plastic trash to throw away.

5. Watch the thermostat.

That's something Nicki and I are constantly doing. Our home is definitely not an icebox during the torrid Florida summers. We keep the thermostat between 76–78 degrees inside the house, which does feel a tad warm, but we're used to it. It's still cooler than the inferno outside. When we leave the home, even for a few hours, we turn the AC off.

6. Clean out the bathroom cabinet.

I already touched on this in chapter 10, but many personal care products contain parabens, synthetic chemicals used as a preservative. Try out natural products and see if they work for you.

7. Unplug cell phone chargers when not in use.

Most people—including myself—were not aware that electrical devices continue to draw electricity when plugged in. I'm talking about plasma screens, DVD players, and even cell phone chargers. It's not practical to unplug every electronic device in the home—who wants to watch a blinking "12:00" on the DVD player—but we can all be mindful of unplugging our chargers for the iPod, cell phone, BlackBerry, and the like.

8. Think green in the laundry room.

Conventional fabric softeners and static cling products use formaldehyde to make clothes softer. You can substitute a half-cup of vinegar to your wash or dip your favorite essential oil on a cloth and dry with your clothes. Seventh Generation produces some great "green" laundry detergents.

9. Check your cookware.

Pots and pans with nonstick coating are popular with the cook and the person doing the clean up. (Nicki says that person is one and the same in our household.) Yet nonstick pans are coated with perfluorooctanoic acid, or PFOA, which has shown up in trace amounts in blood samples taken from people across the country. The Centers for Disease Control estimates that PFOA is in the blood of 95 percent of Americans, and the Environmental Protection Agency advisory panel has labeled PFOA as a likely carcinogen in humans.[4] Environmentally acceptable cookware is stainless steel, ceramic coated, or stoneware.

10. Choose paper products from recycled ingredients.

It's getting easier and easier to find toilet paper, paper towels, and paper napkins made from recycled paper that are either unbleached or nonchlorine bleached to keep dangerous toxins out of the environment and off your skin and your food.

11. Use air filters.

This is another idea to reduce toxins in your home. Since indoor air is three times more polluted than outdoor air, it behooves you to choose an excellent air filter that removes and neutralizes tiny airborne particles of dust, soot, pollen, mold, and dander. I have set up four high-quality air purifiers in our home that scrub harmful impurities out of the air. We also open up our doors and windows to freshen the air.

12. Start your own compost pile.

All you need is some unwanted space in the backyard, and you can set up a handy compost pile. It sure worked for my grandpa!

Become a Green Patriot by David Steinman

As the author of *Safe Trip to Eden: Ten Steps to Save the Planet From the Global Warming Meltdown*, I make the case that one of the benefits of environmentalism is taking steps to reduce our dependence upon foreign oil, which can strengthen America's national security. That's why I'm trying to field an army of Green Patriots (check out www.greenpatriot.us) who can help spread the message that our individual shopping choices truly have a profound impact on change.

When consumers choose healthy, organic foods and emphasize a more plant-based diet with organic fresh produce and foods that are minimally processed, not only are they improving their personal health, but they are also taking weight off the planet.

That's because organic foods are grown without the use of petrochemical pesticides and fertilizers, which are linked to a myriad of health defects, including cancer, reproductive toxicity, and neurological damage. So one of the best decisions you can make for your personal health just happens to be one of the best decisions you can make for improving our planetary health.

Also, when consumers consume meat from animals that were grass-fed and fish caught sustainably, once again, they are doing something that's important for both their health and for the planet. When you choose grass-fed beef, for example, you're putting a value on grass management, which is synonymous with wildlife habitat. Grass-fed animals spend most of their time in open pastures, where ecology is critical. Mel Coleman, founder of Coleman Purely Natural Products, once told me that all ranchers are really grass managers and that America's private grasslands, when taken in total, are among the key habitat areas for many of America's most vulnerable animal species.

So instead of choosing antibiotic-riddled animals, or those that have been given growth-stimulating hormones, choose meat from grass-fed animals. You are voting not only for better health for yourself but also for a healthier planet.

The Maker's Diet for Weight Loss Recap: Take Weight Off Your World

1. Think green. Our objective should to be to minimize our disruptive lifestyles that threaten the sustainability of nature's cycles.
2. Do your best to eat locally, organically, and sustainably.
3. Take steps to adopt a green lifestyle in your home. Switch to fluorescent lighting, unplug appliances not in use, and recycle paper and plastic waste.
4. Carbon offsets—also called renewable energy certificates and "green tags"—represent the reduction of CO_2 in one location to offset the CO_2 produced in another, like your home or car. Carbonfund.org reduces CO_2 for just $5.50 per ton, if you are interested in offsetting your climate footprint by supporting wind, efficiency, and other climate-friendly projects.

thirteen

The Results Are In...

I DECIDED EARLY ON that I couldn't release *The Maker's Diet for Weight Loss* without testing the principles behind the program, so we conducted or partnered in four health initiatives around the country.
The four initiatives were:

1. "Healthy Toledo," based at The Church on Strayer in Maumee, Ohio, a Toledo suburb where 126 church members completed an abbreviated eleven-week program.

2. "Sky Angel," in which two dozen employees of the Sky Angel cable network channel in Cleveland, Tennessee, followed the weight-loss program for sixteen weeks.

3. "Metro Health Initiative," which was a twelve-week program at Metro Christian Academy in Tulsa, Oklahoma, involving thirty-four administrators, teachers, and parents.

4. "Progressive Medical Centers Initiative," which was a study with one hundred patients at the Progressive Medical Centers of America located in Atlanta.

Our biggest test was Healthy Toledo, and let me tell you how that happened. Based upon the success of *The Maker's Diet* book, I received dozens of invitations to speak at churches around the country. When Pastor Tony Scott of The Church on Strayer in Maumee, Ohio, invited me to speak to his congregation about good health a couple of years ago, I discovered a like-minded pastor who's been practicing what he preaches about staying away from junk foods and eating right for twenty years. Pastor Tony, who's in his early sixties, has a flat belly and looks like he could run the New York Marathon tomorrow.

I had heard that many living in the Toledo area, which is known as the "crossroads of America" since the metropolis lies at the busy intersection of Interstate 90 and Interstate 75, were overweight, out of shape, and in poor health. This heavily blue-collar city, where Jeep vehicles have rolled off the assembly line since 1941, was ranked by *Men's Health* magazine as the ninety-eighth out of the one hundred worst cities for men after crunching numbers in twenty-four categories, including life-and-death data on cancer, heart disease, and strokes.[1] *Men's Health* also ran a "sweat check," looking at how often, how long, and how intensely men exercise, but from what people were telling me, pubs and sports bars far outnumbered fitness centers. The joke around town was that the only heavy lifting Toledo guys did following work was raising a cold longneck after a long day on the factory floor.

With its basement ranking, Pastor Tony was quite interested in opening up his church to a "Healthy Toledo" initiative. A couple of months later, we launched the program by conducting sign-ups and objective health screenings so that we could scientifically quantify the improvement in their health before and after Healthy Toledo.

While I designed the Maker's Diet for Weight Loss program to span sixteen weeks, Pastor Tony and I agreed that we would use its principles but shorten the duration of Healthy Toledo to eleven weeks in order to share the results with the Toledo community at Freedom Fest, a part Fourth of July celebration and part health fair to be held at The Church on Strayer on the Saturday night before the Fourth of July.

Overall, I was very pleased with Healthy Toledo's weight-loss results and improvement in health markers. The average age of participants was 44.4 years. We had people ranging in age from 18 to 80. Eighty of the 126 participants had BMIs putting them in the "obese" or "overweight" category, so we categorized this group as well. Here are some interesting statistics:

Weight loss

- The top 3 each lost an average of 43.7 pounds.
- The top 25 lost an average of 28.7 pounds.
- The top 50 lost an average of 23 pounds.
- The 126 participants lost an average of 13.5 pounds.

Body fat

The average body fat loss for the 126 individuals was 4.3 percentage points, or a 14.9 percent improvement. As an example, this means that an individual with 34.3 percent body fat at the initial weigh-in dropped to 30 percent body fat eleven weeks later. We also found that men were more likely than women to see a greater reduction in body fat. Guys won the category hands down because women, on average, have 11 percent more body fat and 8 percent less muscle mass than men.

Inches off the waist

- The 126 individuals in Healthy Toledo lost an average of 3.15 inches.
- The 80 overweight individuals lost an average of 3.6 inches.

Blood pressure

Two numbers are used to describe blood pressure: systolic pressure and diastolic pressure. The systolic pressure, which is always higher and listed first, measures the force that blood exerts on the arterial walls as the heart pumps blood through the body's cardiovascular system. The diastolic pressure, which is always lower and called out second, is the measurement of force as the heart relaxes to allow blood to flow back into the heart. Of the 126 Healthy Toledo participants, 77 percent showed a reduction in systolic, diastolic, or both readings. The average reduction was 9.6 mmHg in systolic and 11.2 mmHg in diastolic readings

A systolic blood pressure reading higher than 120 is viewed as an indicator of heart troubles down the road. A diastolic blood pressure reading higher than 80 is a predictor of heart attacks and strokes in young adults or people of any age suffering from hypertension. Optimal blood pressure is anything below 120/80, and normal blood pressure is between 120/80 and 130/85. Anything above those numbers is considered high blood pressure.

Blood pressure often decreases when weight decreases, and the greater the weight loss, the greater the reduction in blood pressure. In essence, due to weight loss and better food choices, Healthy Toledo participants lost around 10 points in their systolic and diastolic pressure readings, and 25 percent saw their blood pressure fall below 140/90, which signifies hypertension or high blood pressure.

Women power

Since 70 of the 126 participants were women, or 55 percent, we separated their results by gender. These women lost, on average:

- 10.8 pounds in approximately eleven weeks (1 pound per week)
- 3.2 inches off their waist
- 2.2 inches off their hips

Women also lost, on average, 4.1 percent of body fat.

My view

A few observations are in order. First, more than one-third of the test group lost 23 pounds, which is 2 pounds a week. Twenty-three pounds is significant: for men, that usually means two waist sizes (like from a size 38 to 36); for women, 23 pounds usually results in a loss of two or three dress sizes.

Some other comments:

- The average drop in body weight percentile was 9.3 percent, which was a good number after only eleven weeks.

- Twenty-six percent of the participants lost at least 10 percent of their body weight, meaning one-fourth of the Healthy Toledo participants made significant strides toward reaching their ideal weight.

- The average number of inches lost off waists was 3.15 inches, but 28 percent lost at least 5 inches off their waist. When going through the data, we determined that women were more likely than men to see a reduction in their waist measurements.

We also analyzed the answers on the health questionnaire. Not everyone completed the questionnaire, but just over 100 people gave us these observations:

- Sixty-five percent reported an increase in energy.
- Fifty percent reported they were happier.
- Seventy-five percent reported that they were healthier.
- Forty-two percent reported a decrease in occasional heartburn.
- Forty-three percent reported a decrease in symptoms of abdominal distension, such as gas or bloating.
- Forty-three percent reported that it was easier for them to fall asleep.
- Sixty-nine percent reported feeling more refreshed upon waking.

I am extremely pleased with these results, although I will not rest until 100 percent report that they are healthier, happier, and have more energy.

SKY ANGEL SOARS

Healthy Toledo was the first but not the last place we tested the concept for the Maker's Diet for Weight Loss program. At the Sky Angel corporate offices in Cleveland, Tennessee, around two dozen employees committed to following the program for sixteen weeks. This was a corporate endeavor where a group of employees could count on the support of their leadership team, championed by Ken Douglas. Sky Angel paid half the cost for the nutritional supplements and health snacks, while the employees paid the other half.

The Sky Angel employees were "cute" in the way they worked together. One day, one would bring healthy snacks into work, or another would organize a potluck featuring foods found in Phase I. Another would fire up the blender in the break room and make healthy smoothies.

When all was said and done, twenty-three participants attended the final health assessments and completed at least some aspect of the required essay and survey tasks. Of those, eighteen participants (nine men and nine women) were in the overweight or obese category based on body fat, age, and sex and therefore had weight-loss goals or realized weight loss in moving toward their ideal weight.

Here is a summary of their impressive results:

- Average waist circumference reduction (inches, at navel): 3.2 inches
- Average weight loss: 15.4 pounds
- One participant lost over 26.2 pound, five participants lost 20–25 pound, three participants lost 15–20 pound, and six participants lost 10–15 pounds.
- Average body fat percentage reduction: 2 percentage points
- Average body mass index reduction: 2.2 m/kg^2
- Average total cholesterol reduction: 13.2 mg/dL
- Average triglycerides reduction: 48.6 mg/dL

Here is some general feedback: two participants mentioned sleeping better; one participant mentioned loss of knee pain; one participant said his spouse lost 40 pounds by joining in and supporting him; one participant held off taking a new job to finish the program at Sky Angel. Many participants said they are now working out or exercising regularly, while others said they've permanently shifted their eating habits.

The Sky Angel participants also took a Patient Reported Outcome/Quality of Life Survey designed by QualityMetric. QualityMetric is the leading provider of health outcomes measurement surveys and real-time delivery systems that use proprietary methodologies and data assets to produce actionable health information. The survey, called the SF-36v2, is a thirty-six question, comprehensive short-form questionnaire that generates a health profile consisting of eights scales and two summary measures describing health-related quality of life.

This survey asks several questions about physical health, including how well the participant can perform basic physical activities. It asks questions about mental or emotional health and focuses on feelings of well-being. The health survey also asks questions about function, what your patient can do. Do they have health problems that limit them at work, school, or other daily activities?

Ten participants completed both an initial and final SF-36v2 survey. These participants, based on the survey, experienced more than a 25 percent increase in general health and more than a 25 percent increase in vitality.

Furthermore, the survey indicated that the average reduction in monthly medical costs could be projected to be over $67 per month per participant! Considering that the initial average estimated monthly expenses was $202, that is over a 33 percent decrease in monthly medical expenditures! I know we talk a lot about weight and health, but eating right and getting in shape affects the pocketbook too.

METRO HEALTH INITIATIVE

After I spoke at Metro Christian School in Tulsa, Oklahoma, a committee of administration staff and parents were interested in starting the Metro Health Initiative, which greatly excited me because I wanted to develop a relationship within the academic community. The connection between nutrition and academic performance is one that's been long overlooked, even though teachers will tell you that it takes ten minutes to settle down kids after recess or lunch. That's because they're hopped up from eating a bag of M&Ms or drinking soft drinks like Mountain Dew and Surge, which deliver a sweetened caffeine punch—92 milligrams per 20-ounce drink, or the equivalent of a 5-ounce cup of brewed coffee. Sugar and caffeine cause nervousness, irritability, restlessness, and fidgetiness, which impacts classroom discipline and performance.

Headmaster Tom Cameron and the Metro Health Initiative team, which included Health and Safety Director Dody Patrock and parents Alene Davis and Patricia Jones, set out to change that. While they've taken important steps to improve nutrition in the school, the adults also knew they had to lead the way for their students and children. "They took the initiative, no pun intended, on this one," said Stephen Nepa, who worked closely with the administration and parents. "They have the passion and desire to live healthy, balanced lives in their community."

The program ran for twelve weeks and ended in late May 2008. Thirty-four participants completed the program. Of those, twenty-two participants had stated weight loss goals or were in the overweight/obese category based on body fat, age, and sex, and therefore had weight-loss goals or realized weight loss in moving toward their ideal weight.

For the twenty-two participants who realized weight loss, there were eight men and fourteen women. Here is a summary of their results:

- Average waist circumference reduction: 2.6 inches (at navel)
- Average weight loss: 11.2 pounds
- One participant lost 34.5 pound, six participants lost 15–20 pound, and five participants lost 10–14 pounds.
- Average body fat percentage reduction: 1.6 percentage points
- Average body mass index reduction: 1.6 m/kg^2
- Average blood pressure, systolic/diastolic reduction: 5.4 mmHg / 4.1 mmHg
- Triglycerides reduction: 22.7 mg/dL

One unique aspect about of the Metro Health Initiative was the incredible support we received from the owner, Geof Eng, and trainers at The Grand Health and Racquet Club in Tulsa, Oklahoma. Not only did Geof offer his facility for all of the health assessments, but also the club trainers performed assessments utilizing a unique testing tool that determines a participants' "fitness age." It was a huge blessing to have all of our participants so well hosted during the health assessments.

The Grand Health and Racquet Club and I are happy to report that Metro Health Initiative participants reduced their fitness age on average by 5.6 years! While that might not seem significant, consider that the average age of this group was close to fifty years old. I'm sure that spouses, children, and grandchildren were happy to hear their loved ones were getting younger!

The Metro participants also took the SF-36v2 Patient Reported Outcome/Quality of Life Survey. Twenty-eight participants completed an initial and final SF-36v2 online.

The survey estimated that the Metro group will see a 27 percent decrease in estimated monthly medical expenditures. The survey analysis also showed that the participants experienced over a 15 percent increase in general health, over a 26 percent increase in vitality, and over a 17 percent increase in mental health.

While the Metro Health Initiative was in development, Dody Patrick tried to make some headway in conducting a "whole paradigm shift"—as she called it—in what Metro Christian students ate and how much they exercised. Three years ago, the private school started a "Respect Your Body" week to start the education process with the students, who, during puberty and rapid growth spurts, are getting interested in their bodies, wanting to get bigger and stronger...or thinner. The school tried to have the students focus on the five meals they eat at school each week and get the parents and children to focus on the sixteen meals a week they eat at home.

Toward that end, the school took some active steps. The cafeteria asked the catering company that provided the midday lunch meal for the students and the staff to use whole-wheat bread, whole-wheat tortillas, and whole-wheat pasta. Spinach and other deep-greens were added to salads that were made predominantly with "head lettuce," which is not so green and thus less nutritious. Fries were served once a week; baked potato wedges were served on the other days. There were no more soda pop or boxed "fruit juice" drinks. Instead, the students and staff enjoyed baked tilapia, whole-wheat lasagna, healthy soups, and delicious wraps. "If the kids want junk food, they had to bring it to school," said Dody.

Metro Christian's vending machines got a makeover as well. Banished were Coke and Pepsi; in were bottled water and bottles of 100 percent fruit juice. During my visit, I saw that some of the vending machines were selling healthy items like Garden of Life food bars, Clif bars, 100 percent fruit leathers, and healthy granola bars without hydrogenated oils. I hope they sell like the proverbial hotcakes in the future.

PROGRESSIVE MEDICAL CENTERS INITIATIVE

The last partnership has been very unique as well. After reconnecting with an old friend, Gez Agolli, ND, PhD, on an airplane, we began sharing what was going on in our lives. Dr. Gez had grown his practice, Progressive Medical Centers of America, into the largest integrative medical clinic in the Southeast. I shared with him everything we were doing to spread the message of health and wellness through programs and books like *The Maker's Diet for Weight Loss*. By the time the flight landed, we were discussing the idea of his clinic facilitating an intervention-based nutrition study. I felt it would be groundbreaking to have the chance for the nutrition and lifestyle principles of *The Maker's Diet for Weight Loss* to be put to the test, and Dr. Agolli felt the same way. Not only did he assign key personnel to oversee the project, but Progressive Medical also agreed to underwrite the cost of comprehensive blood work for every participating patient.

Unfortunately, the Progressive Medical Centers Initiative with one hundred patients was not finished in time for this edition of the book. I am very excited to see the results from this study since Dr. Gez and his team will be performing quantitative blood and body composition analysis on those making major lifestyle changes.

FINAL THOUGHT

I'd now like to give the pulpit, so to speak, to Pastor Tony Scott, who didn't officially participate in the eleven-week Maker's Diet program because he's been practicing what he preaches about good health for twenty years. But without him and his incredible energy and dedication to ministering to others, Healthy Toledo never would have happened. Thank you, Pastor Tony, for your leadership.

> Our message has always been living a balanced, disciplined life between spirit, soul, and body. And I started with myself twenty years ago and turned away from junk foods and started eating right, listening to the right people, reading the right books, listening to the right tapes, reading the Bible, and saying, "What should I be eating?"
>
> As a show of support, I followed Healthy Toledo on my own. Well, I lost 10 pounds and 2½ inches off my waist, which I got very excited about it, but here's the important thing that happened to me: Most of my life, I've been a very light sleeper. I go to bed, sleep for two or three hours, wake up, and repeat this pattern. When I was into about the tenth or twelfth day of this program, I woke up one morning, looked at the clock, and realized I'd been asleep for seven and a half hours! That may have been a first in my adult life, sleeping right through for seven and a half hours with no waking up. That pattern has continued. I go to bed now, sleep six, seven, or seven and a half hours, and then wake up feeling refreshed and energetic.
>
> I would say that Jordan Rubin's message is an inspiration to become everything that God created us to be. God wants you to be everything that you can be spiritually, He wants you to be everything that you can be in your soul, and He wants you to be everything that you can be in your body.
>
> There are so many pastors who aren't healthy, who are overweight, who are on high blood pressure medication, and there's no reason for that. God has put the foods in the earth that heal. I've been praying and believing God will spread this message of good health beyond Toledo, so I'm excited to see what happens with Jordan's Maker's Diet for Weight Loss campaign.
>
> —PASTOR TONY SCOTT

fourteen

The Maker's Diet Daily Weight-Loss Plan

Back in chapter 7, I outlined the Weight Loss Eating Plan that was broken down into a sixteen-week, four-phase program. I also asked you to answer the nutritional type questionnaire in chapter 3 on page 66. If you haven't filled out the questionnaire, you should go back and complete it at this time.

You'll see I've incorporated the FIT exercise regimen from chapter 9 and the Healing Codes exercises from chapter 11 into the following plans. If you believe the physical demands of the FIT exercise regimen are too great, pick and choose the exercises you feel comfortable performing.

The following plans are divided by gender and whether you're a meat or a potato type. Here's how they're arranged:

Female Meat Type, Phase I
Female Meat Type, Phase II
Female Meat Type, Phase III

Female Potato Type, Phase I
Female Potato Type, Phase II
Female Potato Type, Phase III

Male Meat Type, Phase I
Male Meat Type, Phase II
Male Meat Type, Phase III

Male Potato Type, Phase I
Male Potato Type, Phase II
Male Potato Type, Phase III

A WORD ABOUT PHASE IV

Regardless of whether you are a female, male, meat type, or potato type, when you reach Phase IV, you have some options. If you are satisfied with your progress, you should continue on the Phase III plan and finish strong. If you feel that your weight loss has slowed or you liked the way you felt on Phase I or II, you are welcome to repeat one of those phases for the final four weeks.

Ready to get started? Then turn to Phase I for your gender and type, and let's get going!

Female Meat Type		
Phase I (Weeks 1–4)		
Upon waking Drink 16–24 ounces of water.		
Spend some time this morning picturing yourself at your ideal weight. See yourself doing the things you think you can't do now or don't do because you're not at your ideal weight. Picture yourself looking great, free from all of the diseases that people said you're at a high risk for. Next, picture yourself at your ideal weight, inspiring your family and friends, who remark how great you look. Now stand in front of the mirror and repeat: *Today I am going to take another positive step toward achieving my ideal weight.*		
Perform the Healing Codes exercise. (You can learn about the Healing Codes exercise on pages 184–185. I recommend that you perform the Healing Codes exercise twice a day—once in the morning and once in the evening—but feel free to try this two-minute exercise three, four, or five times a day.)		
Perform FIT exercises for twenty minutes, choosing from physical activities like sprinting, bodyweight exercises, strength training with bands, medicine balls, dumbbells or kettlebells, stationary bike, or the stair stepper.		
BREAKFAST (7:30 a.m.) **Breakfast Option 1:** Make a smoothie in a blender with the following ingredients: 1 cup plain whole-milk yogurt or kefir; 1 tsp. organic flaxseed oil; 1 tsp. organic extra-virgin coconut oil; 1 Tbsp. organic raw honey; 1 cup organic fruit, fresh or frozen (berries, peaches, pineapple, etc.); 1 scoop goat's milk protein powder (see Appendix C for recommendations); dash of vanilla extract (optional).	**Breakfast Option 2:** Two eggs any style, cooked in extra-virgin coconut oil (see Appendix C for recommended products) Stir-fried onions, mushrooms, and peppers One grapefruit	**Breakfast Option 3:** 6 ounces of organic whole-milk yogurt or cottage cheese with fruit (pineapple, peaches, or berries), honey, and a dash of vanilla extract Handful of raw almonds
Drink 8–12 ounces of water.		
Take two or three whole-food multivitamin caplets and one to four capsules of concentrated fucoxanthin. (See Appendix C for recommended products.)		
10:00 a.m. **Morning Snack Option 1:** One whole-food nutrition bar (see Appendix C for recommended products)	**Morning Snack Option 2:** One serving of whole-food meal supplement with native whey protein and glucomannan fiber mixed with 12 ounces of water	
Drink 8–12 ounces of water.		

	Female Meat Type
	Phase I (Weeks 1–4)

LUNCH (12:30 p.m.)	Toss a large green salad with mixed greens, avocado, carrots, cucumbers, celery, tomatoes, red cabbage, red peppers, red onions, sprouts, 2 ounces of canned beans (black, garbanzo, or pinto), and two hard-boiled omega-3 eggs. (Option 1: substitute 3 ounces of cold, poached, or canned wild salmon in place of hard-boiled eggs. Option 2: substitute 2 ounces of low-mercury, high-omega-3 canned tuna in place of hard-boiled eggs.)
	For the salad dressing, mix extra-virgin olive oil, apple-cider vinegar or lemon juice, naturally brewed soy sauce, liquid aminos, sea salt, herbs, and spices, or mix 1 tablespoon of extra-virgin olive oil with 1 tablespoon of a healthy store-bought dressing. (See Appendix C for recommended brands.)
	One piece of fruit in season
	Drink 12–16 ounces of water.
	Take two or three whole-food multivitamin caplets and one to three capsules of concentrated fucoxanthin.

3:30 p.m.	**Afternoon Snack Option 1:** One whole-food nutrition bar (see Appendix C for recommended products)	**Afternoon Snack Option 2:** One whole-food meal supplement with native whey protein mixed with 12 ounces of water
	Drink 8–12 ounces of water.	

DINNER (6:15 p.m., but try to finish eating by 7:00 p.m.)	**Dinner Option 1:** Baked, poached, or grilled wild-caught salmon Steamed broccoli	**Dinner Option 2:** Roasted organic chicken Cooked vegetables (carrots, onions, peas, etc.)	**Dinner Option 3:** Red meat steak or ground meat (beef, buffalo, or venison) Steamed broccoli Baked winter squash with butter
	Toss a green salad with mixed greens, avocado, carrots, cucumbers, celery, tomatoes, red cabbage, red peppers, red onions, and sprouts.		
	For the salad dressing, mix extra-virgin olive oil, apple-cider vinegar or lemon juice, naturally brewed soy sauce, liquid aminos, sea salt, herbs, and spices, or mix 1 tablespoon of extra-virgin olive oil with 1 tablespoon of a healthy store-bought dressing. (See Appendix C for recommended brands.)		
	Drink 12–16 ounces of water.		
	Take two or three whole-food multivitamin caplets, one to three capsules of concentrated fucoxanthin, and 1 to 3 teaspoons (or three to nine capsules) of a high omega-3 cod liver oil complex. (See Appendix C for recommended products.)		

Before Bed	Perform the Healing Codes exercise on pages 184–185.
	Drink 8–12 ounces of water (optional).
	Perform five minutes of deep-breathing exercises by taking a slow, five-second breath in through your nose (inhale), holding for one second, followed by a forceful quick exhale through your mouth, completely emptying your lungs with each exhalation and completely filling your lungs with each inhalation. Repeat for two to five minutes.
	Go to bed by 10:30 p.m.

Female Meat Type
Phase II (Weeks 5–8)

Upon waking	Drink 16–24 ounces of water.
	Spend some time this morning picturing yourself at your ideal weight. See yourself doing the things you think you can't do now or don't do because you're not at your ideal weight. Picture yourself looking great, free from all of the diseases that people said you're at a high risk for. Next, picture yourself at your ideal weight, inspiring your family and friends, who remark how great you look. Now stand in front of the mirror and repeat: *Today I am going to take another positive step toward achieving my ideal weight.*
	Perform the Healing Codes exercise. (You can learn about the Healing Codes exercise on pages 184–185. I recommend that you perform the Healing Codes exercise twice a day—once in the morning and once in the evening—but feel free to try this two-minute exercise three, four, or five times a day.)
	Perform FIT exercises for twenty minutes, choosing from physical activities like sprinting, bodyweight exercises, strength training with bands, medicine balls, dumbbells or kettlebells, stationary bike, or the stair stepper.

BREAKFAST (7:30 a.m.)	**Breakfast Option 1:** 4–6 ounces of yogurt or cottage cheese with raw honey, berries, sliced almonds, 1 teaspoon of flax seed oil (optional), and a dash of vanilla extract	**Breakfast Option 2:** Two or three eggs any style, cooked in extra-virgin coconut oil (see Appendix C for recommended products) One orange	**Breakfast Option 3:** 6 ounces of organic whole-milk yogurt or cottage cheese with fruit (pineapple, peaches, or berries), honey, and a dash of vanilla extract Handful of raw almonds
	Drink 8–12 ounces of water.		
	Take two or three whole-food multivitamin caplets and one to four capsules of concentrated fucoxanthin. (See Appendix C for recommended products.)		

10:00 a.m.	**Morning Snack Option 1:** One whole-food nutrition bar (see Appendix C for recommended products)	**Morning Snack Option 2:** One serving of whole-food meal supplement with native whey protein and glucomannan fiber mixed with 12 ounces of water
	Drink 8–12 ounces of water.	

LUNCH (12:30 p.m.)	Toss a large green salad with mixed greens, avocado, carrots, cucumbers, celery, tomatoes, red cabbage, red peppers, red onions, sprouts, 2 ounces of canned beans (black, garbanzo, or pinto), and two hard-boiled omega-3 eggs. (Option 1: substitute 3 ounces of cold, poached, or canned wild salmon in place of hard-boiled eggs. Option 2: substitute 2 ounces of low-mercury, high-omega-3 canned tuna in place of hard-boiled eggs.)
	For the salad dressing, mix extra-virgin olive oil, apple-cider vinegar or lemon juice, naturally brewed soy sauce, liquid aminos, sea salt, herbs, and spices, or mix 1 tablespoon of extra-virgin olive oil with 1 tablespoon of a healthy store-bought dressing. (See Appendix C for recommended brands.)
	One piece of fruit in season
	Drink 12–16 ounces of water.
	Take two or three whole-food multivitamin caplets and one to three capsules of concentrated fucoxanthin.

3:30 p.m.	**Afternoon Snack Option 1:** One whole-food nutrition bar (see Appendix C for recommended products)	**Afternoon Snack Option 2:** One whole-food meal supplement with native whey protein mixed with 12 ounces of water
	Drink 8–12 ounces of water.	

Female Meat Type		
Phase II (Weeks 5–8)		
Dinner Option 1: 4–6 oz. ground meat burger (beef, buffalo, venison) Sautèed mushrooms and onions	**Dinner Option 2:** Grilled chicken breast Grilled peppers, onions, and pineapple	**Dinner Option 3:** Red meat steak or ground meat (beef, buffalo, or venison) Sautèed spinach Baked sweet potato with butter
Toss a green salad with mixed greens, avocado, carrots, cucumbers, celery, tomatoes, red cabbage, red peppers, red onions, and sprouts.		
For the salad dressing, mix extra-virgin olive oil, apple-cider vinegar or lemon juice, naturally brewed soy sauce, liquid aminos, sea salt, herbs, and spices, or mix 1 tablespoon of extra-virgin olive oil with 1 tablespoon of a healthy store-bought dressing. (See Appendix C for recommended brands.)		
Drink 12–16 ounces of water.		
Take two or three whole-food multivitamin caplets, one to three capsules of concentrated fucoxanthin, and 1 to 3 teaspoons (or three to nine capsules) of a high omega-3 cod liver oil complex. (See Appendix C for recommended products.)		
Perform the Healing Codes exercise on pages 184–185.		
Drink 8–12 ounces of water (optional).		
Perform five minutes of deep-breathing exercises by taking a slow, five-second breath in through your nose (inhale), holding for one second, followed by a forceful quick exhale through your mouth, completely emptying your lungs with each exhalation and completely filling your lungs with each inhalation. Repeat for two to five minutes.		
Go to bed by 10:30 p.m.		

DINNER (6:15 p.m., but try to finish eating by 7:00 p.m.) — *Before Bed*

Female Meat Type		
Phase III (Weeks 9–12)		
Drink 16–24 ounces of water.		
Spend some time this morning picturing yourself at your ideal weight. See yourself doing the things you think you can't do now or don't do because you're not at your ideal weight. Picture yourself looking great, free from all of the diseases that people said you're at a high risk for. Next, picture yourself at your ideal weight, inspiring your family and friends, who remark how great you look. Now stand in front of the mirror and repeat:		
Today I am going to take another positive step toward achieving my ideal weight.		
Perform the Healing Codes exercise. (You can learn about the Healing Codes exercise on pages 184–185. I recommend that you perform the Healing Codes exercise twice a day—once in the morning and once in the evening—but feel free to try this two-minute exercise three, four, or five times a day.)		
Perform FIT exercises for twenty minutes, choosing from physical activities like sprinting, bodyweight exercises, strength training with bands, medicine balls, dumbbells or kettlebells, stationary bike, or the stair stepper.		

Upon waking

	Female Meat Type		
	Phase III (Weeks 9–12)		
BREAKFAST (7:30 a.m.)	**Breakfast Option 1:** Make a smoothie in a blender with the following ingredients: 1 cup plain whole-milk yogurt or kefir; 1 tsp. organic flaxseed oil; 1 tsp. organic extra-virgin coconut oil; 1 Tbsp. organic raw honey; 1 cup organic fruit, fresh or frozen (berries, banana, peaches, pineapple, etc.); 2 scoops goat's milk protein powder (see Appendix C for recommendations); dash of vanilla extract (optional).	**Breakfast Option 2:** Egg and cheese omelet, cooked in extra-virgin coconut oil One piece of sprouted or yeast-free toast with butter and 1 ounce of raw cheese	**Breakfast Option 3:** 6 ounces of organic whole-milk cottage cheese with fruit (pineapple, peaches, or berries), honey, and a dash of vanilla extract
	Drink 8–12 ounces of water.		
	Take two or three whole-food multivitamin caplets and one to four capsules of concentrated fucoxanthin. (See Appendix C for recommended products.)		
10:00 a.m.	**Morning Snack Option 1:** One whole-food nutrition bar (see Appendix C for recommended products)		**Morning Snack Option 2:** One serving of whole-food meal supplement with native whey protein and glucomannan fiber mixed with 12 ounces of water
	Drink 8–12 ounces of water.		
LUNCH (12:30 p.m.)	Toss a large green salad with mixed greens, avocado, carrots, cucumbers, celery, tomatoes, red cabbage, red peppers, red onions, sprouts, 2 ounces of canned beans (black, garbanzo, or pinto), and two hard-boiled omega-3 eggs. (Option 1: substitute 3 ounces of cold, poached, or canned wild salmon in place of hard-boiled eggs. Option 2: substitute 2 ounces of low-mercury, high-omega-3 canned tuna in place of hard-boiled eggs.)		
	For the salad dressing, mix extra-virgin olive oil, apple-cider vinegar or lemon juice, naturally brewed soy sauce, liquid aminos, sea salt, herbs, and spices, or mix 1 tablespoon of extra-virgin olive oil with 1 tablespoon of a healthy store-bought dressing. (See Appendix C for recommended brands.)		
	One piece of fruit in season		
	Drink 12–16 ounces of water.		
	Take two or three whole-food multivitamin caplets and one to three capsules of concentrated fucoxanthin.		
3:30 p.m.	**Afternoon Snack Option 1:** One whole-food nutrition bar (see Appendix C for recommended products)		**Afternoon Snack Option 2:** One whole-food meal supplement with native whey protein mixed with 12 ounces of water
	Drink 8–12 ounces of water.		

	Female Meat Type		
	Phase III (Weeks 9–12)		
DINNER (6:15 p.m., but try to finish eating by 7:00 p.m.)	**Dinner Option 1:** Meatloaf Roasted veggies (peas, carrots, and potatoes) Toss a green salad with mixed greens, avocado, carrots, cucumbers, celery, tomatoes, red cabbage, red peppers, red onions, and sprouts.	**Dinner Option 2:** Broiled or sautèed white fish Cooked vegetables (carrots, onions, peas, etc.) Small serving of whole grain (brown rice, quinoa, millet, amaranth, buckwheat)	**Dinner Option 3:** Red meat and bean chili Flax crackers, whole-grain crackers, or baked corn chips Toss a green salad with mixed greens, avocado, carrots, cucumbers, celery, tomatoes, red cabbage, red peppers, red onions, and sprouts.
	For the salad dressing, mix extra-virgin olive oil, apple-cider vinegar or lemon juice, naturally brewed soy sauce, liquid aminos, sea salt, herbs, and spices, or mix 1 tablespoon of extra-virgin olive oil with 1 tablespoon of a healthy store-bought dressing. (See Appendix C for recommended brands.)		
	Drink 12–16 ounces of water.		
	Take two or three whole-food multivitamin caplets, one to three capsules of concentrated fucoxanthin, and 1 to 3 teaspoons (or three to nine capsules) of a high omega-3 cod liver oil complex. (See Appendix C for recommended products.)		
Before Bed	Perform the Healing Codes exercise on pages 184–185.		
	Drink 8–12 ounces of water (optional).		
	Perform five minutes of deep-breathing exercises by taking a slow, five-second breath in through your nose (inhale), holding for one second, followed by a forceful quick exhale through your mouth, completely emptying your lungs with each exhalation and completely filling your lungs with each inhalation. Repeat for two to five minutes.		
	Go to bed by 10:30 p.m.		

	Female Potato Type
	Phase I (Weeks 1–4)
Upon waking	Drink 16–24 ounces of water.
	Spend some time this morning picturing yourself at your ideal weight. See yourself doing the things you think you can't do now or don't do because you're not at your ideal weight. Picture yourself looking great, free from all of the diseases that people said you're at a high risk for. Next, picture yourself at your ideal weight, inspiring your family and friends, who remark how great you look. Now stand in front of the mirror and repeat: *Today I am going to take another positive step toward achieving my ideal weight.*
	Perform the Healing Codes exercise. (You can learn about the Healing Codes exercise on pages 184–185. I recommend that you perform the Healing Codes exercise twice a day—once in the morning and once in the evening—but feel free to try this two-minute exercise three, four, or five times a day.)
	Perform FIT exercises for twenty minutes, choosing from physical activities like sprinting, bodyweight exercises, strength training with bands, medicine balls, dumbbells or kettlebells, stationary bike, or the stair stepper.

	Female Potato Type
	Phase I (Weeks 1–4)

BREAKFAST (7:30 a.m.)	**Breakfast Option 1:** Make a smoothie in a blender with the following ingredients: 1 cup plain whole-milk yogurt or kefir; 1 tsp. organic extra-virgin coconut oil; 2 Tbsp. organic raw honey; 1 cup organic fruit, fresh or frozen (berries, peaches, pineapple, etc.); 1 scoop goat's milk protein powder (see Appendix C for recommendations); dash of vanilla extract (optional).	**Breakfast Option 2:** Two eggs any style, cooked in extra-virgin coconut oil Stir-fried onions, mushrooms, and peppers One serving of grapes	**Breakfast Option 3:** 4 to 8 ounces of organic whole-milk yogurt with fruit (pineapple, peaches, or berries), honey, and a dash of vanilla extract Handful of raw almonds

Drink 8–12 ounces of water.

Take two or three whole-food multivitamin caplets and one to four capsules of concentrated fucoxanthin. (See Appendix C for recommended products.)

10:00 a.m.	**Morning Snack Option 1:** One whole-food nutrition bar (see Appendix C for recommended products)	**Morning Snack Option 2:** One serving of whole-food meal supplement with native whey protein and glucomannan fiber mixed with 12 ounces of water

Drink 8–12 ounces of water.

LUNCH (12:30 p.m.)

Toss a large green salad with mixed greens, avocado, carrots, cucumbers, celery, tomatoes, red cabbage, red peppers, red onions, sprouts, 2 ounces of canned beans (black, garbanzo, or pinto), and two hard-boiled omega-3 eggs. (Option 1: substitute 3 ounces of cold, poached, or canned wild salmon in place of hard-boiled eggs. Option 2: substitute 2 ounces of low-mercury, high-omega-3 canned tuna in place of hard-boiled eggs.)

For the salad dressing, mix extra-virgin olive oil, apple-cider vinegar or lemon juice, naturally brewed soy sauce, liquid aminos, sea salt, herbs, and spices, or mix 1 tablespoon of extra-virgin olive oil with 1 tablespoon of a healthy store-bought dressing. (See Appendix C for recommended brands.)

One apple with skin (or one piece of fruit in season)

Drink 12–16 ounces of water.

Take two or three whole-food multivitamin caplets and one to three capsules of concentrated fucoxanthin.

3:30 p.m.	**Afternoon Snack Option 1:** One whole-food nutrition bar (see Appendix C for recommended products)	**Afternoon Snack Option 2:** One whole-food meal supplement with native whey protein mixed with 12 ounces of water

Drink 8–12 ounces of water.

Female Potato Type		
Phase I (Weeks 1–4)		
Dinner Option 1: Baked, poached, or grilled wild-caught salmon Peas and carrots	**Dinner Option 2:** Roasted organic chicken Cooked vegetable (carrots, onions, peas, etc.)	**Dinner Option 3:** Red meat steak (beef, buffalo, or venison) Steamed broccoli
Toss a green salad with mixed greens, avocado, carrots, cucumbers, celery, tomatoes, red cabbage, red peppers, red onions, and sprouts.		
For the salad dressing, mix extra-virgin olive oil, apple-cider vinegar or lemon juice, naturally brewed soy sauce, liquid aminos, sea salt, herbs, and spices, or mix 1 tablespoon of extra-virgin olive oil with 1 tablespoon of a healthy store-bought dressing. (See Appendix C for recommended brands.)		
Drink 12–16 ounces of water.		
Take two or three whole-food multivitamin caplets, one to three capsules of concentrated fucoxanthin, and 1 to 3 teaspoons (or three to nine capsules) of a high omega-3 cod liver oil complex. (See Appendix C for recommended products.)		

DINNER (6:15 p.m., but try to finish eating by 7:00 p.m.)

Before Bed

Perform the Healing Codes exercise on pages 184–185.

Drink 8–12 ounces of water (optional).

Perform five minutes of deep-breathing exercises by taking a slow, five-second breath in through your nose (inhale), holding for one second, followed by a forceful quick exhale through your mouth, completely emptying your lungs with each exhalation and completely filling your lungs with each inhalation. Repeat for two to five minutes.

Go to bed by 10:30 p.m.

Female Potato Type
Phase II (Weeks 5–8)
Drink 16–24 ounces of water.
Spend some time this morning picturing yourself at your ideal weight. See yourself doing the things you think you can't do now or don't do because you're not at your ideal weight. Picture yourself looking great, free from all of the diseases that people said you're at a high risk for. Next, picture yourself at your ideal weight, inspiring your family and friends, who remark how great you look. Now stand in front of the mirror and repeat: *Today I am going to take another positive step toward achieving my ideal weight.*
Perform the Healing Codes exercise. (You can learn about the Healing Codes exercise on pages 184–185. I recommend that you perform the Healing Codes exercise twice a day—once in the morning and once in the evening—but feel free to try this two-minute exercise three, four, or five times a day.)
Perform FIT exercises for twenty minutes, choosing from physical activities like sprinting, bodyweight exercises, strength training with bands, medicine balls, dumbbells or kettlebells, stationary bike, or the stair stepper.

Upon waking

Female Potato Type		
Phase II (Weeks 5–8)		
BREAKFAST (7:30 a.m.) **Breakfast Option 1:** Make a smoothie in a blender with the following ingredients: 1 cup plain whole-milk yogurt or kefir; 1 tsp. organic extra-virgin coconut oil; 2 Tbsp. organic raw honey; 1 cup organic fruit, fresh or frozen (berries, banana, peaches, pineapple, etc.); 1 scoop goat's milk protein powder (see Appendix C for recommendations); dash of vanilla extract (optional).	**Breakfast Option 2:** 2 ounces of raw almonds One banana	**Breakfast Option 3:** 4 to 8 ounces of organic whole-milk yogurt with fruit (banana, pineapple, peaches, or berries), honey, and a dash of vanilla extract Handful of raw almonds
Drink 8–12 ounces of water.		
Take two or three whole-food multivitamin caplets and one to four capsules of concentrated fucoxanthin. (See Appendix C for recommended products.)		
10:00 a.m. **Morning Snack Option 1:** One whole-food nutrition bar (see Appendix C for recommended products)		**Morning Snack Option 2:** One serving of whole-food meal supplement with native whey protein and glucomannan fiber mixed with 12 ounces of water
Drink 8–12 ounces of water.		
LUNCH (12:30 p.m.) Toss a large green salad with mixed greens, avocado, carrots, cucumbers, celery, tomatoes, red cabbage, red peppers, red onions, sprouts, 2 ounces of canned beans (black, garbanzo, or pinto), and two hard-boiled omega-3 eggs. (Option 1: substitute 3 ounces of cold, poached, or canned wild salmon in place of hard-boiled eggs. Option 2: substitute 2 ounces of low-mercury, high-omega-3 canned tuna in place of hard-boiled eggs.)		
For the salad dressing, mix extra-virgin olive oil, apple-cider vinegar or lemon juice, naturally brewed soy sauce, liquid aminos, sea salt, herbs, and spices, or mix 1 tablespoon of extra-virgin olive oil with 1 tablespoon of a healthy store-bought dressing. (See Appendix C for recommended brands.)		
One piece of fruit in season or organic grapes		
Drink 12–16 ounces of water.		
Take two or three whole-food multivitamin caplets and one to three capsules of concentrated fucoxanthin.		
3:30 p.m. **Afternoon Snack Option 1:** A piece of fruit or cacao chocolate (see Appendix C for recommended products)		**Afternoon Snack Option 2:** One whole-food meal supplement with native whey protein mixed with 12 ounces of water
Drink 8–12 ounces of water.		

Female Potato Type
Phase II (Weeks 5–8)

DINNER (6:15 p.m., but try to finish eating by 7:00 p.m.)			
	Dinner Option 1: Broiled fish	**Dinner Option 2:** Grilled chicken	**Dinner Option 3:** Red meat chili
	Sautéed spinach	Grilled vegetables (onions, peppers, and zucchini)	Roasted potatoes
	Toss a large green salad with mixed greens, avocado, carrots, cucumbers, celery, tomatoes, red cabbage, red peppers, red onions, and sprouts.	Baked sweet potato with butter	Toss a green salad with mixed greens, avocado, carrots, cucumbers, celery, tomatoes, red cabbage, red peppers, red onions, and sprouts.

For the salad dressing, mix extra-virgin olive oil, apple-cider vinegar or lemon juice, naturally brewed soy sauce, liquid aminos, sea salt, herbs, and spices, or mix 1 tablespoon of extra-virgin olive oil with 1 tablespoon of a healthy store-bought dressing. (See Appendix C for recommended brands.)

Drink 12–16 ounces of water.

Take two or three whole-food multivitamin caplets, one to three capsules of concentrated fucoxanthin, and 1 to 3 teaspoons (or three to nine capsules) of a high omega-3 cod liver oil complex. (See Appendix C for recommended products.)

Before Bed

Perform the Healing Codes exercise on pages 184–185.

Drink 8–12 ounces of water (optional).

Perform five minutes of deep-breathing exercises by taking a slow, five-second breath in through your nose (inhale), holding for one second, followed by a forceful quick exhale through your mouth, completely emptying your lungs with each exhalation and completely filling your lungs with each inhalation. Repeat for two to five minutes.

Go to bed by 10:30 p.m.

Female Potato Type
Phase III (Weeks 9–12)

Upon waking

Drink 16–24 ounces of water.

Spend some time this morning picturing yourself at your ideal weight. See yourself doing the things you think you can't do now or don't do because you're not at your ideal weight. Picture yourself looking great, free from all of the diseases that people said you're at a high risk for. Next, picture yourself at your ideal weight, inspiring your family and friends, who remark how great you look. Now stand in front of the mirror and repeat:

Today I am going to take another positive step toward achieving my ideal weight.

Perform the Healing Codes exercise. (You can learn about the Healing Codes exercise on pages 184–185. I recommend that you perform the Healing Codes exercise twice a day—once in the morning and once in the evening—but feel free to try this two-minute exercise three, four, or five times a day.)

Perform FIT exercises for twenty minutes, choosing from physical activities like sprinting, bodyweight exercises, strength training with bands, medicine balls, dumbbells or kettlebells, stationary bike, or the stair stepper.

Female Potato Type		
Phase III (Weeks 9–12)		
BREAKFAST (7:30 a.m.)	**Breakfast Option 1:** Old-fashioned oatmeal with honey, cinnamon, and raisins 2 ounces of cottage cheese and blueberries	**Breakfast Option 2:** Two eggs any style, cooked in 1 tablespoon of extra-virgin coconut oil One slice of sprouted or yeast-free whole-grain bread with almond butter and honey	**Breakfast Option 3:** Organic sprouted dry cereal (see Appendix C for recommended brands) or ½ cup of old-fashioned oats, whole corn grits, or seven-grain porridge 4 ounces of organic whole-milk yogurt or cottage cheese with fruit (pineapple, peaches, or berries), honey, and a dash of vanilla extract
	Drink 8–12 ounces of water.		
	Take two or three whole-food multivitamin caplets and one to four capsules of concentrated fucoxanthin. (See Appendix C for recommended products.)		
10:00 a.m.	**Morning Snack Option 1:** One whole-food nutrition bar (see Appendix C for recommended products)	**Morning Snack Option 2:** One serving of whole-food meal supplement with native whey protein and glucomannan fiber mixed with 12 ounces of water	
	Drink 8–12 ounces of water.		
LUNCH (12:30 p.m.)	**Lunch Option 1:** Roasted chicken, turkey, or roast beef with lettuce, cheese tomato, sprouts, and organic mayo (soy oil, not canola) on sprouted or yeast-free whole-grain bread (see Appendix C for recommended brands) One apple with skin	**Lunch Options 2 and 3:** Toss a large green salad with mixed greens, avocado, carrots, cucumbers, celery, tomatoes, red cabbage, red peppers, red onions, sprouts, and 2 ounces of canned beans (black, garbanzo, or pinto). (Option 1: include 3 ounces of cold, poached, or canned wild salmon. Option 2: include 2 ounces of low-mercury, high-omega-3 canned tuna.) One piece of fruit in season or organic grapes	
	For the salad dressing, mix extra-virgin olive oil, apple-cider vinegar or lemon juice, naturally brewed soy sauce, liquid aminos, sea salt, herbs, and spices, or mix 1 tablespoon of extra-virgin olive oil with 1 tablespoon of a healthy store-bought dressing. (See Appendix C for recommended brands.)		
	Drink 12–16 ounces of water.		
	Take two or three whole-food multivitamin caplets and one to three capsules of concentrated fucoxanthin.		
3:30 p.m.	**Afternoon Snack Option 1:** A piece of fruit or cacao chocolate	**Afternoon Snack Option 2:** One whole-food meal supplement with native whey protein mixed with 12 ounces of water	
	Drink 8–12 ounces of water.		
DINNER (6:15 p.m., but try to finish eating by 7:00 p.m.)	**Dinner Option 1:** Baked, poached, or grilled wild-caught salmon Peas and carrots	**Dinner Option 2:** Grilled chicken kabobs with pineapple, peppers, onions, and zucchini	**Dinner Option 3:** Red meat chili Steamed quinoa, peas, and carrots
	Toss a green salad with mixed greens, avocado, carrots, cucumbers, celery, tomatoes, red cabbage, red peppers, red onions, and sprouts.		
	For the salad dressing, mix extra-virgin olive oil, apple-cider vinegar or lemon juice, naturally brewed soy sauce, liquid aminos, sea salt, herbs, and spices, or mix 1 tablespoon of extra-virgin olive oil with 1 tablespoon of a healthy store-bought dressing. (See Appendix C for recommended brands.)		
	Drink 12–16 ounces of water.		
	Take two or three whole-food multivitamin caplets, one to three capsules of concentrated fucoxanthin, and 1 to 3 teaspoons (or three to nine capsules) of a high omega-3 cod liver oil complex. (See Appendix C for recommended products.)		

Female Potato Type
Phase III (Weeks 9–12)

Before Bed	Perform the Healing Codes exercise on pages 184–185.
	Drink 8–12 ounces of water (optional).
	Perform five minutes of deep-breathing exercises by taking a slow, five-second breath in through your nose (inhale), holding for one second, followed by a forceful quick exhale through your mouth, completely emptying your lungs with each exhalation and completely filling your lungs with each inhalation. Repeat for two to five minutes.
	Go to bed by 10:30 p.m.

Male Meat Type
Phase I (Weeks 1–4)

Upon waking	Drink 16–24 ounces of water.
	Spend some time this morning picturing yourself at your ideal weight. See yourself doing the things you think you can't do now or don't do because you're not at your ideal weight. Picture yourself looking great, free from all of the diseases that people said you're at a high risk for. Next, picture yourself at your ideal weight, inspiring your family and friends, who remark how great you look. Now stand in front of the mirror and repeat:
	Today I am going to take another positive step toward achieving my ideal weight.
	Perform the Healing Codes exercise. (You can learn about the Healing Codes exercise on pages 184–185. I recommend that you perform the Healing Codes exercise twice a day—once in the morning and once in the evening—but feel free to try this two-minute exercise three, four, or five times a day.)
	Perform FIT exercises for twenty minutes, choosing from physical activities like sprinting, bodyweight exercises, strength training with bands, medicine balls, dumbbells or kettlebells, stationary bike, or the stair stepper.

BREAKFAST (7:30 a.m.)	**Breakfast Option 1:** Make a smoothie in a blender with the following ingredients: 1 cup plain whole-milk yogurt or kefir; 1 tsp. organic flaxseed oil; 1 tsp. organic extra-virgin coconut oil; 1 Tbsp. organic raw honey; 1 cup organic fruit, fresh or frozen (berries, peaches, pineapple, etc.); 1 scoop goat's milk protein powder (see Appendix C for recommendations); dash of vanilla extract (optional).	**Breakfast Option 2:** Eat three eggs any style, cooked in extra-virgin coconut oil (see Appendix C for recommended products) Stir-fried onions, mushrooms, and peppers One grapefruit	**Breakfast Option 3:** 8 ounces of organic whole-milk yogurt or cottage cheese with fruit (pineapple, peaches, or berries), honey, and a dash of vanilla extract Handful of raw almonds

	Drink 8–12 ounces of water.
	Take two or three whole-food multivitamin caplets and one to four capsules of concentrated fucoxanthin. (See Appendix C for recommended products.)

10:00 a.m.	**Morning Snack Option 1:** One whole-food nutrition bar (see Appendix C for recommended products)	**Morning Snack Option 2:** One serving of whole-food meal supplement with native whey protein and glucomannan fiber mixed with 12 ounces of water
	Drink 8–12 ounces of water.	

	Male Meat Type
	Phase I (Weeks 1–4)

LUNCH (12:30 p.m.)	Toss a large green salad with mixed greens, avocado, carrots, cucumbers, celery, tomatoes, red cabbage, red peppers, red onions, sprouts, 2 ounces of canned beans (black, garbanzo, or pinto), and two hard-boiled omega-3 eggs. (Option 1: substitute 3 ounces of cold, poached, or canned wild salmon in place of hard-boiled eggs. Option 2: substitute 2 ounces of low-mercury, high-omega-3 canned tuna in place of hard-boiled eggs.)
	For the salad dressing, mix extra-virgin olive oil, apple-cider vinegar or lemon juice, naturally brewed soy sauce, liquid aminos, sea salt, herbs, and spices, or mix 1 tablespoon of extra-virgin olive oil with 1 tablespoon of a healthy store-bought dressing. (See Appendix C for recommended brands.)
	One piece of fruit in season
	Drink 12–16 ounces of water.
	Take two or three whole-food multivitamin caplets and one to three capsules of concentrated fucoxanthin.

3:30 p.m.	**Afternoon Snack Option 1:** One whole-food nutrition bar (see Appendix C for recommended products)	**Afternoon Snack Option 2:** One whole-food meal supplement with native whey protein mixed with 12 ounces of water
	Drink 8–12 ounces of water.	

DINNER (6:15 p.m., but try to finish eating by 7:00 p.m.)	**Dinner Option 1:** Baked, poached, or grilled wild-caught salmon Steamed broccoli	**Dinner Option 2:** Roasted organic chicken Cooked vegetables (carrots, onions, peas, etc.)	**Dinner Option 3:** Red meat steak or ground meat (beef, buffalo, or venison) Steamed broccoli Baked winter squash with butter
	Toss a green salad with mixed greens, avocado, carrots, cucumbers, celery, tomatoes, red cabbage, red peppers, red onions, and sprouts.		
	For the salad dressing, mix extra-virgin olive oil, apple-cider vinegar or lemon juice, naturally brewed soy sauce, liquid aminos, sea salt, herbs, and spices, or mix 1 tablespoon of extra-virgin olive oil with one tablespoon of a healthy store-bought dressing. (See Appendix C for recommended brands.)		
	Drink 12–16 ounces of water.		
	Take two or three whole-food multivitamin caplets, one to three capsules of concentrated fucoxanthin, and 1 to 3 teaspoons (or three to nine capsules) of a high omega-3 cod liver oil complex. (See Appendix C for recommended products.)		

Before Bed	Perform the Healing Codes exercise on pages 184–185.
	Drink 8–12 ounces of water (optional).
	Perform five minutes of deep-breathing exercises by taking a slow, five-second breath in through your nose (inhale), holding for one second, followed by a forceful quick exhale through your mouth, completely emptying your lungs with each exhalation and completely filling your lungs with each inhalation. Repeat for two to five minutes.
	Go to bed by 10:30 p.m.

	Male Meat Type
	Phase II (Weeks 5–8)

Upon waking	Drink 16–24 ounces of water.
	Spend some time this morning picturing yourself at your ideal weight. See yourself doing the things you think you can't do now or don't do because you're not at your ideal weight. Picture yourself looking great, free from all of the diseases that people said you're at a high risk for. Next, picture yourself at your ideal weight, inspiring your family and friends, who remark how great you look. Now stand in front of the mirror and repeat:
	Today I am going to take another positive step toward achieving my ideal weight.
	Perform the Healing Codes exercise. (You can learn about the Healing Codes exercise on pages 184–185. I recommend that you perform the Healing Codes exercise twice a day—once in the morning and once in the evening—but feel free to try this two-minute exercise three, four, or five times a day.)
	Perform FIT exercises for twenty minutes, choosing from physical activities like sprinting, bodyweight exercises, strength training with bands, medicine balls, dumbbells or kettlebells, stationary bike, or the stair stepper.

BREAKFAST (7:30 a.m.)		
Breakfast Option 1: Make a smoothie in a blender with the following ingredients: 1 cup plain whole-milk yogurt or kefir; 1 tsp. organic flaxseed oil; 1 tsp. organic extra-virgin coconut oil; 1 Tbsp. organic raw honey; 1 cup organic fruit, fresh or frozen (berries, peaches, pineapple, etc.); 1 scoop goat's milk protein powder (see Appendix C for recommendations); dash of vanilla extract (optional).	**Breakfast Option 2:** Three eggs any style, cooked in 1 tablespoon of extra-virgin coconut oil Sautèed tomatoes and onions One orange	**Breakfast Option 3:** 6 ounces of organic whole-milk yogurt or cottage cheese with fruit (pineapple, peaches, or berries), honey, and a dash of vanilla extract Handful of raw almonds
Drink 8–12 ounces of water.		
Take two or three whole-food multivitamin caplets and one to four capsules of concentrated fucoxanthin. (See Appendix C for recommended products.)		

10:00 a.m.		
Morning Snack Option 1: One whole-food nutrition bar (see Appendix C for recommended products)	**Morning Snack Option 2:** One serving of whole-food meal supplement with native whey protein and glucomannan fiber mixed with 12 ounces of water	
Drink 8–12 ounces of water.		

LUNCH (12:30 p.m.)	
Toss a large green salad with mixed greens, avocado, carrots, cucumbers, celery, tomatoes, red cabbage, red peppers, red onions, sprouts, 2 ounces of canned beans (black, garbanzo, or pinto), and two hard-boiled omega-3 eggs. (Option 1: substitute 4 ounces of cold, poached, or canned wild salmon in place of hard-boiled eggs. Option 2: substitute 4 ounces of low-mercury, high-omega-3 canned tuna in place of hard-boiled eggs.)	
For the salad dressing, mix extra-virgin olive oil, apple-cider vinegar or lemon juice, naturally brewed soy sauce, liquid aminos, sea salt, herbs, and spices, or mix 1 tablespoon of extra-virgin olive oil with 1 tablespoon of a healthy store-bought dressing. (See Appendix C for recommended brands.)	
One piece of fruit in season	
Drink 12–16 ounces of water.	
Take two or three whole-food multivitamin caplets and one to three capsules of concentrated fucoxanthin.	

3:30 p.m.		
Afternoon Snack Option 1: One whole-food nutrition bar (see Appendix C for recommended products)	**Afternoon Snack Option 2:** One whole-food meal supplement with native whey protein mixed with 12 ounces of water	
Drink 8–12 ounces of water.		

Male Meat Type
Phase II (Weeks 5–8)

DINNER (6:15 p.m., but try to finish eating by 7:00 p.m.)	**Dinner Option 1:** Broiled or steamed fish Sautèed spinach	**Dinner Option 2:** Meatloaf Roasted vegetables (potatoes, carrots, onions, peas, etc.)	**Dinner Option 3:** Red meat steak or ground meat (beef, buffalo, or venison) Steamed broccoli Baked sweet potato with butter
	Toss a green salad with mixed greens, avocado, carrots, cucumbers, celery, tomatoes, red cabbage, red peppers, red onions, and sprouts.		
	For the salad dressing, mix extra-virgin olive oil, apple-cider vinegar or lemon juice, naturally brewed soy sauce, liquid aminos, sea salt, herbs, and spices, or mix 1 tablespoon of extra-virgin olive oil with 1 tablespoon of a healthy store-bought dressing. (See Appendix C for recommended brands.)		
	Drink 12–16 ounces of water.		
	Take two or three whole-food multivitamin caplets, one to three capsules of concentrated fucoxanthin, and 1 to 3 teaspoons (or three to nine capsules) of a high omega-3 cod liver oil complex. (See Appendix C for recommended products.)		
Before Bed	Perform the Healing Codes exercise on pages 184–185.		
	Drink 8–12 ounces of water (optional).		
	Perform five minutes of deep-breathing exercises by taking a slow, five-second breath in through your nose (inhale), holding for one second, followed by a forceful quick exhale through your mouth, completely emptying your lungs with each exhalation and completely filling your lungs with each inhalation. Repeat for two to five minutes.		
	Go to bed by 10:30 p.m.		

Male Meat Type
Phase III (Weeks 9–12)

Upon waking	Drink 16–24 ounces of water.		
	Spend some time this morning picturing yourself at your ideal weight. See yourself doing the things you think you can't do now or don't do because you're not at your ideal weight. Picture yourself looking great, free from all of the diseases that people said you're at a high risk for. Next, picture yourself at your ideal weight, inspiring your family and friends, who remark how great you look. Now stand in front of the mirror and repeat: *Today I am going to take another positive step toward achieving my ideal weight.*		
	Perform the Healing Codes exercise. (You can learn about the Healing Codes exercise on pages 184–185. I recommend that you perform the Healing Codes exercise twice a day—once in the morning and once in the evening—but feel free to try this two-minute exercise three, four, or five times a day.)		
	Perform FIT exercises for twenty minutes, choosing from physical activities like sprinting, bodyweight exercises, strength training with bands, medicine balls, dumbbells or kettlebells, stationary bike, or the stair stepper.		
BREAKFAST (7:30 a.m.)	**Breakfast Option 1:** Three-egg tomato and cheese omelet One piece of sprouted or yeast-free toast with butter	**Breakfast Option 2:** Three eggs any style, cooked in 1 tablespoon of extra-virgin coconut oil 4 ounces cottage cheese, raw honey, and raisins	**Breakfast Option 3:** 8 ounces of organic whole-milk yogurt or cottage cheese with fruit (banana, pineapple, peaches, or berries), honey, and a dash of vanilla extract Handful of raw almonds
	Drink 8–12 ounces of water.		
	Take two or three whole-food multivitamin caplets and one to four capsules of concentrated fucoxanthin. (See Appendix C for recommended products.)		

Male Meat Type
Phase III (Weeks 9–12)

10:00 a.m.	**Morning Snack Option 1:** One whole-food nutrition bar (see Appendix C for recommended products)	**Morning Snack Option 2:** One serving of whole-food meal supplement with native whey protein and glucomannan fiber mixed with 12 ounces of water
	Drink 8–12 ounces of water.	

LUNCH (12:30 p.m.)	**Lunch Option 1:** Red meat chili 1 ounce of raw cheese Whole-grain crackers or baked corn chips	**Lunch Option 2:** Toss a large green salad with mixed greens, avocado, carrots, cucumbers, celery, tomatoes, red cabbage, red peppers, red onions, sprouts, 2 ounces of canned beans (black, garbanzo, or pinto), and 4 ounces of cold, poached, or canned wild salmon.	**Lunch Option 3:** Toss a large green salad with mixed greens, avocado, carrots, cucumbers, celery, tomatoes, red cabbage, red peppers, red onions, sprouts, 2 ounces of canned beans (black, garbanzo, or pinto), and 4 ounces of low-mercury, high-omega-3 canned tuna. (See Appendix C for recommended products.)
	For the salad dressing, mix extra-virgin olive oil, apple-cider vinegar or lemon juice, naturally brewed soy sauce, liquid aminos, sea salt, herbs, and spices, or mix 1 tablespoon of extra-virgin olive oil with 1 tablespoon of a healthy store-bought dressing. (See Appendix C for recommended brands.)		
	One piece of fruit in season		
	Drink 12–16 ounces of water.		
	Take two or three whole-food multivitamin caplets and one to three capsules of concentrated fucoxanthin.		

3:30 p.m.	**Afternoon Snack Option 1:** One whole-food nutrition bar (see Appendix C for recommended products)	**Afternoon Snack Option 2:** One whole-food meal supplement with native whey protein mixed with 12 ounces of water
	Drink 8–12 ounces of water.	

DINNER (6:15 p.m., but try to finish eating by 7:00 p.m.)	**Dinner Option 1:** Baked chicken breast One baked potato with butter	**Dinner Option 2:** Roasted organic chicken Roasted vegetables (potatoes, carrots, onions, peas, etc.)	**Dinner Option 3:** Meatloaf One baked sweet potato with butter Steamed broccoli
	Toss a green salad with mixed greens, avocado, carrots, cucumbers, celery, tomatoes, red cabbage, red peppers, red onions, and sprouts.		
	For the salad dressing, mix extra-virgin olive oil, apple-cider vinegar or lemon juice, naturally brewed soy sauce, liquid aminos, sea salt, herbs, and spices, or mix 1 tablespoon of extra-virgin olive oil with 1 tablespoon of a healthy store-bought dressing. (See Appendix C for recommended brands.)		
	Drink 12–16 ounces of water.		
	Take two or three whole-food multivitamin caplets, one to three capsules of concentrated fucoxanthin, and 1 to 3 teaspoons (or three to nine capsules) of a high omega-3 cod liver oil complex. (See Appendix C for recommended products.)		

Before Bed	Perform the Healing Codes exercise on pages 184–185.
	Drink 8–12 ounces of water (optional).
	Perform five minutes of deep-breathing exercises by taking a slow, five-second breath in through your nose (inhale), holding for one second, followed by a forceful quick exhale through your mouth, completely emptying your lungs with each exhalation and completely filling your lungs with each inhalation. Repeat for two to five minutes.
	Go to bed by 10:30 p.m.

Male Potato Type		
Phase I (Weeks 1–4)		
Upon waking	Drink 16–24 ounces of water.		
	Spend some time this morning picturing yourself at your ideal weight. See yourself doing the things you think you can't do now or don't do because you're not at your ideal weight. Picture yourself looking great, free from all of the diseases that people said you're at a high risk for. Next, picture yourself at your ideal weight, inspiring your family and friends, who remark how great you look. Now stand in front of the mirror and repeat: *Today I am going to take another positive step toward achieving my ideal weight.*		
	Perform the Healing Codes exercise. (You can learn about the Healing Codes exercise on pages 184–185. I recommend that you perform the Healing Codes exercise twice a day—once in the morning and once in the evening—but feel free to try this two-minute exercise three, four, or five times a day.)		
	Perform FIT exercises for twenty minutes, choosing from physical activities like sprinting, bodyweight exercises, strength training with bands, medicine balls, dumbbells or kettlebells, stationary bike, or the stair stepper.		
BREAKFAST (7:30 a.m.)	**Breakfast Option 1:** Make a smoothie in a blender with the following ingredients: 1 cup plain whole-milk yogurt or kefir; 1 tsp. organic extra-virgin coconut oil; 2 Tbsp. organic raw honey; 1 cup organic fruit, fresh or frozen (berries, peaches, pineapple, etc.); 1 scoop goat's milk protein powder (see Appendix C for recommendations); dash of vanilla extract (optional).	**Breakfast Option 2:** Three eggs any style, cooked in 1 tablespoon of extra-virgin coconut oil Stir-fried onions, mushrooms, and peppers One serving of grapes	**Breakfast Option 3:** 4 to 8 ounces of organic whole-milk yogurt with fruit (pineapple, peaches, or berries), honey, and a dash of vanilla extract Handful of raw almonds
	Drink 8–12 ounces of water.		
	Take two or three whole-food multivitamin caplets and one to four capsules of concentrated fucoxanthin. (See Appendix C for recommended products.)		
10:00 a.m.	**Morning Snack Option 1:** One whole-food nutrition bar (see Appendix C for recommended products)	**Morning Snack Option 2:** One serving of whole-food meal supplement with native whey protein and glucomannan fiber mixed with 12 ounces of water	
	Drink 8–12 ounces of water.		
LUNCH (12:30 p.m.)	Toss a large green salad with mixed greens, avocado, carrots, cucumbers, celery, tomatoes, red cabbage, red peppers, red onions, sprouts, 2 ounces of canned beans (black, garbanzo, or pinto), and two hard-boiled omega-3 eggs. (Option 1: substitute 2 ounces of cold, poached, or canned wild salmon in place of hard-boiled eggs. Option 2: substitute 4 ounces of low-mercury, high-omega-3 canned tuna in place of hard-boiled eggs.)		
	For the salad dressing, mix extra-virgin olive oil, apple-cider vinegar or lemon juice, naturally brewed soy sauce, liquid aminos, sea salt, herbs, and spices, or mix 1 tablespoon of extra-virgin olive oil with 1 tablespoon of a healthy store-bought dressing. (See Appendix C for recommended brands.)		
	One apple with skin (or one piece of fruit in season)		
	Drink 12–16 ounces of water.		
	Take two or three whole-food multivitamin caplets and one to three capsules of concentrated fucoxanthin.		
3:30 p.m.	**Afternoon Snack Option 1:** One whole-food nutrition bar (see Appendix C for recommended products)	**Afternoon Snack Option 2:** One whole-food meal supplement with native whey protein mixed with 12 ounces of water	
	Drink 8–12 ounces of water.		

Male Potato Type		
Phase I (Weeks 1–4)		
Dinner Option 1: Baked, poached, or grilled wild-caught salmon Peas and carrots	**Dinner Option 2:** Roasted organic chicken Cooked vegetables (carrots, onions, peas, etc.)	**Dinner Option 3:** Red meat steak (beef, buffalo, or venison) Steamed broccoli
Toss a green salad with mixed greens, avocado, carrots, cucumbers, celery, tomatoes, red cabbage, red peppers, red onions, and sprouts.		
For the salad dressing, mix extra-virgin olive oil, apple-cider vinegar or lemon juice, naturally brewed soy sauce, liquid aminos, sea salt, herbs, and spices, or mix 1 tablespoon of extra-virgin olive oil with 1 tablespoon of a healthy store-bought dressing. (See Appendix C for recommended brands.)		
Drink 12–16 ounces of water.		
Take two or three whole-food multivitamin caplets, one to three capsules of concentrated fucoxanthin, and 1 to 3 teaspoons (or three to nine capsules) of a high omega-3 cod liver oil complex. (See Appendix C for recommended products.)		
Perform the Healing Codes exercise on pages 184–185.		
Drink 8–12 ounces of water (optional).		
Perform five minutes of deep-breathing exercises by taking a slow, five-second breath in through your nose (inhale), holding for one second, followed by a forceful quick exhale through your mouth, completely emptying your lungs with each exhalation and completely filling your lungs with each inhalation. Repeat for two to five minutes.		
Go to bed by 10:30 p.m.		

Left label for DINNER rows: DINNER (6:15 p.m., but try to finish eating by 7:00 p.m.)
Left label for bottom rows: Before Bed

Male Potato Type		
Phase II (Weeks 5–8)		
Drink 16–24 ounces of water.		
Spend some time this morning picturing yourself at your ideal weight. See yourself doing the things you think you can't do now or don't do because you're not at your ideal weight. Picture yourself looking great, free from all of the diseases that people said you're at a high risk for. Next, picture yourself at your ideal weight, inspiring your family and friends, who remark how great you look. Now stand in front of the mirror and repeat: *Today I am going to take another positive step toward achieving my ideal weight.*		
Perform the Healing Codes exercise. (You can learn about the Healing Codes exercise on pages 184–185. I recommend that you perform the Healing Codes exercise twice a day—once in the morning and once in the evening—but feel free to try this two-minute exercise three, four, or five times a day.)		
Perform FIT exercises for twenty minutes, choosing from physical activities like sprinting, bodyweight exercises, strength training with bands, medicine balls, dumbbells or kettlebells, stationary bike, or the stair stepper.		
Breakfast Option 1: 8 ounces of cottage cheese with raw honey and banana	**Breakfast Option 2:** Three eggs any style, cooked in 1 tablespoon of extra-virgin coconut oil 4 ounces of old-fashioned oatmeal with butter, honey, raisins, and cinnamon	**Breakfast Option 3:** 4 to 8 ounces of organic whole-milk yogurt with fruit (pineapple, peaches, or berries), honey, and a dash of vanilla extract Handful of raw almonds and raisins
Drink 8–12 ounces of water.		
Take two or three whole-food multivitamin caplets and one to four capsules of concentrated fucoxanthin. (See Appendix C for recommended products.)		

Left label for top rows: Upon waking
Left label for breakfast rows: BREAKFAST (7:30 a.m.)

Male Potato Type
Phase II (Weeks 5–8)

<table>
<tr><td rowspan="2">10:00 a.m.</td><td colspan="2">Morning Snack Option 1: One whole-food nutrition bar (see Appendix C for recommended products)</td><td colspan="2">Morning Snack Option 2: One serving of whole-food meal supplement with native whey protein and glucomannan fiber mixed with 12 ounces of water</td></tr>
<tr><td colspan="4">Drink 8–12 ounces of water.</td></tr>
<tr><td rowspan="5">LUNCH (12:30 p.m.)</td><td colspan="4">Toss a large green salad with mixed greens, avocado, carrots, cucumbers, celery, tomatoes, red cabbage, red peppers, red onions, sprouts, 2 ounces of canned beans (black, garbanzo, or pinto), and three hard-boiled omega-3 eggs. (Option 1: substitute 4 ounces of cold, poached, or canned wild salmon in place of hard-boiled eggs. Option 2: substitute 4 ounces of low-mercury, high-omega-3 canned tuna in place of hard-boiled eggs.)</td></tr>
<tr><td colspan="4">For the salad dressing, mix extra-virgin olive oil, apple-cider vinegar or lemon juice, naturally brewed soy sauce, liquid aminos, sea salt, herbs, and spices, or mix 1 tablespoon of extra-virgin olive oil with 1 tablespoon of a healthy store-bought dressing. (See Appendix C for recommended brands.)</td></tr>
<tr><td colspan="4">One piece of fruit in season (or organic grapes)</td></tr>
<tr><td colspan="4">Drink 12–16 ounces of water.</td></tr>
<tr><td colspan="4">Take two or three whole-food multivitamin caplets and one to three capsules of concentrated fucoxanthin.</td></tr>
<tr><td rowspan="2">3:30 p.m.</td><td colspan="2">Afternoon Snack Option 1: A piece of fruit or cacao chocolate (see Appendix C for recommended products)</td><td colspan="2">Afternoon Snack Option 2: One whole-food meal supplement with native whey protein mixed with 12 ounces of water</td></tr>
<tr><td colspan="4">Drink 8–12 ounces of water.</td></tr>
<tr><td rowspan="4">DINNER (6:15 p.m., but try to finish eating by 7:00 p.m.)</td><td>Dinner Option 1: Meatloaf</td><td colspan="2">Dinner Option 2: Grilled chicken</td><td>Dinner Option 3: Red meat chili</td></tr>
<tr><td>Mashed potato with butter

Steamed broccoli</td><td colspan="2">Brown rice

Stir-fried vegetables (peppers, onions, mushrooms, etc.)</td><td>Raw cheese

Whole-grain crackers or baked corn chips

Toss a green salad with mixed greens, avocado, carrots, cucumbers, celery, tomatoes, red cabbage, red peppers, red onions, and sprouts.

For the salad dressing, mix extra-virgin olive oil, apple-cider vinegar or lemon juice, naturally brewed soy sauce, liquid aminos, sea salt, herbs, and spices, or mix 1 tablespoon of extra-virgin olive oil with 1 tablespoon of a healthy store-bought dressing. (See Appendix C for recommended brands.)</td></tr>
<tr><td colspan="4">Drink 12–16 ounces of water.</td></tr>
<tr><td colspan="4">Take two or three whole-food multivitamin caplets, one to three capsules of concentrated fucoxanthin, and 1 to 3 teaspoons (or three to nine capsules) of a high omega-3 cod liver oil complex. (See Appendix C for recommended products.)</td></tr>
</table>

	Male Potato Type
	Phase II (Weeks 5–8)
Before Bed	Perform the Healing Codes exercise on pages 184–185.
	Drink 8–12 ounces of water (optional).
	Perform five minutes of deep-breathing exercises by taking a slow, five-second breath in through your nose (inhale), holding for one second, followed by a forceful quick exhale through your mouth, completely emptying your lungs with each exhalation and completely filling your lungs with each inhalation. Repeat for two to five minutes.
	Go to bed by 10:30 p.m.

	Male Potato Type		
	Phase III (Weeks 9–12)		
Upon waking	Drink 16–24 ounces of water.		
	Spend some time this morning picturing yourself at your ideal weight. See yourself doing the things you think you can't do now or don't do because you're not at your ideal weight. Picture yourself looking great, free from all of the diseases that people said you're at a high risk for. Next, picture yourself at your ideal weight, inspiring your family and friends, who remark how great you look. Now stand in front of the mirror and repeat: *Today I am going to take another positive step toward achieving my ideal weight.*		
	Perform the Healing Codes exercise. (You can learn about the Healing Codes exercise on pages 184–185. I recommend that you perform the Healing Codes exercise twice a day—once in the morning and once in the evening—but feel free to try this two-minute exercise three, four, or five times a day.)		
	Perform FIT exercises for twenty minutes, choosing from physical activities like sprinting, bodyweight exercises, strength training with bands, medicine balls, dumbbells or kettlebells, stationary bike, or the stair stepper.		
BREAKFAST (7:30 a.m.)	**Breakfast Option 1:** Make a smoothie in a blender with the following ingredients: 1 cup plain whole-milk yogurt or kefir; 1 tsp. organic extra-virgin coconut oil; 2 Tbsp. organic raw honey; 1 cup organic fruit, fresh or frozen (berries, peaches, pineapple, etc.); 1 scoop goat's milk protein powder (see Appendix C for recommendations); dash of vanilla extract (optional).	**Breakfast Option 2:** Two or three eggs any style, cooked in 1 tablespoon of extra-virgin coconut oil (see Appendix C for recommended products) Stir-fried onions, mushrooms, and peppers One slice of sprouted or yeast-free whole-grain bread with almond butter and honey	**Breakfast Option 3:** Organic sprouted dry cereal (see Appendix C for recommended brands) or ½ cup of old-fashioned oats, whole corn grits, or seven-grain porridge 4 ounces of organic whole-milk yogurt or cottage cheese with fruit (pineapple, peaches, or berries), honey, and a dash of vanilla extract
	Drink 8–12 ounces of water.		
	Take two or three whole-food multivitamin caplets and one to four capsules of concentrated fucoxanthin. (See Appendix C for recommended products.)		
10:00 a.m.	**Morning Snack Option 1:** One whole-food nutrition bar (see Appendix C for recommended products)	**Morning Snack Option 2:** One serving of whole-food meal supplement with native whey protein and glucomannan fiber mixed with 12 ounces of water	
	Drink 8–12 ounces of water.		

	Male Potato Type
	Phase III (Weeks 9–12)

LUNCH (12:30 p.m.)	**Lunch Option 1:** Roasted chicken, turkey, or roast beef with lettuce, cheese, tomato, sprouts, and organic mayo (soy oil, not canola) on sprouted or yeast-free whole-grain bread (see Appendix C for recommended brands)

Lunch Options 2 and 3: Toss a large green salad with mixed greens, avocado, carrots, cucumbers, celery, tomatoes, red cabbage, red peppers, red onions, sprouts, and 2 ounces of canned beans (black, garbanzo, or pinto). (Option 1: include 4 ounces of cold, poached, or canned wild salmon. Option 2: include 4 ounces of low-mercury, high-omega-3 canned tuna.)

For the salad dressing, mix extra-virgin olive oil, apple-cider vinegar or lemon juice, naturally brewed soy sauce, liquid aminos, sea salt, herbs, and spices, or mix 1 tablespoon of extra-virgin olive oil with 1 tablespoon of a healthy store-bought dressing. (See Appendix C for recommended brands.)

One piece of fruit in season (or organic grapes)

Drink 12–16 ounces of water.

Take two or three whole-food multivitamin caplets and one to three capsules of concentrated fucoxanthin.

3:30 p.m.

Afternoon Snack Option 1: A piece of fruit or cacao chocolate

Afternoon Snack Option 2: One whole-food meal supplement with native whey protein mixed with 12 ounces of water

Drink 8–12 ounces of water.

DINNER (6:15 p.m., but try to finish eating by 7:00 p.m.)

Dinner Option 1: Baked, poached, or grilled wild-caught salmon

Peas and carrots

Dinner Option 2: Roasted organic chicken

Cooked vegetable (carrots, onions, peas, etc.)

Dinner Option 3: Red meat steak (beef, buffalo, or venison)

Sautèed spinach

Mashed potatoes with butter

Toss a green salad with mixed greens, avocado, carrots, cucumbers, celery, tomatoes, red cabbage, red peppers, red onions, and sprouts.

For the salad dressing, mix extra-virgin olive oil, apple-cider vinegar or lemon juice, naturally brewed soy sauce, liquid aminos, sea salt, herbs, and spices, or mix 1 tablespoon of extra-virgin olive oil with 1 tablespoon of a healthy store-bought dressing. (See Appendix C for recommended brands.)

Drink 12–16 ounces of water.

Take two or three whole-food multivitamin caplets, one to three capsules of concentrated fucoxanthin, and 1 to 3 teaspoons (or three to nine capsules) of a high omega-3 cod liver oil complex. (See Appendix C for recommended products.)

Before Bed

Perform the Healing Codes exercise on pages 184–185.

Drink 8–12 ounces of water (optional).

Perform five minutes of deep-breathing exercises by taking a slow, five-second breath in through your nose (inhale), holding for one second, followed by a forceful quick exhale through your mouth, completely emptying your lungs with each exhalation and completely filling your lungs with each inhalation. Repeat for two to five minutes.

Appendix A

Recipes From Chef Carol

Y OU READ MUCH of Chef Carol Green's compelling story in chapter 11, "Think for Your Ideal Weight." She was raised on a farm in rural South Africa, surrounded by the rhythms of the seasons. Her budding culinary skills were first professionally put to the test when she followed her spirit of adventure and began cooking onboard megayachts in the Caribbean.

To truly understand the foundation of good food, she took a hiatus and studied the art of French cuisine and *patisserie* at the *Ecole des Arts Culinaires* in Lyon, France. I first met Carol when I was invited to speak in South Africa in 2006 and was told of her great talent in the kitchen. I asked Carol if she would come to the United States and appear on my television show, *Extraordinary Health*, seen weekly on the Trinity Broadcast Network and other cable outlets. We taped a couple of dozen wonderful cooking segments, but the best part was when the cameras were turned off and I got to dig in to the appetizing entrees and dishes that she had prepared.

Below are sixteen examples of delicious and nutritious recipes created by Chef Carol. For products like sea salt, seasoned salt, honey, flaxseed, extra-virgin coconut oil, powdered whole-food meal supplement, and cacao chocolate, please see the Maker's Diet Resource Guide on page 263.

Baked Eggs in Tomato Cups With Sautèed Spinach

4 tomatoes	2 cloves garlic, minced
4 eggs	1 Tbsp. extra-virgin coconut oil
8 Tbsp. Parmesan cheese (raw pecorino)	Seasoned salt, as needed
8 oz. spinach	

SPECIAL EQUIPMENT: Muffin tins

Preheat oven to 400°F. Cut off tops of tomatoes, and scoop out all the flesh with a spoon. Place tomatoes in muffin tins and gently break an egg in each one. Sprinkle with seasoned salt ; then sprinkle 2 tablespoons of cheese over each tomato. Tent the muffin tin with foil and bake for 20 minutes, or until just set.

While eggs are baking, heat a sauté pan over medium heat, and melt the coconut oil. Add the garlic and sauté for a few minutes; then add the spinach and cook, stirring until just wilted. Season with salt and serve as a side to the eggs.

Serves 4.

Chef Carol's comment: "These individual tomato cups look as good as they taste and are easy and quick to prepare. Serve with a side of sautéed spinach or mushrooms."

Nutritional facts per serving: 116 calories; 6 g fat (47.6 percent calories from fat); 9 g protein; 7 g carbohydrate; 1 g dietary fiber; 191 mg cholesterol; 160 mg sodium.

Blueberry Clouds

¼ cup hot water	1 envelope unflavored beef gelatin
1 cup blueberry juice	1 cup ice water
1 cup frozen blueberries	2 scoops powdered whole-food meal supplement
4 Tbsp. fresh blueberries, for garnish	

Pour hot water into cup, and sprinkle the gelatin over; stir to dissolve. Add blueberry juice and refrigerate until "wobbly," about 1 hour. Then place the jelly in blender and blend on high; add ice water and frozen blueberries. Then add the whole-food meal supplement, and blend until fluffy. Serve immediately or pour into individual ramekins and allow to set. Top with reserved fresh blueberries.

Serves 6.

Chef Carol's comment: "The first phase of the Maker's Diet for Weight Loss program is the most challenging. Here is a fluffy and light delicious treat to reward the effort."

Nutritional facts per serving: 114 calories; trace fat (2.8 percent calories from fat); 4 g protein; 24 g carbohydrate; 3 g dietary fiber; 0 mg cholesterol; 53 mg sodium.

Cucumber and Tomato Tzatziki

3 cups Greek yogurt	1 clove garlic, minced
1 cucumber	1 large tomato, chopped fine
3 Tbsp. dill, freshly chopped	Sea salt and pepper as needed

SPECIAL EQUIPMENT: 2 strainers, cheesecloth

Place a strainer over a medium bowl and line with cheesecloth. Spoon yogurt into the lined strainer, and allow to stand at room temperature to drain, about 3 hours. Coarsely grate cucumber, place in another strainer, and let stand at room temperature until most of the liquid drains out, about 3 hours. Discard extra liquids. Mix yogurt and cucumber with dill, garlic, and tomato. Season with salt and pepper.

Serves 6.

Chef Carol's comment: "Diced tomatoes make a colorful addition to this classic Greek yogurt sauce, wonderful when served with fish."

Nutritional facts per serving: 91 calories; 4 g fat (39.9 percent calories from fat); 5 g protein; 9 g carbohydrate; 1 g dietary fiber; 16 mg cholesterol; 63 mg sodium.

―――

Fragrant Chicken and Pineapple Broth Bowl

1 small pineapple	1 stalk lemongrass, crushed
4 cups filtered water	2 skinless boneless chicken breasts, cubed
2 Tbsp. extra-virgin coconut oil	¼ cup tamari soy sauce
½ pounds of shiitake mushrooms, sliced ½-inch thick	2 limes, zested and juiced
2 cloves garlic, minced	½ tsp. stevia
2 Tbsp. roasted red chili paste	1 cup bean sprouts
2 inches fresh ginger, finely grated	½ cup cilantro, rough chopped
3 spring onions, cut on bias	½ cup basil, julienned

Peel and core pineapple; set aside the core and chop the flesh into ¼-inch pieces. Rough chop the core; then place in a blender with 4 cups of water and blend well. Strain through a fine sieve and discard the solids.

Place a stockpot over medium high heat; add the coconut oil and sauté mushrooms and garlic until softened. Add chili paste, ginger, and spring onions; sauté 1 minute more. Add pineapple broth and lemongrass. Bring to a slow simmer, and cook 10 minutes. Add chicken cubes and cook until just done, about 3 minutes. Add tamari sauce, lime juice, and a touch of zest. Sweeten with the herbal supplement stevia and salt to taste. Discard lemongrass stalk. Divide into large, deep soup bowls and heap bean sprouts, cilantro, and basil on top.

Serves 4.

Chef Carol's comment: "Light and satisfying, broths are a great way to assist weight loss. Don't let the long list of ingredients deter you from making this wonderful dish. It takes minutes to assemble and can be made with fewer ingredients."

Nutritional facts per serving: 438 calories; 5 g fat (9.7 percent calories from fat); 46 g protein; 80 g carbohydrate; 13 g dietary fiber; 71 mg cholesterol; 2376 mg sodium.

————

Herbed Pesto

1 cup fresh basil leaves, packed

½ cup parsley leaves, packed

1 Tbsp. fresh thyme leaves

1 Tbsp. fresh oregano leaves

¼ cup fresh mint leaves

½ cup grated Parmesan cheese

1 head garlic, chopped

½ cup pine nuts

½ cup olive oil

SPECIAL EQUIPMENT: Food processor

In food processor, blend all ingredients with a pinch of salt and pepper until smooth. Place in storage container and drizzle a little extra olive oil over the top to keep.

Serves 6.

Chef Carol's comment: "Fresh, bright herb pesto, a versatile ingredient to keep on hand in your refrigerator."

Nutritional facts per serving: 144 calories; 15 g fat (92.4 percent calories from fat); 2 g protein; 1 g carbohydrate; trace dietary fiber; 54 mg cholesterol; 94 mg sodium.

————

Mayan Gold Chocolate Smoothie

4 scoops powdered chocolate whole-food meal supplement

2 cups plain full-fat kefir

2 cups ice water

1 cup ice cubes

1 cup organic fresh squeezed orange juice

3 tsp. orange zest

1 tsp. cinnamon

¼ tsp. nutmeg

Pinch chili powder

Place all ingredients in blender; blend well. Serve immediately.

Serves 4.

Chef Carol's comment: "Delicious smoothie influenced by flavors of the Incas."

Nutritional facts per serving: 184 calories; 5 g fat (14.7 percent calories from fat); 13 g protein; 19 g carbohydrate; trace dietary fiber; 30 mg cholesterol; 6 mg sodium.

———

Roasted Corn and Zucchini Sautè

4 ears sweet corn	¼ tsp. ground cumin
4 Tbsp. extra-virgin coconut oil	¼ tsp. sea salt
½ cup chopped scallions	⅛ tsp. black pepper
½ tsp. garlic, finely chopped	½ cup chopped fresh cilantro
2 medium zucchini, diced	

Rub corn with 2 tablespoons of coconut oil; roast in 400°F oven for 20 to 24 minutes, turning occasionally. Remove corn from oven and let cool. Cut corn from cob, yielding about 2 cups corn. Heat remaining oil in a 12-inch heavy skillet over moderate heat until hot, but not smoking; then cook scallions, stirring occasionally, until softened, about 3 minutes. Add garlic and cook, stirring for 1 minute.

Add corn, zucchini, cumin, salt, and pepper, and cook, stirring occasionally until zucchini is tender, 4–6 minutes. Stir in cilantro and season with salt and pepper.

Serves 4.

Chef Carol's comment: "Quick and easy, roasting the corn makes all the flavor difference."

Nutritional facts per serving: 136 calories; 10 g fat (59.3 percent calories from fat); 3 g protein; 13 g carbohydrate; 2 g dietary fiber; 0 mg cholesterol; 101 mg sodium.

———

Southwest Chopped Chicken Salad With Whole-Grain Mustard Balsamic Dressing

4 single chicken breasts	2 cups cherry tomatoes, halved
2 Tbsp. extra-virgin coconut oil	¼ cup green onions, minced
½ cup balsamic vinegar	3 Tbsp. cilantro, rough chopped
½ cup corn kernels	3 Tbsp. peppadew, finely chopped
1½ cups black beans	2 cups romaine lettuce, shredded
¾ cup celery, diced	1 jalapeño chili pepper, finely diced

BEFORE BEGINNING: Peppadew is a pepper native to South Africa; it's available pickled in supermarkets across the United States.

Sauté chicken breasts in a little coconut oil over medium high heat. When almost cooked through, add balsamic vinegar to pan; allow to reduce to a syrupy consistency, turning chicken often. Remove to plate and allow to cool. Cube chicken. Toss together remaining ingredients and chicken. Serve with whole-grain balsamic dressing on the side.

For the Whole-Grain Mustard Balsamic Dressing, whisk 3 tablespoons lemon juice, 2 tablespoons whole-grain mustard, ½ cup olive oil, and 1 teaspoon honey.

Serves 4.

Chef Carol's comment: "I fell in love with Tex-Mex flavors living in Texas, flavors that challenge and wake up the palate, as in this chopped salad."

Nutritional facts per serving with the dressing: 509 calories; 25 g fat (83.7 percent calories from fat); 32 g protein; 43 g carbohydrate; 9 g dietary fiber; 62 mg cholesterol; 84 mg sodium.

——

Grilled Chicken and Pineapple Salad With Basil and Mint

Fresh mayonnaise dressing

4 egg yolks, raw or from three-minute hard-boiled eggs

3 Tbsp. Dijon mustard

Pinch sea salt

Pinch cayenne pepper

3 Tbsp. lemon juice

1 cup extra-virgin olive oil

2 Tbsp. raw honey

Marinade

4 Tbsp. lemon juice

2 Tbsp. Dijon mustard

3 Tbsp. olive oil

2 Tbsp. raw honey

1 Tbsp. seafood seasoning

8 chicken breasts, boned and skinned

¼ cup green onion, chopped

3 pineapples

1 red bell pepper

½ cup celery, diced

¼ cup basil leaf, julienned

3 Tbsp. mint, chopped

SPECIAL EQUIPMENT: Food processor

To make the mayonnaise: Place egg yolks, mustard, salt, cayenne pepper, and half the lemon juice in food processor. Blend just enough to combine ingredients; then, with machine running, add olive oil in slow stream. Add remaining lemon juice and honey. The mayonnaise will be very runny, as it is mayonnaise dressing. Pour in container and store in refrigerator until needed.

Combine all marinade ingredients and whisk together. Butterfly the chicken breasts to allow for even cooking, cover in marinade, and refrigerate overnight. Halve the pineapples, with tops intact, and scoop out the flesh in two or three large chunks using a grapefruit knife or curved paring knife. Discard the core and cut remaining pieces in ½-inch chunks. Set aside scooped out pineapple halves for use later as serving bowls.

Heat grill on high, and grill chicken breasts. Allow to cool. Then cut into 1-inch pieces and dress with mayonnaise dressing. Lightly toss chicken pieces with pineapple chunks and remaining salad ingredients. Scoop evenly into pineapple boats and serve.

Serves 6.

Chef Carol's comment: "Grilling the chicken adds a new dimension to this flavorful salad with fresh mayonnaise. Presented in pineapple boats, it is perfect for summer outdoor entertaining."

Nutritional facts per serving: 556 calories; 37 g fat (59.1 percent calories from fat); 28 g protein; 30 g carbohydrate; 3 g dietary fiber; 184 mg cholesterol; 218 mg sodium.

Blended Chocolate Mocha Mousse

½ cup strong coffee, organic, fresh-brewed, and hot

1 envelope beef gelatin

2 oz. dark chocolate bar, 80 percent cacao, finely chopped

3 egg whites

2 scoops powdered chocolate whole-food meal supplement

¾ cup heavy cream

2 oz. cacao chocolate

½ cup ice water

1 tsp. stevia

Pour hot coffee in small bowl; sprinkle the gelatin over it. Stir to dissolve. Add chopped chocolate. Stir to dissolve; then allow to cool. Pour coffee and chocolate mixture into blender. Add egg whites and blend on high for two minutes.

With the blender running, slowly add the powdered whole-food meal supplement, ice water, and stevia. Add ½ cup of the heavy cream and blend to a soft creamy texture; do not overwhip, as it will clot. Pour into individual ramekins, and allow to set in refrigerator to firm. Whip remaining cream. Top each ramekin with a spoonful, and then sprinkle with cacao chocolate.

Serves 4.

Chef Carol's comment: "I have a terrible sweet tooth, and this quick, easy, and very luxurious dessert is a great treat. Be sure to use good quality 80 percent cacao for full flavor."

Nutritional facts per serving: 269 calories; 16 g fat (70.5 percent calories from fat); 12 g protein; 20 g carbohydrate; 5 g dietary fiber; 11 mg cholesterol; 75 mg sodium.

Baked Herbed Eggplant With Tomatoes and Caramelized Onions

2 large eggplants (approximately 3 lbs.)

Sea salt, sprinkled

⅓ cup extra-virgin coconut oil, as needed

2 medium yellow onions, halved and sliced

4 cloves garlic, minced

15 oz. fresh tomato, red ripe, chopped

4 Tbsp. fresh parsley, finely chopped

½ cup whole-milk yogurt

½ cup crème fraîche

2 Tbsp. fresh dill, finely chopped

¼ cup Parmesan cheese (raw pecorino), grated

2 Tbsp. chives, snipped

Pinch sea salt and fresh ground pepper

Slice eggplant into ¾-inch rounds. Lay in a colander, and sprinkle liberally with salt. Allow to rest for 30 minutes until beads appear on the flesh. Rinse lightly and pat dry. (Salting the eggplant and allowing the bitter juices to degorge also allow less oil to be used in cooking. The eggplant will cook through properly in the baking process and soak up the wonderful flavors from the tomato and onions.)

While the eggplant is resting, heat a heavy-bottom pan over medium heat; add just enough coconut oil to lightly coat the bottom. Add onions and cook, stirring occasionally, scraping the bottom of the pan with a flat wooden spoon. (This is a patient process, but it's worth it as the onions begin to caramelize in their own natural sugars.)

Remove the onions to a plate and heat a ¼-inch depth of coconut oil in the pan. Fry the eggplant slices, a few at a time, turning until golden brown. Drain on kitchen paper. Heat a little more coconut oil in another pan and sauté the garlic for a few minutes. Add the tomatoes and simmer on low heat for 15 minutes. Season with salt and pepper. Reserving half the parsley, stir together the yogurt, crème fraîche, and herbs, and season to taste.

Preheat the oven to 350°F. Line the bottom of a medium ovenproof dish with a thin layer of tomatoes. Top with a layer of eggplant, followed by onions and eggplant again. Top with the remaining tomato sauce and finish off with the yogurt sauce. Sprinkle the cheese on top and bake for 20 to 25 minutes. Scatter remaining parsley and chives on top.

Serves 4.

Chef Carol's comment: "Rich and colorful, this fabulous dish is a wonderful accompaniment to fish or alone as a main dish with a side salad. Slowly caramelizing the onions is time consuming, but it imparts a rich flavor to this dish."

Nutritional facts per serving: 290 calories; 23 g fat (65.9 percent calories from fat); 6 g protein; 20 g carbohydrate; 6 g dietary fiber; 26 mg cholesterol; 105 mg sodium.

Herb-Crusted Rack of Lamb With Port Shallot Gravy

Gravy

12 small shallots	3 Tbsp. extra-virgin olive oil
6 cloves garlic	3 cups lamb stock
¼ cup balsamic vinegar	½ cup ruby port
1 tsp. raw sugar	

Herb-Crusted Rack of Lamb

2 1¼-lb. racks of lamb, French trimmed	4 small sprigs rosemary
½ cup Dijon mustard	4 small sprigs thyme
2 cloves garlic	½ cup grated pecorino cheese
2 cups yeast-free sourdough bread crumbs	¼ cup olive oil
½ cup fresh basil leaves	Sea salt and pepper to taste
½ cup fresh parsley leaves	

SPECIAL EQUIPMENT: Instant red meat thermometer, food processor, and stick immersion blender

Preheat oven to 425°F.

To prepare gravy: Combine shallots, garlic, balsamic vinegar, raw sugar, and 2 tablespoons olive oil in a shallow baking pan. Roast until shallots are caramelized, stirring a few times, about 20–30 minutes. In a pan, bring port and lamb stock to a boil; simmer until reduced by half, and season. Add caramelized shallots and garlic, and blend with a stick blender. Strain and set aside.

To prepare the lamb: In food processor, mince garlic; add sourdough crumbs and grated pecorino cheese. Then add herbs, using on/off turns. With machine running, slowly add olive oil, just enough to bind the mixture together. Season with a little salt and pepper. Brush lamb with Dijon mustard; then press the crumb mixture evenly over the lamb, keeping the bones clean to prevent them from burning. Arrange bone side down on a baking sheet and roast until meat thermometer inserted into center of lamb registers 135°F for medium rare, about 25 minutes. Let lamb rest for 15 minutes; then transfer to cutting board, and cut into individual or double chops. Serve with Port Shallot gravy.

Serves 6.

Chef Carol's comment: "For an elegant presentation, ask your butcher to 'French' the rack of lamb, which is trimming the fat from the end of the bones. With an herb crust and oven roasted, this dish has rich flavor and tender consistency, and is Jordan's favorite dish I have made to date!"

Nutritional facts per serving: 748 calories; 63 g fat (74.9 percent calories from fat); 29 g protein; 19 g carbohydrate; 1 g dietary fiber; 117 mg cholesterol; 568 mg sodium.

Butternut Orange Soup

2 Tbsp. clarified butter (ghee)	2 large butternut squash, peeled, rough cubed
1 yellow onion, rough diced	1 large sweet potato, peeled and cubed
2 medium carrots, rough chopped	4 cups fresh squeezed orange juice
2 celery ribs, chopped	½ gallon chicken stock
4 cloves garlic, minced	Sea salt and pepper, to taste
1 tsp. nutmeg	1 cup heavy cream
3 tsp. cinnamon	Chives or parsley, for garnish

Heat 1 tablespoon butter in large stockpot over medium heat. Add the onions, and slow cook until caramelized. Add remaining butter, carrots, celery, and garlic; cook approximately 15 more minutes. Add spices, and cook a few minutes. Add butternut squash, sweet potato, and chicken stock. Simmer approximately 1 hour until all are tender. Purée soup, add orange juice, and adjust seasoning to taste. Serve, garnished with a swirl of cream and chopped chives or parsley.

Serves 4.

Chef Carol's comment: "Warming winter soup with a new twist."

Nutritional facts per serving: 400 calories; 28 g fat (62.8 percent calories from fat); 11 g protein; 27 g carbohydrate; 4 g dietary fiber; 34 mg cholesterol; 435 mg sodium.

Cardamom Poached Pear With Chocolate Glaze and Crème Fraîche

4 pears, slightly under ripe	¼ cup raw honey
1 cup pear juice	4 oz. dark chocolate bar, 80 percent cacao, grated
¼ cup white balsamic vinegar	
4 pods cardamom	½ cup crème fraîche

Keeping the stalks intact, peel pears with a vegetable peeler. Set pears aside. Stir together pear juice, vinegar, cardamom, and honey in saucepan just big enough to hold the pears on their side. Bring the liquid to a boil; then add pears to the pan. Cover and reduce heat. Simmer, turning pears twice with a rubber spatula, until they are tender, about 8 minutes. Remove pears from pan; then stand up in individual serving dishes.

Whisk chocolate into sauce until melted. Pour over pears. Serve with crème fraîche on the side.

Serves 4.

Chef Carol's comment: "An elegant dinner party dessert, the chocolate melted in the poaching liquid makes for an instant sauce."

Nutritional facts per serving: 427 calories; 18 g fat (34.9 percent calories from fat); 3 g protein; 73 g carbohydrate; 7 g dietary fiber; 27 mg cholesterol; 25 mg sodium.

Beef Tenderloin Salad With Pomegranate and Avocado

Marinade and dressing

2 Tbsp. pomegranate syrup*	1 Tbsp. Dijon mustard
½ cup pomegranate juice	2 tsp. red pepper flakes
3 Tbsp. tamari soy sauce	Sea salt and pepper
½ cup extra-virgin olive oil	1 Tbsp. extra-virgin coconut oil

*Note: Pomegranate syrup can be bought at specialty stores. If you can't find it, boil down pomegranate juice and reduce it to about a third of the original volume.

1½ lbs. beef tenderloin steak, grass fed

Salad

3 cups lettuce, mâche

3 cups lettuce, spring mix

8 oz. spinach, baby leaves

3 avocados, sliced

½ cup spring onion, minced

1 cup feta cheese

1 cup sunflower sprouts

1½ cups pomegranate seeds

Combine all marinade ingredients and whisk together.

Heat grill or a grill pan to high heat. Season beef steaks with salt and pepper. Add coconut oil to pan, and grill beef steaks on high, 2–3 minutes per side, until still very rare in the middle. Remove to a plate, allow to cool, and slice thinly. Spoon just enough marinade over to coat; allow to marinate for several hours.

To assemble, toss salad leaves with just enough dressing to coat. Pile on serving plate, and place beef on top. Surround with avocado slices, and sprinkle feta, sprouts, and pomegranate seeds over the top.

Serves 6.

Chef Carol's comment: "A luxurious and beautiful salad; grass-fed beef steak in a tangy pomegranate marinade, thinly sliced and served with avocado and pomegranate jewels. The marinade 'cooks' the beef, so be sure not to overcook it when searing."

Nutritional facts per serving: 605 calories; 52 g fat (74.8 percent calories from fat); 21 g protein; 18 g carbohydrate; 4 g dietary fiber; 70 mg cholesterol; 626 mg sodium.

Fettuccine With Creamy Wild Mushroom Sauce

1 cup hot water

¼ cup dried porcini mushrooms

2 lbs. mushrooms, variety

3 Tbsp. clarified butter (ghee)

2 shallots, finely chopped

2 cloves garlic, minced

¼ cup dry white wine

½ cup chicken stock

1 cup crème fraîche

12 oz. fettuccine (whole-wheat, spelt, or sprouted pasta)

½ cup Parmesan cheese, grated

Chives, for garnish

Sea salt and pepper to taste

Pour cup hot water over porcini mushrooms and allow to soak for an hour. Remove mushrooms and strain, soaking liquid through cheesecloth to remove impurities. Set aside mushroom broth for use later. Finely mince porcini mushrooms.

Slice your other mushroom selection. Heat a large heavy-bottomed pan over high heat. Add a little butter and sauté mushrooms in batches. Remove from pan and set aside.

Reduce heat and sauté shallots, garlic, and porcini mushrooms until softened. Turn heat up to medium high; add white wine and reduce down to a syrupy consistency. Add chicken stock and mushroom broth; simmer until reduced by half. Return mushrooms to the pan. Add crème fraîche, season, and allow to simmer gently for 10 minutes. In the meantime, cook pasta in salted water to tender. Drain pasta, then toss through the sauce. Serve topped with Parmesan and snipped chives.

Serves 4.

Chef Carol's comment: "The yacht I cooked for docked in Portland, Maine, one summer, and I discovered a fabulous market with the most gorgeous and exotic mushrooms I had ever seen! After provisioning, I went back onboard and created this pasta dish for very happy guests and crew. When selecting fresh mushrooms, they should be firm to the touch and not spongy. Look out for an exotic blend readily available at many markets, such as portabella, shiitake, cremini, oyster, and maitake."

Nutritional facts per serving: 595 calories; 22 g fat (41.1 percent calories from fat); 20 g protein; 80 g carbohydrate; 5 g dietary fiber; 57 mg cholesterol; 427 mg sodium.

Appendix B

Snacks From Chef Mandy

OUR SNACK RECIPES come from Mandilyn Canistelle, a graduate of Living Light Culinary Arts Institute in Fort Bragg, California, where she received her certification as a raw food chef and instructor. Mandy teaches raw culinary arts classes in Edmond, Oklahoma, where she's a mother of five. Like Chef Carol Green, Chef Mandy has appeared on my weekly television series, *Extraordinary Health*, in a segment called, "Snack in a Minute," where Mandy shares recipes for quick raw snacks on the go.

Many of these recipes entail using a dehydrator, a small home appliance for drying fresh food yourself. They come in a variety of sizes and work by very gently heating the air and blowing throughout the food drying area. They generally cost a couple of hundred dollars and up.

For more information about Mandilyn Canistelle and her booklet, *Raw Fast Food*, go online to www.chefmandy.com. For products like sea salt, honey, flaxseed, extra-virgin coconut oil, powdered whole-food meal supplement, and protein powder, please see the Maker's Diet Resource Guide on page 263.

Asian Nori Crackers

Asian Nori Crackers can be made from the leftover Sunny Sunflower Pâté (page 250) by adding chickpea miso paste and spreading the mixture onto Nori sea vegetable sheets. Below is the actual recipe.

2 cups sunflower seeds, soaked overnight

1 apple, chopped

½ red onion, chopped

3 stalks celery, chopped

6 organic dill pickles or a handful of fresh dill, chopped

¼ cup any chickpea miso paste

¼ cup whole dulse

2 Tbsp. lemon juice

2 Tbsp. dulse granules

2 tsp. wasabi

¼ cup any variety of miso paste

1 package dried Nori sheets

2 cups sesame seeds

SPECIAL EQUIPMENT: Dehydrator

Soak sunflower seeds for 8 hours in filtered water. Prepare ingredients. Process all ingredients, except for Nori sheets and sesame seeds, in food processor. Spread on Nori sheets, sprinkle with sesame seeds, and dehydrate at 105°F until dry. Cut into desired shapes. Store in the freezer to keep on hand.

Makes 8–10 full sheets of Nori.

Avocado Rice Boats

Cauliflower, a member of the cruciferous family, is a vegetable that is often overlooked. It is an excellent source of fiber that helps to improve colon health.

Cauliflower rice

1 head cauliflower, chopped

1 cup pine nuts

1 tsp. sea salt

Boat ingredients

8 avocados, diced with reserved shells

4 ears of corn, kernelled

4 tomatoes, seeded, and diced

SPECIAL EQUIPMENT: Food processor

Wash and chop cauliflower. Place rice ingredients in food processor and blend until mixture is slightly crumbly and slightly sticky. Prepare boat ingredients and toss with cauliflower rice. Fill each shell and serve on a large serving platter to accommodate eight to sixteen people. Only half of the meat of each avocado will be used in this recipe. The other half can be made into guacamole for another snack.

Serves 8–16.

Fruit Roll-Ups

Fruit roll-ups can be made from leftover fresh fruit smoothies by simply adding more fruit and agave to the mixture. Below is the actual recipe for fruit roll-ups, thicker and sweeter than a typical fruit smoothie.

1 cup fresh squeezed orange juice

2 cups grapes

2 fresh bananas

¼ cup agave

1 cup desired chopped fruit: peaches, nectarines, pineapple, blueberries, strawberries, mango, etc.

SPECIAL EQUIPMENT: Vita-Mix blender

Prepare orange juice and fruit. Blend ingredients in a Vita-Mix blender until smooth and creamy. Pour nine small disks for each solid dehydrator sheet without spreading or smoothing them and dehydrate at 105°F until completely dry. Flipping the roll-up is not necessary. Peel the roll-up from the solid sheet when completely dry. If roll-up does not peel easily, continue drying and check every 2 hours. Fruit roll-ups can be rolled, or cookie cutouts can entertain children with dried sheets of fruit. Store in the freezer until ready to eat.

Makes 5 trays of roll-ups.

Easy Guacamole

The U.S. government recently revised its official nutrition guidelines to urge all of us to eat more avocados because the "good" fat in avocado helps to lower cholesterol levels. The avocado is also full of vitamin E, which is wonderful for the skin.

1 Tbsp. lime juice, from fresh lime

8 ripe avocados

1 tsp. garlic powder

1 tsp. onion powder

½ tsp. ground cumin

½ tsp. sea salt

¼ tsp. celery seed (optional)

SPECIAL EQUIPMENT: Juicing gadget, bowl, and fork

Juice lime. Mash flesh of avocados, leaving some chunky bits to add texture. Combine remaining ingredients. Serve on a top a bed of organic mixed greens with flax chips or cut-up veggies.

Makes 1 pint.

Fresh Fruit Smoothies

One of the most popular fruits, the orange is a delightful snack or recipe ingredient. Oranges are known as an excellent source of vitamin C. In addition, they contain 170 different phytonutrients.

4 cups fresh squeezed orange juice

2 cups grapes

2 cups packaged frozen tropical fruit
(pineapple, 2 frozen bananas, blueberries,
and/or strawberries)

Powdered whole-food meal supplement

SPECIAL EQUIPMENT: Vita-Mix blender

Peel and freeze bananas. Blend ingredients in a Vita-Mix until smooth and creamy. Serve in a tall glass with any desired fruit toppings.

Serves 8.

Key Lime Mousse

Limes are an excellent source of vitamin C and have antioxidant and anticancer properties. They help to build a strong immune system.

3 avocados

½ cup raw agave

½ cup lime juice

2 Tbsp. lime zest

Dash sea salt

3 kiwis

3 bananas

6 raspberries

6 lime wedges

SPECIAL EQUIPMENT: Vita-Mix blender

Process all ingredients—except kiwis, bananas, raspberries, and lime wedges—in a Vita-Mix. Serve in a small glass dessert bowl and garnish with fruit toppings.

Serves 6.

Key Lime Tart

Key Lime Tart can be made from the leftover Key Lime Mousse by adding extra-virgin coconut oil and creamy raw honey. Below is the actual recipe for this delicious dessert.

Crust

1 cup macadamia nuts

1 cup shredded coconut

2 Tbsp. agave

1 teaspoon sea salt

Mousse

3 avocados

¾ cup raw agave

½ cup lime juice

2 Tbsp. lime zest

2 Tbsp. extra-virgin coconut oil

1 Tbsp. creamy raw honey

Dash sea salt

Filtered water, small amount only if needed to blend

Toppings

8 kiwis

1 cup mixture of fruit compote (bananas, lime, strawberries)

SPECIAL EQUIPMENT: Vita-Mix blender and food processor

To make the crust, grind macadamia nuts with the coconut in a food processor until crumbly. Add agave and salt while the machine is running. Do not overprocess to a mush state. Remove and press into small spring form tartlets.

To make the mousse, process all ingredients in a Vita-Mix blender. Pour the mixture into the tartlets and freeze until ready to serve.

When ready to serve, pop out of the spring form tart immediately from the freezer. Do not thaw. Serve on a white plate with layered kiwis and fruit compote.

Serves 8.

Oatmeal Raisin Cookies

Oatmeal Raisin Cookies can be made from the leftover Nutty Dates (below) by adding a ripe plantain or banana and whole oats or quinoa flakes. Dates are valuable for their tonic effect. Being easily digested, they are very useful for supplying energy and treating occasional constipation since the roughage stimulates sluggish bowels.

1 cup nuts (walnuts, pecans, and/or almonds)	1 cup raisins
1 cup macadamia nuts	1 tsp. cinnamon
1 cup coconut	½ tsp. Celtic Sea Salt
1 cup dates, soaked	1 cup whole oats or quinoa flakes
2 Tbsp. creamy raw honey	¼ cup protein powder (optional)
1 very ripe plantain or banana	

SPECIAL EQUIPMENT: Food processor

Process walnuts, pecans, and/or almonds in food processor until crumbly. Remove to large mixing bowl.

Process macadamia nuts and coconut until crumbly. Add to the nut mixture. Process dates, honey, and plantain (or banana) until creamy. Add to the nut mixture. Add remaining ingredients and mix well with hands until thoroughly blended. Drop by tablespoon onto a solid sheet and dehydrate at 105°F until a crust forms. Flip and crust the bottom side. Cookies will have a moist, chewy, fresh-out-of-the-oven taste on the inside with a crust on the outside.

Serve on a wooden plate surrounded by other dehydrated fruit, or they can be frozen or used for a quick, easy, satisfying snack later.

Makes 2 dozen.

Nutty Dates

Macadamias contain a significant amount of protein comprising all the essential amino acids.

1 cup nuts (walnuts, pecans, and/or almonds)

1 cup macadamia nuts

1 cup shredded coconut

1 cup pitted dates, soaked

2 Tbsp. creamy raw honey

1 cup raisins

1½ tsp. Celtic Sea Salt

1 Tbsp. orange zest (optional)

1 tsp. cinnamon (optional)

¼ cup ground-up flaxseed (optional)

Coating

1 cup sesame seeds

1 cup finely ground coconut

SPECIAL EQUIPMENT: Food processor and zester

Process walnuts, pecans, and/or almonds in food processor until crumbly. Remove to large mixing bowl. Process macadamia nuts and coconut until crumbly. Add to the nut mixture. Process dates and honey until creamy. Add to the nut mixture. Add remaining ingredients and mix well with hands until thoroughly blended. Shape into small balls and roll in sesame seeds and/or finely ground coconut.

These little morsels are wonderful to freeze and make for a quick, easy, satisfying snack.

Makes 40–50.

Pastel Parfaits

They say money doesn't grow on trees? In some islands earlier in history, whole coconuts were used as currency for the purchase of goods. Coconuts are the fruit of the coconut palm.

Creamy Coconut Sauce

2 cups young Thai coconut meat, chopped

2 Tbsp. lemon juice

2 Tbsp. raw cashew butter

2 Tbsp. creamy raw honey

2 Tbsp. extra-virgin coconut oil

1 tsp. vanilla

¼ tsp. Celtic Sea Salt

Fruit toppings

1 cup chopped strawberries for bottom layer

1 cup chopped bananas for middle layer

1 cup chopped peaches for top layer

1 cup cluster of blueberries to top

1 cup shredded coconut for garnish

SPECIAL EQUIPMENT: Juicing gadget, bowl, and fork

Open enough young Thai coconuts for approximately 2 cups chopped coconut meat. Reserve the coconut water, if needed, for blending. Juice lemons to get 2 tablespoons lemon juice. Process sauce ingredients in Vita-Mix blender until smooth and creamy. Layer parfaits with 2 tablespoons each of strawberries, bananas, and peaches. Drizzle ¼ cup of the cream sauce over fruit. Top with 2 tablespoons each of blueberries and shredded coconut. Serve parfaits in crystal goblets.

Serves 8.

Sherbet Sundaes

Sherbet Sundaes can be made by freezing the leftovers from the Pastel Parfait sauce. Below is an actual recipe for Sherbet Sundaes with all the toppings.

Sherbet

2 cups young Thai coconut meat, chopped	2 Tbsp. extra-virgin coconut oil
2 Tbsp. lemon juice	1 tsp. vanilla
2 Tbsp. raw cashew butter	¼ tsp. Celtic Sea Salt
2 Tbsp. creamy raw honey	4 bananas, peeled and frozen

Strawberry Agave Sauce

2 cups chopped strawberries

¼ cup agave

Toppings

A variety of chopped nuts

Shredded coconut

Medley of fresh berries

SPECIAL EQUIPMENT: Vita-Mix blender, citrus juicer, any Twin Gear or Champion juicer

To make the sherbet, open enough young Thai coconuts for approximately 2 cups chopped coconut meat. Reserve the coconut water, if needed, for blending. Juice lemons to get 2 tablespoons lemon juice.

Process sherbet ingredients, except for bananas, in a Vita-Mix blender until smooth and creamy. Freeze in ice cube trays. Run through a juicer with a blank screen with frozen bananas.

To make the strawberry agave sauce, blend ingredients in a Vita-Mix until smooth. Serve sherbet in small dessert dishes with toppings and strawberry agave sauce.

Serves 8.

Sliced Apples With Cheese

Cheeses can be made from leftover dips and dressings. The Dilly Dip (page 252) makes a great cheese by simply adding nutritional yeast flakes, miso, flax meal, and turmeric to the dip recipe. Below is the actual recipe for a cheese. The dill has also been omitted from the recipe.

¼ cup golden flaxseeds, ground up

2 Tbsp. lemon juice

½ cup raw tahini

2 zucchini, peeled and chopped

1 cup chopped celery

1 clove garlic, pressed

1 pitted date, soaked

½ cup nutritional yeast flakes

2 Tbsp. chickpea miso

1 tsp. onion powder

1 tsp. Celtic Sea Salt

1 tsp. turmeric

¼ cup protein powder (optional)

SPECIAL EQUIPMENT: Vita-Mix blender, coffee grinder, and citrus juicer

Grind golden flaxseeds in a coffee grinder to make flax meal, or use flaxseeds already ground up. Juice lemons. Prepare vegetables. Blend ingredients, except flax meal, until smooth and creamy. Pulse flax meal at the end. Pour small disks onto solid dehydrator sheets and dehydrate at 105°F until dry. Serve with an array of fresh cut-up apples.

Serves 8.

Sunny Sunflower Pâté

Sunflower seeds are an excellent natural source of vitamin E.

2 cups sunflower seeds, soaked 8 hrs.

1 apple, chopped

½ red onion, chopped

3 stalks celery, chopped

6 organic dill pickles or a handful of fresh dill, chopped

¼ cup chickpea miso paste

¼ cup whole dulse

2 Tbsp. lemon juice

2 Tbsp. dulse granules

2 tsp. wasabi (optional)

Garnish

Ground-up flaxseeds, sprinkled

6 tomatoes, 3 large slices per person

1 cup alfalfa sprouts

2 cucumbers, sliced

24 lemon swirls, or 3 per person, made from cutting a lemon slice ¾ of the way through and twisting to sit on a plate

SPECIAL EQUIPMENT: Food processor

Soak sunflower seeds for eight hours in filtered water. Prepare and process ingredients in a food processor.

Serve 3 small scoops of Sunny Sunflower Pâté on each tomato with garnishes.

Serves 8.

Taco Lettuce Wraps

Walnuts are one of the best plant sources of protein and omega-3 fatty acids. They are rich in fiber, B vitamins, magnesium, and antioxidants such as vitamin E. Walnuts also aid in the lowering of LDL cholesterol.

Taco "meat"

2 cups walnuts, soaked

1 bunch cilantro

⅓ cup wheat-free tamari soy sauce

1 Tbsp. cumin powder

½ Tbsp. coriander powder

Taco wraps and toppings

1 head romaine lettuce

3 avocados, sliced

3 tomatoes, sliced

Sea salt to taste

SPECIAL EQUIPMENT: Food processor

In the afternoon of the day before, soak walnuts overnight in filtered water. On the day of, process taco "meat" ingredients in a food processor until the mixture resembles ground taco meat. Stop to scrape sides. Remove and set aside. Wash and choose firm crispy lettuce leaves for taco wraps. Slice avocados and tomatoes. Fill lettuce cavities with taco "meat" and top with toppings. Serve two tacos on a white salad plate with a favorite Mexican seasoning on top.

Serves 8.

Veggies With Dilly Dip

Tahini is made from sesame seed kernels. Not only are sesame seeds a good source of manganese and copper, but they are also an excellent source of calcium, magnesium, iron, phosphorous, vitamin B_1, zinc, and dietary fiber.

Dilly Dip

½ cup raw tahini

2 zucchini, peeled and chopped

1 cup chopped celery

1 clove garlic, pressed

2 Tbsp. lemon juice

2 pitted dates, soaked

1 tsp. onion powder

1 tsp. Celtic Sea Salt

¾ cup fresh dill

1 Tbsp. protein powder (optional)

Veggies

4 celery stalks, julienned

4 carrots, julienned

2 cucumbers, sliced

2 red bell peppers, circles

1 yellow squash, julienned

1 head broccoli spears

1 cup mushrooms, sliced

A handful of snow peas

SPECIAL EQUIPMENT: Vita-Mix blender and citrus juicer

Juice lemons. Blend Dilly Dip ingredients, except fresh dill, until smooth and creamy. Add dill and pulse until mixed throughout. Refrigerate for an hour to thicken and cool. Serve with an array of fresh cut-up vegetables.

Serves 8.

Veggie Patties

Veggie patties can be made from the leftovers of Taco Lettuce Wraps (page 251) by adding a few ingredients. These make great raw meals to store in the freezer for a quick dinner to warm in the dehydrator and throw on a salad.

Taco "meat"

2 cups walnuts, soaked

1 bunch cilantro

⅓ cup wheat-free tamari soy sauce

1 Tbsp. cumin powder

½ Tbsp. coriander powder

¼ cup first cold-pressed olive oil

½ cup flax meal

2 Tbsp. barbeque seasoning

Marinated veggies

2 Tbsp. wheat-free tamari soy sauce

¼ cup cold-pressed olive oil

1 Tbsp. lemon juice

2 cups variety of chopped veggies (red bell pepper, cremini mushrooms, red onions, and broccoli)

Toppings

1 head green leaf lettuce leaves

3 slices of colored bell peppers (per person)

1 slice cheese (per person)

2 Tbsp. sprouts (per person)

3 red onion rings (per person)

1 large slice of tomato (per person)

3 slices of small cucumbers (per person)

.1 dollop of guacamole (per person; see recipe on page 245)

1 radish flower for garnish (per person)

SPECIAL EQUIPMENT: Food processor

Soak walnuts in filtered water for 8 hours. Combine marinated veggie ingredients and let set in refrigerator for 4 hours. Process "meat" ingredients in a food processor until the mixture resembles ground taco meat. Remove and mix with the veggies. Form into patties and dehydrate at 105°F for 4 hours. Flip for 2–4 more hours. Patties will be moist inside and have a crust on the outside. Serve on a white dinner plate with all the toppings.

Serves 8.

Shiitake Chow Mein

The Orient is known for healthy low-fat dishes. This one is no exception. If noodles symbolize long lifespan in the Orient, then this raw version rivals the classic one not only in taste but also in promoting longevity filled with live nutrients, enzymes, and fiber.

Noodles

2 parsnips, spiralized

2 carrots, spiralized

1 zucchini, spiralized

1 cup Mung bean sprouts

½ cup julienne jicama

Shiitake

2 cups sliced shiitake mushrooms

2 Tbsp. poultry seasoning

Sea salt to taste (optional)

Fresh ground pepper, to taste (optional)

Oriental Dressing

1 green onion, chopped

3 sprigs cilantro leaves

2 Tbsp. minced scallion

1 Tbsp. minced cilantro

2 Tbsp. wheat-free tamari soy sauce

1½ Tbsp. lemon juice

1 Tbsp. raw honey

1 tsp. minced ginger

2 Tbsp. toasted sesame oil

1 Tbsp. raw sesame oil

Seed garnish

2 Tbsp. hulled sesame or hemp seeds

2 Tbsp. ground-up flaxseeds

SPECIAL EQUIPMENT: Vita-Mix, chef knife, peeler or paring knife, spiralizer, shredder or kitchen shears

To make noodles, spiralize, combine, and cut long noodles; then set aside in mixing bowl. To make shiitake, combine ingredients and toss with noodles. To make the dressing, blend ingredients in a Vita-Mix and coat the noodles. Serve on a bowl of noodles garnished with hemp seeds and sesame seeds.

Serves 8.

Vietnamese Spring Rolls

Vietnamese Spring Rolls are fun to create and a beautiful way to present a salad.

Vegetable filling

2 cups Shiitake Chow Mein

3 green onions, slivered

4 cups Mung bean sprouts

1 cup fresh mint leaves

1 small bunch cilantro

2 heads Napa cabbage

Mock chicken filling

2 cups sliced shiitake mushrooms

2 Tbsp. poultry seasoning

Celtic Sea Salt, to taste

Fresh ground pepper, to taste

Other ingredients

8 Vietnamese wrappers

1 cup Oriental Dressing (above)

1 cup Tahini Ginger Sauce (page 255)

SPECIAL EQUIPMENT: Chef knife, spiralizer, or shredder

Prepare vegetable ingredients and create an assembly line for quick stacking. Dip wrapper in a tray of filtered water. Lay the wrapper on a flat, clean surface. Lay two Napa leaves on the bottom half of the rice wrapper. Layer ingredients inside the leaves. Fold in the sides and tightly roll the wrapper, being careful not to rip the wrapper. Slant cut the roll and stack the two halves on top of one another. Serve stacked on top of each other with a side of Oriental Dressing and Tahini Ginger Sauce.

Serves 8.

Tahini Ginger Sauce

Tahini is a source of calcium, protein, B vitamins, and essential fatty acids, which help to maintain healthy skin. It is a wonderful alternative to peanut butter.

½ cup raw tahini

¼ cup filtered water

2 Tbsp. lemon juice

2 cloves garlic, pressed

2 Tbsp. raw honey

2 Tbsp. wheat-free tamari soy sauce

1 Tbsp. minced ginger

SPECIAL EQUIPMENT: Vita-Mix blender

Blend all ingredients until smooth. Add more filtered water if needed. Dip Vietnamese Spring Rolls into this sauce that rivals the classic peanut sauce.

Serves 8.

Clean Green Sweep

Green smoothies are an excellent meal choice because they provide healthy carbohydrates, vitamins, minerals, phytochemicals, and chlorophyll. They are also an excellent source of fiber. Favorite nutritious powders can be added for cleansing and extra nutrition.

Green Smoothie Base

2 bananas, peeled and frozen

2 cups green grapes

2 cups fresh pineapple

1 small cucumber, chopped

1 cup green chard

Crushed ice, as needed

SPECIAL EQUIPMENT: Vita-Mix blender

Peel and freeze bananas the night before. Blend all ingredients in a Vita-Mix until smooth and creamy. Serve in a tall glass with a straw.

Serves 8.

Beautiful Bread

Beautiful Bread can be made from leftover Clean Green Sweep (page 255).

2 cups Clean Green Sweep

¼ cup ground-up flaxseeds

SPECIAL EQUIPMENT: Vita-Mix blender or fork or spoon to mix

Mix or blend the ingredients until mixture is a batter texture. Spread a ¼-inch thick layer of batter on solid sheet and dehydrate at 105°F for 4 hours. Flip and continue drying. Bread will be moist. Slice into sandwich slices and store in the freezer until ready to eat.

Serves 8.

Apple Pear Sauce

An apple a day truly keeps the doctor away. Apples help weight control, provide insoluble and soluble fiber, and help relieve occasional constipation. The pectin in apples reduces cholesterol. This is a fresher, tastier applesauce to encourage eating apples.

2 cups apples, peeled and chopped

2 cups pears, peeled and chopped

1 banana, peeled and sliced

1 tsp. lemon juice

Cinnamon, sprinkled to taste

SPECIAL EQUIPMENT: Vita-Mix blender or food processor

Process ingredients in food processor until desired texture is achieved. Refrigerate until ready to serve. Sprinkle with cinnamon. Serve as a comfort healthy snack, especially in fall or winter.

Makes 1 quart.

Apple Spice Cake

Apple Spice Cake can be made from leftover Apple Pear Sauce.

Cake layers

2 cups Apple Pear Sauce

1 cup soaked and dried pecans, ground

6 dates, soaked, or ⅓ cup date paste

1 scoop ground-up flaxseeds

1 Tbsp. cinnamon

1 Tbsp. vanilla

½ tsp. Celtic Sea Salt

Icing

2 cups pine nuts, soaked

2 pears, peeled and chopped

¼ cup raw honey

2 Tbsp. extra-virgin coconut oil

Topping

1 cup pecans and walnuts, mixed, chopped

¼ cup raw honey

1½ tsp. cinnamon

½ tsp. Celtic Sea Salt

Garnish

1 full slice of pear with stem and seeds (per person)

Cinnamon sprinkles (per person)

SPECIAL EQUIPMENT: Vita-Mix blender or food processor

Blend cake layer ingredients until smooth. Spread 2 cups cake batter on a solid sheet and dehydrate at 105°F for four hours. Flip and continue until dry. Blend icing ingredients in Vita-Mix blender until smooth, reserving some for garnishing slices. Place in freezer to firm up while layers are drying. Assemble cake, alternating between cake layers and icing until 3–4 inches in height. Freeze and slice for a quick healthy dessert to serve. Combine topping and place in freezer to firm. When ready to serve, remove cake and slice while frozen to reveal the beautiful layers.

Sprinkle Apple Spice Cake with topping, and garnish with a slice of pear and sprinkled cinnamon. Drizzle with reserved icing.

Serves 8.

Sunny Bunny

Sunny Bunny is the perfect juice to introduce any age to the world of juicing. Oranges and carrots are sweet and supply vitamin C, beta-carotene, and antioxidants.

16 carrots, peeled and chopped

8 oranges, juiced

SPECIAL EQUIPMENT: Twin Gear juicer and/or citrus juicer

Push ingredients separately through juicer to extract the juice. Keep carrot pulp separate to make other recipes. Optional method would be to juice the oranges in a citrus juicer.

Serve fresh squeezed juice in an elegant glass and sip slowly.

Serves 8.

Salmon Pâté

Salmon Pâté may look like a lot of work, but this tasty treat is worth it. This recipe can be made from leftover Sunny Bunny for a new creation.

Flaxnaise

1 cup filtered water

¼ cup lemon juice

2 tsp. ground mustard powder

1 Tbsp. raw honey

¼ cup golden flaxseeds, soaked, or ground-up

½ tsp. Celtic Sea Salt

Pâté

1½ cups carrot pulp

¾ cup Flaxnaise (from recipe above)

¾ cup minced onion

1 cup chopped dill

2 Tbsp. minced garlic

1 Tbsp. dulse

SPECIAL EQUIPMENT: Vita-Mix blender

To make Flaxnaise, grind flaxseeds to a meal or use flaxseeds already ground up. Blend soaked seeds with lemon juice in a Vita-Mix blender until whipped to a cream. Add filtered water, if needed, to prevent thickening. Texture should be smooth, not jellylike. Add remaining ingredients, and mix until blended.

To make pâté, prepare ingredients and combine in a mixing bowl. Refrigerate to chill. Serve pâté with flax crackers or flat bread, wrapped in a romaine leaf or a Nori sheet.

Serves 8.

Salmon Sushi

Salmon Sushi can be made from leftover Salmon Pâté for a new creation.

Rolls

2 cups Salmon Pâté (above)

2 red bell peppers, julienned

2 carrots, shredded or julienned

2 avocados, julienned

2 cups alfalfa sprouts, or any variety sprouts

2 cucumbers, seeded and thinly sliced

2 mangos, julienned

8 Nori seaweed sheets

Condiments

Wheat-free tamari

Pickled ginger

Wasabi

SPECIAL EQUIPMENT: Food processor

Prepare ingredients. To assemble rolls, lay one sheet of Nori, shiny side down. Layer ingredients stacked atop 2–3 rows on one-third of the Nori sheet closest to you. To roll the sushi, grip the edge of the Nori sheet with your thumbs and forefingers. Press the filling back with your other fingers. Roll the front end of the Nori over the filling. Pull the Nori back with your fingers, giving the roll a tight squeeze, and continue rolling. Seal the edge with water and set seam side down. Cut the roll into 8 pieces with a sharp knife.

Serve sushi with condiments for a satisfying flavorful snack or light meal.

Serves 8.

Break-Fast Salad

This salad is a great way to break a liquid fast. Dressing is not needed or missed because it satisfies every taste bud. The salad can be eaten any time during the day and can even replace a typical breakfast. Keep prepared ingredients refrigerated for easy assembly.

2 green leaf lettuce leaves, shredded	¼ cup raisins
1 slice red cabbage, shredded	2 bananas, diced
1 carrot, shredded	8 dates, diced
1 tomato, diced	4 small radishes, diced
1 stalk celery, diced	1 apple, shredded
1 plum or pear, diced	1 avocado, diced
1 peach or persimmon, diced	½ cup walnuts, chopped

SPECIAL EQUIPMENT: Chef knife

Layer ingredients in listed order, going from left to right. Arrange salad to include all the ingredients for a colorful display on a white dinner plate.

Serves 8.

Zucchini Bisque

This soup is a rich and creamy soup without the extra fat. Zucchini contains large amounts of folate, potassium, and magnesium.

6 zucchini, peeled and chopped	¼ cup lemon juice, from fresh lemon
6 stalks celery, chopped	¼ cup chickpea miso
3 cloves garlic, pressed	3 cups water, add to thin

Garnish

4 tomatoes, seeded and diced

Extra-virgin coconut oil, drizzled

SPECIAL EQUIPMENT: Citrus juicer and Vita-Mix blender

Juice lemon and prepare vegetables. Blend first six ingredients in Vita-Mix blender until smooth. Chill to refrigerate or warm on a stovetop to 100°, stirring constantly. Serve soup with diced tomatoes and extra-virgin coconut oil.

Serves 8.

———

Bounty Bars

Bounty Bars can be made from leftover Break-Fast Salad for a new creation.

2 cups Break-Fast Salad (page 259)

½ Tbsp. Celtic Sea Salt

1 cup soaked pitted dates or date paste

1 cup raisins or other choice of dried fruit

2 Tbsp. cinnamon

4 packages of cacao chocolate

2 cups mixture of seeds, soaked (sesame, flax, sunflower, and pumpkin)

SPECIAL EQUIPMENT: Dehydrator with solid and mesh sheets, and metal spatula

To make date paste, process or mash pitted and soaked dates to form a paste. Mix everything in a large mixing bowl with hands. Spread 6 cups of the mixture onto a solid dehydrator sheet. Smooth with a metal spatula and score into bars. Dehydrate at 105°F for four hours. Flip and continue until dry. Store bars in freezer container and keep frozen until ready to snack.

Serves 8.

———

ALT

ALTs (avocado, lettuce, and tomatoes) are made with zucchini wraps.

Flaxnaise

¼ cup golden flaxseeds, ground up

¼ cup lemon juice

1 cup filtered water

1 Tbsp. raw honey

2 tsp. ground mustard powder

½ tsp. Celtic Sea Salt

Filling

2 avocados, sliced

2 cups mixed greens

1 cup alfalfa sprouts

2 tomatoes, sliced

Mrs. Dash seasoning, to taste

SPECIAL EQUIPMENT: Dehydrator, coffee grinder, or Vita-Mix blender

Prepare filling ingredients. To make Flaxnaise, grind flaxseeds to a meal or use flaxseeds already ground up. Blend ingredients in a Vita-Mix blender. Texture should be smooth and not a jelly texture. Add more filtered water to prevent thickening. Fill wraps with filling and drizzle immediately with Flaxnaise.

Serve wraps as a light meal or quick snack.

Serves 8.

―――――

Tomatillo Salsa

This unique low-fat salsa explodes with flavor, using only fresh vegetables and herbs. *Tomatillo* means "little tomato" in Spanish. They are rich in potassium and have only 11 calories. In addition, tomatillos contain vitamins C and A, calcium, and folic acid.

6 tomatillos, chopped

3 red peppers, chopped

1 yellow sweet onion, chopped

1 anise bulb, chopped

2 Tbsp. ginger, minced

1 clove garlic, minced

¼ cup mixture of freshly minced thyme, basil, rosemary, and sage

SPECIAL EQUIPMENT: Food processor or chef knife

Pulse-chop all ingredients in food processor to reach a fresh salsa texture. Alternate method: dice all ingredients and toss. Refrigerate to blend flavors. Serve with fresh corn chips in a wooden chip and dip bowl.

Makes 1 pint.

―――――

Kim-Chi

Kim-Chi is made from leftover Tomatillo Salsa. Fermented foods are full of live enzymes and healthy flora to help digestion.

1 large head of cabbage, shredded with
several reserved

½ cup mixture of freshly minced thyme, basil,
rosemary, outside leaves and sage

1 head broccoli, chopped

1 cup chopped dandelion greens

1–2 cups lemon juice

2 Tbsp. ginger, pressed

2 cups Tomatillo Salsa (page 261)

2 cloves garlic, minced

1 Tbsp. celery seed

4 carrots, chopped

SPECIAL EQUIPMENT: Chef knife and/or food processor and citrus juicer

Slice cabbage, carrots, broccoli, and dandelion greens through a food processor using the slicing attachment. Juice lemons. Combine remaining ingredients and massage to wilt. Place slaw halfway full in a clean glass jar(s). Cover slaw and juices with reserved cabbage leaves to prevent spoilage. Place a smaller jar full of water with a lid inside to weigh down the slaw. Be careful to completely cover the mixture with the juices to prevent spoilage. Cover with a clean food cloth and place in a dark area such as an unused oven. Allow to ferment for 3 to 7 days. Daily check slaw for liquid coverage. Slaw will expand. Refrigerate when desired fermentation has been achieved.

Serve on a wooden dish along side flax crackers and a raw soup for a simple lunch.

Serves 8.

Korean Flax Crackers

Korean Flax Crackers are made from leftover Kim-Chi with flaxseed added.

2 cups Kim-Chi (above)

2 cups flaxseeds, soaked

¼ cup flaxseeds, ground-up

1 tsp. Celtic Sea Salt

SPECIAL EQUIPMENT: Chef knife, spatula, dehydrator, and solid and mesh sheet

Combine ingredients and spread 3 cups mixture onto a solid sheet. Dehydrate at 105°F for four hours and flip. Continue drying until crispy. Korean Flax Crackers can be stored in the pantry or freezer.

Serves 8.

Appendix C

The Maker's Diet for Weight Loss Resource Guide

THIS RESOURCE SECTION contains contact information for manufacturers and distributors of products recommended in *The Maker's Diet for Weight Loss*. To the best of our abilities, we are suggesting well-established companies whose health goals match up with ours. Please note, however, that we cannot be held responsible for any possible consequences relating to the eating or ingestion of foods and/or supplements.

You will note that products from Garden of Life are recommended. In the interest of full disclosure, Jordan Rubin founded this company following his illness when he had trouble finding the nutritional supplements and superfoods that his body needed. Using his knowledge gained from years of studying health and wellness, Jordan set out to create high-quality functional foods, nutritional supplements, and educational resources to help you on your road to optimal health. All other products are recommended without compensation.

We believe that no matter which company you choose to purchase from, you will be well served on your road to vibrant health. Keep in mind that if you don't find these foods, supplements, or products in your local supermarket, natural-food store, or vitamin store, you can purchase them by mail order or through online retailers. Also, if you have any questions, many of these companies can be reached via e-mail, usually through the company's Web site or by typing info@ plus the company's Web site (example: info@gardenoflife.com).

The importance of shopping for locally grown organic fruits, vegetables, and dairy cannot be underestimated. Several Web sites are tremendous resources:

- www.localharvest.org
- www.eatwild.com
- www.realmilk.com

BREADS AND OTHER GRAIN PRODUCTS

Food for Life Baking Co.
P. O. Box 1434
Corona, CA 92878
(800) 797-5090
www.foodforlife.com

Food for Life, makers of Ezekiel 4:9 breads, English muffins, and tortillas, is an excellent supplier of grain products. Easily digestible, well tolerated by many who suffer from digestive ailments and allergies, and high in protein and fiber, Food for Life products truly provide the bread of life.

French Meadow Bakery
1000 Apollo Rd.
Eagan, MN 55121
(651) 286-7861
www.frenchmeadow.com

Food for Life and French Meadow products are found in natural-food stores and grocery stores nationwide.

WHOLE-FOOD NUTRITION BARS

Perfect Weight America Bars by Garden of Life
(866) 465-0051
www.gardenoflife.com

Perfect Weight America Bars are made with organic foods such as chia seeds, raw honey, nuts, coconut oil, and high-quality protein. Perfect Weight America Bars contain fucoxanthin, which has been shown to support fat loss and increase metabolism, and they are high in fiber and protein.

Available in natural-food stores nationwide and via mail-order catalogs and online retailers nationwide.

Living Foods Nutrition Bars by Garden of Life
(866) 465-0051
www.gardenoflife.com

Living Foods Nutrition Bars are made with organic foods such as sprouted grains and seeds, raw honey, dates, cultured vegetables, nuts, berries, green foods, and coconut. Living Foods Nutrition Bars contain beta glucans from soluble oat fiber, high-quality protein, live probiotics, antioxidants, and more.

Living Foods Nutrition Bars are great for all ages and support overall health by supporting healthy serum cholesterol and triglycerides, promoting maintenance of healthy blood sugar levels, supporting healthy immune function, and aiding in maintenance of healthy body weight.

Available in natural-food stores nationwide and via mail-order catalogs and online retailers nationwide.

CACAO CHOCOLATE/TRAIL MIX

Rainforest Cacao by Garden of Life
(866) 465-0051
www.gardenoflife.com

Rainforest Cacao Chocolate is all-natural, roasted cacao beans harvested from the Ecuadorian Amazon. These all-natural beans are treated with extreme care at the time of harvest and then undergo minimal processing to ensure they maintain their maximum nutritional values, which includes heart-healthy antioxidants.

Available in natural-food stores nationwide and via mail-order catalogs and online retailers nationwide.

WHOLE-FOOD MEAL SUPPLEMENTS

Perfect Meal by Garden of Life
(866) 465-0051
www.gardenoflife.com

Perfect Meal is a delicious and satisfying high-protein and high-fiber drink designed to be used as a meal supplement. Available in two healthy and delicious flavors: creamy vanilla and milk chocolate. As part of a healthy diet and exercise program, Perfect Meal will help you successfully manage your weight by naturally curbing your appetite.

Available in natural-food stores nationwide and via mail-order catalogs and online retailers nationwide.

DAIRY PRODUCTS

The following companies produce natural and organic milk, butter, cheese, cream, cottage cheese, yogurt, kefir, soft cheese, and buttermilk that are either available in natural-food stores or by mail order.

Old Chatham Sheepherding Company
155 Shaker Museum Rd.
Old Chatham, NY 12136
(888) SHEEP-60 (743-3760)
www.blacksheepcheese.com

Old Chatham makes the finest quality sheep's milk yogurt and cheese. This is the yogurt favored by the Rubin family. Available via mail order or in select natural-food stores.

Amaltheia Dairy
3380 Penwell Bridge Rd.
Belgrade, MT 59714
(406) 388-5950
www.amaltheiadairy.com

Grade A goat's cheeses. Available via mail order and in select natural-food stores.

Organic Pastures Dairy Co.
7221 South Jameson Ave.
Fresno, CA 93706
(877) RAW-MILK (729-6455)
www.organicpastures.com

Coconut Milk

Simply Asia Foods, Inc.
Thai Kitchen Coconut Milk
2342 Shattuck Ave.
PMB 322
Berkely, CA 94704
(800) 967-8424
www.thaikitchen.com

Thai Kitchen products are available in natural-food stores nationwide.

Eggs

Gold Circle Farms
310 N. Harbor Blvd., Suite 205
Fullerton, CA 92832
(888) 599-4DHA (599-4342)
www.goldcirclefarms.com

DHA omega-3 eggs available in natural-food stores and grocery stores nationwide.

Organic Valley
One Organic Way
La Farge, WI 54639
(888) 444-6455
www.organicvalley.coop

Certified organic high omega-3 eggs. Available in natural-food stores and grocery stores nationwide.

RED MEATS

Maverick Ranch Natural Meats
5360 North Franklin St.
Denver, CO 80216
(800) 497-2624
www.maverickranch.com

Natural beef, chicken, lamb, and buffalo. Available in grocery stores nationwide.

Coleman Purely Natural Products
1767 Denver West Marriott Rd., Suite 200
Golden, CO 80401
(800) 442-8666
www.colemannatural.com

Naturally raised, hormone- and antibiotic-free beef products. Available in natural-food stores nationwide.

Northstar Bison
1936 28th Ave.
Rice Lake, WI 54868
(888) 295-6332
www.northstarbison.com

One hundred percent grass-fed and finished bison meat.

CHICKEN

Oaklyn Plantation
1312 Oaklyn Rd.
Darlington, SC 29532
(843) 395-0793
www.freerangechicken.com

Free-range chickens and chicken feet (hormone and antibiotic free). Available via mail order.

Bell & Evans
154 W. Main St. Fredericksburg, PA 17026
(717) 865-6626
www.bellandevans.com

Fresh and frozen natural poultry products. Available in natural-food stores and grocery stores nationwide.

DELI MEAT

Applegate Farms
750 Rt. 202 South, Suite 300
Bridgewater, NJ 08807
(866) 587-5858
www.applegatefarms.com

Packaged meats and deli slices (nitrate and nitrite free). Available in natural-food stores and grocery stores nationwide.

FROZEN FISH

Ecofish, Inc.
340 Central Ave.
Dover, NH 03820
(877) 214-3474
www.ecofish.com

Ocean-caught salmon, tuna, and other fish. Available in natural-food stores and grocery stores nationwide.

Vital Choice Seafood
605 30th St.
Anacortes, WA 98221
(800) 608-4825
www.vitalchoice.com

Available in natural-food stores nationwide.

Crown Prince
18581 Railroad Street
City of Industry, CA 91748
(626) 912-3700
www.crownprince.com

Canned sardines, salmon, tuna, and other fish. Available in natural-food stores and grocery stores nationwide.

SWEETENERS

Honey

Hawaiian Lehua Honey by Garden of Life
(866) 465-0051
www.gardenoflife.com

This certified organic honey comes from the island of Hawaii. Hawaiian Lehua Honey contains antioxidants, enzymes, vitamins, and minerals, providing all of the benefits that make honey a superfood from the hive. This raw, unheated honey is the original sweetener used for thousands of years and is a superb resource to sweeten smoothies, yogurt, tea, and coffee. This honey is also an important ingredient in many of the delicious recipes you'll find in this book.

Available in natural-food stores nationwide and via mail-order catalogs and online retailers nationwide.

Rapadura Whole Cane Sugar

Rapunzel
260 Lake Road
Dayville, CT 06241
www.rapunzel.com

SALAD MIXES (PREWASHED)

Earthbound Farm
1721 San Juan Highway
San Juan Bautista, CA 95045
(800) 690-3200
www.ebfarm.com

Fresh, packaged organic produce available in natural-food stores and grocery stores nationwide.

VEGETABLES (INCLUDING RAW FERMENTED)

Earthbound Farm
1721 San Juan Highway
San Juan Bautista, CA 95045
(800) 690-3200
www.ebfarm.com

Fresh, organic produce available in natural-food stores and grocery stores nationwide.

Rejuvenative Foods
P. O. Box 8464
Santa Cruz, CA 95061
(800) 805-7957
www.rejuvenative.com

Rejuvenative Foods produces high-quality raw foods such as sauerkraut, kim-chi, "live" salsas, nut and seed butters, chocolate spreads, raw oils, and more. Available in some grocery and health food stores, and online via mail order.

FROZEN FRUITS AND VEGETABLES

Small Planet Foods
Cascadian Farms
P. O. Box 9452
Minneapolis, MN 55440
(800) 624-4123
www.cfarm.com

Frozen, packaged organic fruits and vegetables, including berries. Available in health food and grocery stores nationwide.

PROTEIN POWDER (FROM GOAT'S MILK)

Goatein by Garden of Life
(866) 465-0051
www.gardenoflife.com

Goatein, an exceptional goat's milk protein powder, is a source of eight essential amino acids crucial to good health.

Easy to digest, Goatein is well tolerated by those who cannot digest cow's milk.

Available in natural-food stores nationwide and via mail-order catalogs and online retailers nationwide.

EXTRA-VIRGIN COCONUT OIL

Extra-Virgin Coconut Oil by Garden of Life
(866) 465-0051
www.gardenoflife.com

Once thought to be a "bad" fat, coconut oil has been shown to be a stable, healthy saturated fat. In fact, extra-virgin coconut oil is one of the healthiest and most versatile unprocessed dietary oils in the world. Garden of Life Extra-Virgin Coconut Oil is an unprocessed culinary oil full of natural coconut flavor and aroma.

Available in natural-food stores nationwide and via mail-order catalogs and online retailers nationwide.

SALAD DRESSINGS AND VINEGARS

Salad Dressings

Bragg Live Foods
Box 7
Santa Barbara, CA 93102
(800) 446-1990
www.bragg.com

Paul C. Bragg and his daughter Patricia have been health pioneers for decades. Bragg Organic Vinaigrette and Ginger & Sesame salad dressings bring you a healthy alternative with all the best of the Bragg tradition of healthy eating and living. Available in natural-food stores, mail-order catalogs, and online retailers nationwide.

Apple-Cider, Organic Balsamic, or Other Vinegars

Bragg Live Foods
Box 7
Santa Barbara, CA 93102
(800) 446-1990
www.bragg.com

Apple-cider vinegar made from organically grown apples, as well as other natural products. Available in health food and grocery stores nationwide.

NUTS AND SEEDS

Living Nutz
P. O. Box 365
Bowdoinham, ME 04008
(207) 780-1101
www.livingnutz.com

Variety of low-temperature-dried sprouted nuts available in select natural-food stores and via mail order.

NUT AND SEED BUTTERS

Rejuvenative Foods
P. O. Box 8464
Santa Cruz, CA 95061
(800) 805-7957
www.rejuvenative.com

The highest-quality, best-tasting raw organic nut and seed butters, including those made from almond, sesame, pumpkin, cashew, and sunflower seeds. Available in some grocery and health food stores, by mail order, or through online merchants.

TEA

Living Foods Teas by Garden of Life
(866) 465-0051
www.gardenoflife.com

Green and black tea delivered in convenient liquid-packs. Wellness Tea is great as hot or iced tea and comes in many flavors, including unflavored lemon green tea and coffee-flavored black tea. Living Foods Teas are loaded with antioxidants and the exciting compound epigallocatechin gallate (EGCG). Available with or without caffeine.

Available in natural-food stores nationwide and via mail-order catalogs and online retailers nationwide.

SEA SALT

Celtic Sea Salt

The Grain & Salt Society
Four Celtic Dr.
Arden, NC 28704
(800) 867-7258
www.celticseasalt.com

Celtic Sea Salt (coarse and fine) is available in some health food stores and grocery stores.

Redmond RealSalt
475 West 910 South
Heber City, UT 84032
(800) FOR-SALT (367-7258)
www.realsalt.com

RealSalt is mined in central Utah and is available in health food and grocery stores.

Herbamare Organic Herb Seasoning Salt
www.veganessentials.com

The Spice Hunter, Inc.
(800) 444-3061
P. O. Box 8110
San Luis Obispo, CA 93403

ORGANIC SPICES

Frontier Natural Products Co-op
Simply Organic
P. O. Box 299
Norway, IA 52318
(800) 669-3275
www.frontiercoop.com

Packaged organic spices in glass jars.

CONDIMENTS

Spectrum Organic Products
1105 Industrial Avenue
Petaluma, CA 94954
(800) 995-2705
www.spectrumorganics.com

Healthy, organic omega-3 mayonnaise using expeller-pressed soy and flaxseed oils. Available in some health food stores and grocery stores.

Westbrae Natural Foods
4600 Sleepytime Drive
Boulder, CO 80301
(800) 434-4246
www.westbrae.com

Natural ketchup and mustard, available in some health food stores and grocery stores.

FLAXSEED OIL

Barlean's Organic Oils
4936 Lake Terrell Rd.
Ferndale, WA 98248
(360) 384-0485
www.barleans.com

Organic high-lignan flaxseed oil and borage seed oil, as well as flaxseed fiber. Available at health food stores nationwide.

ORGANIC VEGETABLE OILS

Garden of Life
(866) 465-0051
www.gardenoflife.com

High-quality organic oils, including extra-virgin olive oil. Available in natural-food stores nationwide and via mail-order catalogs and online retailers nationwide.

Bionaturae
5 Tyler Drive
North Franklin, CT 06254
(860) 642-6996
www.bionaturae.com

Organic extra-virgin olive oil.

Bariani Olive Oil
1330 Waller St.
San Francisco, CA 94117
(415) 864-1917
www.barianioliveoil.com

Organic extra-virgin olive oil.

RAW ALMOND OIL, EVENING PRIMROSE OIL, SUNFLOWER OIL, AND POPPY SEED OIL

Raw Oils from Rejuvenative Foods
P. O. Box 8464
Santa Cruz, CA 95061
(800) 805-7957
www.rawoils.com

ORGANIC CHOCOLATE SPREADS

Rejuvenative Foods
P. O. Box 8464
Santa Cruz, CA 95061
(800) 805-7957
www.rejuvenative.com

Healthy organic chocolate spreads, great for all ages.

MACAROONS

Jennies Macaroons
Red Mill Farms, Inc.
290 South 5th Street
Brooklyn, NY 11211
(888) 294-1164
www.macaroonking.com

A personal favorite of the Rubin family, Jennies Macaroons coconut-rich macaroon treats are a wonderful dessert treat.
Available in natural-food stores or from online retailers.

FLAXSEED CRACKERS

Glaser Organic Farms
19100 SW 137th Ave.
Miami, FL 33177
(305) 238-7747
www.glaserorganicfarms.com

FOOD PREPARATION/UTENSILS

Mercola.com
www.mercola.com

Provides food preparation tools such as juicers and convection ovens. Available online.

Vita-Mix Blender
8615 Usher Rd.
Cleveland, OH 44138
(800) 848-2649
www.vitamix.com

High-quality durable blender excellent for smoothies and soups. A must-have for every health-conscious family.

For more information on eating to live, visit www.BiblicalHealthInstitute.com.

NUTRITIONAL SUPPLEMENTS

Fucoxanthin Products

fücoTHIN by Garden of Life
(866) 465-0051
www.gardenoflife.com

fücoTHIN is a natural, whole food-based supplement that is made with a proprietary concentration of 5 percent fucoxanthin combined with pomegranate seed oil for a patent-pending formula that is naturally thermogenic. Available in natural-food stores nationwide and via mail-order catalogs and online retailers nationwide.

sea-Thin by Specialty Nutrition Products, LLC
www.sea-thin.com

sea-Thin, a formulation of concentrated fucoxanthin made from strains of undaria (wakame) and laminaria (kombu) grown in unpolluted waters, is available nationwide at better pharmacies, grocery stores, and select price clubs.

Whole-Food Multivitamins

Living Multi by Garden of Life
(866) 465-0051
www.gardenoflife.com

Living Multi is a complete vitamin and mineral supplement that delivers superfoods to support your demanding nutritional needs. This comprehensive whole-food multi-nutrient formula contains fruits, vegetables, ocean plants, tonic mushrooms, botanicals, and ionic minerals including enzymes, antioxidants, amino acids, and homeostatic nutrient complexes. Living Multi is available in natural-food stores, mail-order catalogs, and online retailers nationwide.

Omega-3 Cod Liver Oil

Olde World Icelandic Cod Liver Oil by Garden of Life
(866) 465-0051
www.gardenoflife.com

Olde World Icelandic Cod Liver Oil is one of nature's richest sources of vitamins A and D, which can play an important role in supporting cardiovascular health. To ensure that its naturally occurring ingredients remain intact, Olde World Icelandic

Cod Liver Oil is always harvested from the pure cold waters of Iceland and is cold-processed using traditional methods. Olde World Icelandic Cod Liver Oil is available in natural-food stores, mail-order catalogs, and online merchants nationwide.

CODmega by Garden of Life
(866) 465-0051
www.gardenoflife.com

Don't like the taste of cod liver oil on your spoon? CODmega offers EPA and DHA omega-3 fatty acids as well as vitamins A and D in a new capsule form. Available in natural-food stores, mail-order catalogs, and online merchants nationwide.

Green Food/Fiber Blend

Perfect Food by Garden of Life
(866) 465-0051
www.gardenoflife.com

Perfect Food is a green superfood containing organic ingredients, including cereal grass juices, microalgaes, vegetable juice concentrates, sprouts, and seeds. Perfect Food provides antioxidants, enzymes, chlorophyll, and trace minerals. Available in natural-food stores and through online retailers.

Super Seed by Garden of Life
(866) 465-0051
www.gardenoflife.com

Super Seed is a whole-food fiber blend containing organic ingredients, including sprouted and fermented seeds, grains, and legumes. Super Seed is available in natural-food stores, mail-order catalogs, and online retailers nationwide.

Probiotics and Enzymes

Primal Defense Ultra
(800) 622-8986
www.gardenoflife.com

Primal Defense Ultra contains probiotics and prebiotics in a blend that promotes overall wellness and is available in natural-food stores, mail-order catalogs, and online retailers nationwide.

Ω-Zyme Ultra by Garden of Life
(866) 465-0051
www.gardenoflife.com

Ω-Zyme (pronounced omega-zyme) is a whole-food digestive enzyme blend that supports gastrointestinal health, carbohydrate digestion, and normal bowel function. Available in natural-food stores, from mail-order catalogs, and through online retailers.

Digestive Complex by TriVita
TriVita, Inc.
16100 N Greenway Hayden Loop, Suite 950
Scottsdale, AZ 85260
(480) 991-6535
www.trivita.com

A digestive formula containing enzymes and probiotics to support digestion and elimination.

DIGESTIVE CLEANSES

Perfect Cleanse by Garden of Life
(866) 465-0051
www.gardenoflife.com

A ten-day Perfect Cleanse will leave you feeling lighter on your feet and with a brighter outlook in just ten days. This cleanse works in harmony with your body to naturally release and remove toxins so that you will feel like a better you. The Perfect Cleanse system involves following three simple steps:

1. Perfect Cleanse Purify. Your body is constantly working to eliminate toxins via the lungs, kidneys, and particularly the liver. Every minute, around the clock, a properly functioning liver eliminates small amounts of toxins, heavy metals, bacteria, and other impurities from the blood before returning the life-sustaining substance to the rest of the body.

2. Perfect Cleanse Capture. Capturing and binding toxins secreted through the bile for transport out of the body is crucial for effective support of the body's normal internal detox and cleansing functions.

3. Perfect Cleanse Remove. The third and final step is Perfect Cleanse Remove, which works by assisting the trapped toxins to move smoothly through the digestive track, gently sweeping the colon of accumulated waste.

FITNESS PRODUCTS

Functional Fitness DVD by Garden of Life
(866) 465-0051
www.gardenoflife.com

Experience the energizing, enjoyable world of functional fitness exercise. Functional exercise teaches you to train whole body movements, not just isolated muscles. Increase fitness, coordination, flexibility, and agility. Decrease your chances of injury during daily activity. Functional fitness is great for people of any age or skill level. This functional fitness DVD features fun and easy routines that can be performed anywhere and anytime. Call the toll-free number or visit the Web site for more information.

Kingdom Conditioning with Ron Kardashian
www.kingdomconditioning.com

Ron Kardashian has more than 12,000 hours of personal training under his belt and travels around the country as a much-in-demand speaker and trainer.

Russian Kettlebells
www.dragondoor.com

The Russians are coming! The Russians are coming! Pavel Tsatsouline and Dragon Door have spearheaded the kettlebell invasion of the United States. You can achieve power, strength, and conditioning by going to their Web site at www.dragondoor.com.

Institute of Human Performance
1950 NW Boca Raton Blvd.
Boca Raton, FL 33432
(561) 620-9556
www.ihpfit.com

The Institute of Human Performance in Boca Raton, Florida, is where fitness professionals from all over the world come to learn the latest training methods from Juan Carlos Santana and the IHP staff. Santana is one of the world's leading authorities on training and performance.

Perform Better
P. O. Box 8090
Cranston, RI 02920
(888) 556-7464
www.performbetter.com

If you're looking to "get functional," go with the experts in functional training and rehabilitation done through stabilization, plyometric, speed and agility, and strength and conditioning exercises.

Mini-trampolines/Rebounders

Rebound Air
993 North 450 West
Springville, UT 84663
(888) 464-JUMP (5867)
www.reboundair.com

Supplier of rebounders, which are great for low-impact exercise.

Lympholine
Life Source International
1112 Montana Ave., Suite 125
Santa Monica, CA 90403
(310) 284-3565
www.lympholine.com

The Lympholine rebounder activates the lymphatic system to purify the body.

Needak Manufacturing
120 W Douglas Street
O'Neill, NE 68763
(800) 232-5762
www.needak-rebounders.com

SKIN AND BODY CARE

Aubrey Organics
4419 N. Manhattan Ave.
Tampa, FL 33614
(800) 282-7394
www.aubrey-organics.com

Aubrey Hampton, the founder of Aubrey Organics, has been formulating and manufacturing skin and body care products for thirty years. Aubrey produces hundreds of products, including skin care, hair care, soaps and cleansers, toothpaste, natural hair color, and perfumes and colognes.

COSMETICS

Peacekeeper Cosmetics
50 Lexington Ave., #22G
New York, NY 10010
(866) 732-2336
www.iamapeacekeeper.com

In addition to using quality ingredients, the company donates all profits, after taxes, to support women's health advocacy and human rights issues.

CLEANING SUPPLIES

PerfectClean Ultramicrofiber Mops, Wipes, and Dusters
SixWise.com
655 Deerfield Rd.
Suite 100, Box 123
Deerfield, IL 60015
www.SixWise.com

Indoor pollution has become one of the leading causes of disease. A main health risk is dust, which commonly contains over twenty toxins such as heavy metals, PCBs, viruses, bacteria, and allergens. Throw away your mops, sponges, and wipers that require the use of chemical cleaners and that only introduce more toxins into your environment while doing a remarkably poor job of eliminating dust and biological contaminants.

Instead, try the PerfectClean line of mops, wipes, and dusters. They are available exclusively at one of my favorite Web sites, www.SixWise.com. PerfectClean's innovative "ultramicrober" construction means that with just the use of water—no chemical cleaners required—the surfaces in your home will become clean down to the microscopic level, eliminating even the biological contaminants that no other cleaning tool or solution can touch. PerfectClean lasts for hundreds of uses, so it's also economical. PerfectClean products are available online at www.SixWise.com.

Bi-O-Kleen Industries, Inc.
P. O. Box 820689
Vancouver, WA 98682
(800) 477-0188
www.biokleenhome.com

Try Turbo Plus Ceramic Laundry Discs and Flora Brite papaya enzyme laundry additive and whitener.

Orange TKO
3395 S. Jones Blvd. #221
Las Vegas, NV 89146
(800) 995-2463
www.tkoorange.com

All-purpose cleaner, stain remover, and odor remover made from organic orange oil.

Seventh Generation, Inc.
60 Lake Street
Burlington, VT 05401
(800) 456-1191
www.seventhgeneration.com

AIR PURIFIERS

Pionair
HealthQuest Technologies, LLC
P. O. Box 400
Kathleen, GA 31047
(866) PIONAIR (746-6247)
www.pionair.net

The Pionair air purification system enhances the quality of air in the home and reduces harmful toxins such as yeast, mold, bacteria, and debris. Available in select health stores and via mail order.

WATER PURIFIERS

New Wave Enviro Products
P. O. Box 4146
Englewood, CO 80155
(303) 221-3232
www.newwaveenviro.com

Water purifiers and shower filters remove harmful toxins, including chlorine.

PRODUCE WASH

Veggie Wash
Beaumont Products
1560 Big Shanty Dr.
Kennesaw, GA 30144
(800) 451-7096
www.citrusmagic.com

Made 100 percent with natural ingredients derived from citrus fruit, corn, and coconut, Veggie Wash aids in the removal of pesticides, germs, and toxins from fruits and produce.

PAPER PRODUCTS

Seventh Generation
60 Lake Street
Burlington, VT 05401
(800) 456-1191
www.seventhgeneration.com

Unbleached paper towels, napkins, toilet paper, and tissue.

NOTES

INTRODUCTION
WHAT THE MAKER'S DIET FOR WEIGHT LOSS IS ALL ABOUT

1. Carol Sorgen, "Fad Diets: Weight Loss Magic or Myth?" FOXNews.com, August 31, 2006, http://www.foxnews.com/story/0,2933,211597,00.html?sPage=fnc.health/nutrition (accessed August 27, 2008).

2. Chelsea Martinez, "Quitting All at Once," *Los Angeles Times*, June 18, 2007, http://www.latimes.com/features/health/la-he-capsule-18jun18,1,6491724.story?coll=la -headlines-health&ctrack=2&cset=true (accessed August 27, 2008).

CHAPTER 1 GLOBESITY

1. Associated Press, "Obesity an 'International Scourge,'" CBSNews.com, September 3, 2006, http://www.cbsnews.com/stories/2006/09/03/health/main1962961.shtml (accessed August 28, 2008).

2. Dr. Joseph Mercola, "The Global Obesity Epidemic Is More Harmful Than Malnutrition," Mercola.com, November 16, 2006, http://v.mercola.com/blogs/public_blog/The-Global-Obesity-Epidemic-is-More-Harmful-Than-Malnutrition-1810.aspx (accessed August 28, 2008).

3. Worldpress.org, "Obesity: A Worldwide Issue," October 24, 2004, http://www .worldpress.org/Africa/1961.cfm (accessed August 28, 2008).

4. Associated Press, "European Nations Sign Anti-Obesity Charter," CBSNews.com, November 15, 2006, http://www.cbsnews.com/stories/2006/11/16/world/main2188875 .shtml (accessed August 28, 2008).

5. Associated Press, "Japanese Bingeing on Krispy Kremes," MSNBC.com, April 3, 2007, http://www.msnbc.msn.com/id/17933328/ (accessed August 28, 2008).

6. "Obesity Is Going to Extremes, Study Reports," *Los Angeles Times*, October 14, 2003, http://articles.latimes.com/2003/oct/14/science/sci-obesity14 (accessed August 28, 2008).

7. Reuters.com, "Study Predicts 75 Percent Overweight in US by 2015," July 19, 2007, http://www.reuters.com/article/health-SP-A/idUSN1841918320070719 (accessed August 28, 2008).

8. Elisabeth Kübler-Ross, *On Death and Dying* (New York: Scribner, 1997).

9. Abby Ellin, "Fat Studies Gain Weight in Class," *San Diego Union-Tribune*, December 10, 2006, http://www.signonsandiego.com/uniontrib/20061210/news_1c10fat.html (accessed August 28, 2008).

10. PRWeb.com, "U.S. Weight Loss Market to Reach $58 Billion in 2007," April 19, 2007, http://www.prweb.com/releases/2007/4/prweb520127.htm (accessed August 28, 2008).

11. Tani Shaw, "Celebrities Increase Popularity of Gastric Bypass Surgery," http://ezinearticles.com/?Celebrities-Increase-Popularity-of-Gastric-Bypass-Surgery&id=94828 (accessed August 28, 2008); Associated Press, "Star Jones: I Had Gastric Bypass Surgery," USAToday.com, July 31, 2007, http://usatoday.com/life/television/2007-07
-31-864625929_x.htm (accessed August 28, 2008).

12. Herb Weisbaum, "Finally, These Diet Pill Pushers Get Pushed Back," MSNBC.com, January 15, 2007, http://www.msnbc.msn.com/id/16491115 (accessed August 28, 2008).

13. NewsReleaseWire.com, "Passenger Obesity as a Contributing Factor in Commuter Airline Crashes," August 28, 2006, http://www.expertclick.com/NewsReleaseWire/default.cfm?Action=ReleaseDetail&ID=13628 (accessed August 28, 2008).

14. Beverly Beyette, "Airline Seats Getting Even Smaller," Los Angeles Times, March 30, 2007, http://article.wn.com/view/2007/03/31/Airline_seats_getting_even_smaller/ (accessed August 28, 2008).

15. HarrisInteractive.com, "The High Correlation Between Obesity, Illness and Poor Health," January 11, 2005, http://www.harrisinteractive.com/news/allnewsbydate
.asp?NewsID=880 (accessed August 28, 2008).

16. National Center for Health Statistics, "Americans Slightly Taller, Much Heavier Than Four Decades Ago," October 27, 2004, http://www.cdc.gov/nchs/pressroom/04news/americans.htm (accessed August 28, 2008).

17. Ibid.

18. Ibid.

19. Ibid.

20. Rob Stein, "Obesity Passing Smoking as Top Avoidable Cause of Death," Washington Post, March 10, 2004, A1, http://www.washingtonpost.com/ac2/wp-dyn/A43253-2004Mar9?language
=printer (accessed August 28, 2008).

21. WebMD.com, "Weight Loss: Health Risks Associated with Obesity," http://www
.webmd.com/cholesterol-management/obesity-health-risks (accessed August 28, 2008).

22. Jane E. Brody, "Personal Health: Another Study Finds a Link Between Excess Weight and Cancer," New York Times, May 6, 2003, http://query.nytimes.com/gst/fullpage.html?sec=health
&res=9403EFDE143CF935A35756C0A9659C8B63 (accessed August 28, 2008).

23. Harvard School of Public Health, "Volume I: Human Causes of Cancer," Harvard Reports on Cancer Prevention, in Cancer Causes and Control 7 (Supplement) (November 1996): http://www.hsph.harvard.edu/cancer/resources_ materials/reports/HCCPreport_1.htm (accessed August 21, 2007).

24. Alex Barnum, "Major Obesity Threat Seen for Life Expectancy," WorldHealth.net, http://www.worldhealth.net/p/286,6703.html (accessed August 28, 2008).

25. S. J. Olshansky et al., "A Potential Decline in Life Expectancy in the United States in the 21st Century," New England Journal of Medicine 352, no. 11 (2005): 1138–1145.

26. David Hawkins, MH, CNC, "Obesity and Weight Management," MotherEarthWorks.com, http://motherearthworks.com/articles_dave_hawkins/obesity_and_weight_management.htm (accessed August 28, 2008).

27. Barnum, "Major Obesity Threat Seen for Life Expectancy."

28. Agency for Healthcare Research and Quality, "Obesity Contributes to Early-Onset Heart Problems and Longer Hospital Stays," U.S. Department of Health and Human Services, http://www.ahrq.gov/research/dec04/1204RA21.htm (accessed August 28, 2008).

29. Peter Kessler, "Phil Mickelson Interview," GolfOnline.com, March 2003, http://www.golfonline.com/golfonline/features/kessler/columnist/0,17742,468530,00.html (accessed August 28, 2008).

30. Peggy Peck, "High-Fat Diets Ups Dangerous 'Hidden' Fat," WebMD.com, March 31, 2003, http://www.webmd.com/diet/news/20030331/high-fat-diet-ups-dangerous -hidden-fat (accessed August 28, 2008).

31. Associated Press, "Thin People Can Be Fat on the Inside," MSNBC.com, May 11, 2007, http://www.msnbc.msn.com/id/18594089/ (accessed August 28, 2008).

32. Christian Nordqvist, "Dangerous Visceral Fat Builds Up If You Don't Exercise, Can Go Down If You Do," MedicalNewsToday.com, http://www.medicalnewstoday .com/healthnews.php?newsid=30641 (accessed August 28, 2008).

33. Pew Research Center, "In the Battle of the Bulge, More Soldiers Than Successes," Pew Research Center Publications, April 26, 2006, http://pewresearch.org/pubs/310/in -the-battle-of-the-bulge-more-soldiers-than-successes (accessed August 28, 2008).

CHAPTER 2 WHAT ARE YOU FAILING FOR?

1. ScienceDaily.com, "Dieting Does Not Work, Researchers Report," http://www .sciencedaily.com/releases/2007/04/070404162428.htm (accessed August 28, 2008).

2. North Dakota State University Extension News, "Fad Diets Popular but Have Major-League Failure Rate," Agriculture Communication, July 8, 1999, http://www .ext.nodak.edu/extnews/newsrelease/1999/070899/04faddie.htm (accessed August 28, 2008).

3. Elaine Magee, "Your 'Hunger Hormones,'" MedicineNet.com, http://www .onhealth.com/script/main/art.asp?articlekey=55992 (accessed on August 29, 2008).

4. Gary Taubes, "What if It's All Been a Big Fat Lie?" *New York Times Magazine*, July 2, 2002, 22.

5. Leonard Pitts Jr., "Search for Ideal Body Takes Toll," LJWorld.com, February 6, 2003, http://www2.ljworld.com/news/2003/feb/06/search_for_ideal/ (accessed August 29, 2008).

6. CommonSenseMedia.org, "What's the Skinny on the Media and Weight?" September 26, 2006, http://www.commonsensemedia.org/news/press-releases.php?id=29 (accessed August 29, 2008); and Mark Hyman, MD, *Ultrametabolism: The Simple Plan for Automatic Weight Loss* (New York: Scribner, 2006), 14–15.

7. Hyman, *Ultrametabolism: The Simple Plan for Automatic Weight Loss*, 14–15.

8. E. J. Mundell, "Furor Over Anorexic Models Hits U.S. Fashion Week," *Washington Post*, February 2, 2007, http://www.washingtonpost.com/wp-dyn/content/article/2007/02/02/AR2007020200500.html (accessed August 29, 2008).

9. Domino's Pizza Press Release, "Domino's Pizza Gets Ready to Kick-off for the Big Game," PRNewswire, January 31, 2007, http://phx.corporate-ir.net/phoenix .zhtml?c=135383&p=irol-newsArticle&ID=956166&highlight= (accessed August 29, 2008).

10. Associated Press, "Role of TV Ads in Kids' Obesity? FCC to Study," MSNBC.com, September 27, 2006, http://www.msnbc.msn.com/id/15035381/from/ET (accessed August 29, 2008).

11. CommonSenseMedia.org, "What's the Skinny on the Media and Weight?"

12. Judith A. Shinogle, Maria F. Owings, and Lola Jean Kozak, "Gastric Bypass as Treatment for Obesity: Trends, Characteristics, and Complications," *Obesity Research* 13 (2005): 2202–2209.

13. Robin Blackstone, David Engstrom, and Lisa Rivera, "Patients in Despair: Weight Regain After a Primary Bariatric Surgery Procedure," BariatricTimes.com, April 2007, http://bariatric-times.com/2007/04/26/patients-in-despair-weight-regain-after-a-primary -bariatric-surgery-procedure/ (accessed August 29, 2008).

14. EmpowerFoods.com, "Self-Image," http://www.empowerfoods.com.au/news/?article_id=11 (accessed August 29, 2008).

CHAPTER 3 EAT FOR YOUR IDEAL WEIGHT

1. *Toledo: Treasures and Tradition* (Memphis, TN: Towery Publishing, Inc., 2001), 17.

2. Judy Sarles, "McAlister's Deli to Expand With Brentwood Franchise," *Nashville Business Journal*, February 3, 2006, http://nashville.bizjournals.com/nashville/stories/2006/02/06/story6. html (accessed August 29, 2008).

3. Craig Lambert, "The Way We Eat Now," *Harvard Magazine*, May–June 2004, http://www. harvardmagazine.com/on-line/050465.html (accessed August 29, 2008).

4. Hyman, *Ultrametabolism: The Simple Plan for Automatic Weight Loss*, 60.

5. Patrik Jonsson, "Is Eating Out Cheaper?" *Christian Science Monitor*, 2006, http://articles. moneycentral.msn.com/SavingandDebt/SaveMoney/IsEatingOutCheaperThan Cooking.aspx (accessed April 20, 2007).

6. Hyman, *Ultrametabolism: The Simple Plan for Automatic Weight Loss*, 60.

7. Sasha Nemecek, "Does the World Need GM Foods? Interview With Margaret Mellon," *Scientific American*, March 27, 2001, as viewed at http://www.mindfully.org/GE/World-Need-GM-Mellon.htm (accessed August 29, 2008).

8. Rick Weiss, "Americans Fuzzy on Biotech Foods," *Los Angeles Times*, December 11, 2006, F9.

9. Elisabeth Leamy, "Secrets in Your Food," ABCNews.com, August 21, 2006, http:// abcnews.go.com/gma/story?id=2337731&page=1 (accessed August 29, 2008).

10. Kathleen Kiley, "Private Label Meets Organic Food," *KPMG Consumer Markets Insider*, October 6, 2006, and Parija Bhatnagar, "Wal-Mart's Next Conquest: Organics," CNNMoney. com, May 1, 2006, at http://money.cnn.com/2006/05/01/news/companies/walmart_organics/ (accessed August 29, 2008).

11. WholeFoodMarkets.com, "Organic Foods Continue to Grow in Popularity According to Whole Foods Market Survey," October 21, 2004, http://www.whole foodsmarket.com/cgi-bin/print10pt.cgi?url=/company/pr_10-21-04.html (accessed April 26, 2007).

12. Don Lee, "China's Additives on Menu in U.S." *Los Angeles Times*, May 18, 2007, A1.

13. MayoClinic.com, "Exchange List: Fruits," http://www.mayoclinic.com/health/diabetes-diet/DA00070 (accessed April 29, 2008).

14. Julian Dibbell, "The Fast Supper," *New York* magazine, October 24, 2006.

15. WebMd.com, "Healthy Eating for Weight Loss," http://my.webmd.com/content/article/46/2731_1670 (accessed August 29, 2008).

16. Brenda Watson, *The Fiber35 Diet* (New York: Free Press, 2007).

17. Continuum Health Partners, Inc., "Dietary Fiber and Bowel Function," http://www.wehealny.org/healthinfo/dietaryfiber/fibercontentchart.html (accessed Jung 26, 2007).

18. Lavon J. Dunne, *Nutrition Almanac*, fifth edition (New York: McGraw-Hill, 2001), 5–6.

19. Hyman, *Ultrametabolism: The Simple Plan for Automatic Weight Loss*, 51.

20. Ibid., 70–71.

21. Jaye Lewis, "The Food Pyramid: Its History, Purpose, and Effectiveness," Health .LearningInfo.org, http://health.learninginfo.org/food-pyramid.htm (accessed August 29, 2008).

22. Hyman, *Ultrametabolism: The Simple Plan for Automatic Weight Loss*, 70.

23. William Wolcott, *The Metabolic Typing Diet* (New York: Broadway Books, 2002).

24. Anahad O'Connor, "The Claim: C.L.A. Supplements Can Help You Lose Weight," *New York Times*, May 29, 2007.

25. Thomas L. Halton and Frank B. Hu, "The Effects of High Protein Diets on Thermogenesis, Satiety and Weight Loss: A Critical Review," *Journal of the American College of Nutrition* 23, no. 5 (October 2004): 373–385, http://www.jacn.org/cgi/content/full/23/5/373 (accessed August 29, 2008).

26. Framingham Heart Study, "History of the Framingham Heart Study," http://www .framinghamheartstudy.org/about/history.html (accessed August 24, 2007).

27. G. V. Mann, ed., *Coronary Heart Disease: The Dietary Sense and Nonsense* (London, England: Janus Publishing Company, 1993), in Christian B. Allan, PhD, and Wolfgang Lutz, MD, *Life Without Bread: How a Low-Carbohydrate Diet Can Save Your Life* (Chicago: Keats Publishing, 2000), 83.

28. Diana Schwarzbein, MD, *The Schwarzbein Principle: The Truth About Losing Weight, Being Healthy, and Feeling Younger* (Deerfield Beach, FL: HCI Publishing, 1999).

29. Ibid., 253.

30. Ibid., 254.

31. Netfit.Co.Uk., "Food Combining," http://www.netfit.co.uk/fatcom.htm (accessed September 2, 2008).

32. Wolfgang Puck, "Changing Tastes," *Newsweek*, http://www.newsweek.com/id/34658 (accessed September 2, 2008).

33. United States Department of Agriculture, "Profiling Food Consumption in America," *Agriculture Fact Book, 2001–2002,* http://www.usda.gov/factbook/chapter2 .htm (accessed August 15, 2007).

34. Ann Louise Gittleman, MS, CNS, *How to Stay Young and Healthy in a Toxic World* (Chicago, IL: Keats Publishing, 1999), 19.

35. Ibid., 21.

36. Sally Squires, "High-Fructose Corn Syrup May Act More Like Fat Than Sugar in the Body," *Washington Post,* March 11, 2003, H1, and Dr. Joseph Mercola with Rachael Droege, "Six Reasons Why Corn Is Making You Fat," http://www.mercola .com/2004/apr/10/corn_fat.htm (accessed April 26, 2007).

37. Patricia King, "Blaming It on Corn Syrup," *Los Angeles Times,* March 24, 2003, F1.

38. George A. Bray, Samara Joy Nielsen, and Barry M. Popkin, "Consumption of High-Fructose Corn Syrup in Beverages May Play a Role in the Epidemic of Obesity," *American Journal of Clinical Nutrition* 79, no. 4 (April 2004): 537–543.

39. Jerry Hirsch, "Food Prices Continue to Rise," *Los Angeles Times,* May 15, 2007.

40. Ibid.

41. T. L. Davidson and S. E. Swithers, "A Pavlovian Approach to the Problem of Obesity," *International Journal of Obesity* 28, no. 7 (July 2004): 933–935.

42. FOXNews.com, "Diet Soda Dangerous?" partial transcript from March 19, 2004, *The O'Reilly Factor,* posted March 24, 2004, http://www.foxnews.com/story/0,2933,114880,00.html (accessed on September 2, 2008).

43. Daniel Engber, "The Scarlet Batter: Why Our Aversion to Artificial Coloring Makes No Sense," Slate.com, March 14, 2007, http://www.slate.com/id/2161806/ (accessed September 2, 2008).

44. Michael Pollan, "Discover How Your Beef Is Really Raised," *New York Times,* March 31, 2002.

45. Ibid.

46. Marian Burros, "Veal to Love, Without the Guilt," *New York Times,* April 18, 2007.

47. Ibid.

48. Ibid.

49. Russ Parsons, "New Rite of Spring," *Los Angeles Times,* April 4, 2007, F1.

50. Mary Shomon, *The Thyroid Diet* (New York: HarperCollins, 2004).

CHAPTER 4 DRINK FOR YOUR IDEAL WEIGHT

1. Jerry Adler, "Attack of the Diet Cokes," *Newsweek,* May 14, 2007.

2. Andrew Martin, "Want Vitamins and Minerals With That Soda?" HamptonRoads.com, March 14, 2007, http://hamptonroads.com/node/236241 (accessed September 2, 2008).

3. H. J. Roberts, *The Aspartame Problem,* Statement for Committee on Labor and Human Resources, U.S. Senate Hearing on NutraSweet—Health and Safety Concerns, November 3, 1987, 83–178 (Washington DC: U.S. Government Printing Office, 1988), 466–467.

4. "Study First to Confirm Drinking Water Could Help You Lose Weight," Children's Hospital and Research Center in Oakland, California, December 14, 2006, http://www.childrenshospitaloakland.org/about/press_releases/Waterweightloss.asp (accessed September 2, 2008).

5. Environmental Protection Agency, "130 Cities Exceed Lead Levels for Drinking Water," *Environmental News*, October 1992.

6. R. J. Ignelzi, "Flow Chart: Don't Count on Those 'Eight Glasses' to Determine Your Proper Fluid Intake," *San Diego Union-Tribune*, February 20, 2007, E1.

7. Salynn Boyles, "Drinking Water May Speed Weight Loss," WebMD.com, January 5, 2004, http://www.webmd.com/diet/news/20040105/drinking-water-may-speed -weight-loss (accessed September 2, 2008).

8. F. Batmanghelidj, MD, *Water: For Health, for Healing, for Life* (New York: Warner Books, 2003), 161, 225–226.

9. F. Batmanghelidj, MD, *Your Body's Many Cries for Water* (Vienna, VA: Global Health Solutions, Inc., 1997), 110–111.

10. Stephen Daniells, "Do Antioxidants Make Tea Healthier Than Water?" NutraIngredients-USA.com, August 28, 2006, http://www.nutraingredients-usa.com/news/ ng.asp?n=70121-tea-polyphenols-antioxidants (accessed September 2, 2008).

11. Nubella.com, "Stressed Out? Try a Cup of Black Tea," http://nubella.com/content/ view/2277/62/ (accessed September 2, 2008).

12. GreenTeaAndCLL.com, "Health Benefits of Green Tea—Fact or Fairytale?" May 18, 2007, http://greenteaandcll.com/2007/05/18/ (accessed September 2, 2008).

13. Siobhan Roth, "Kombucha Fermenting a Revolution in Health Drinks," *Pittsburgh Post-Gazette*, June 7, 2007.

Chapter 5 Snack for Your Ideal Weight

1. BBC News, "Chocolate Better Than Kissing," April 16, 2007, http://news.bbc .co.uk/1/hi/health/6558775.stm (accessed September 2, 2008).

2. Cybele May, "Hands Off My Chocolate, FDA!" *Los Angeles Times*, April 19, 2007, http:// www.latimes.com/news/opinion/la-oe-may19apr19,0,4511657.story?coll=la -opinion-rightrail (accessed August 27, 2007).

3. NutraIngredients-USA.com, "The Sum of Chocolate," December 20, 2005, http://www. nutraingredients-usa.com/news/ng.asp?n=64689-chocolate-cocoa-flavonoids (accessed September 2, 2008).

4. David Wolfe and Shazzie, *Naked Chocolate* (San Diego, CA: Maui Brothers Publishing, 2005), 6.

5. Ibid., 65.

6. Richard and Rachel Heller, *The Carbohydrate Addict's Diet* (New York: Signet, 2000), 96–97.

CHAPTER 6 SUPPLEMENT FOR YOUR IDEAL WEIGHT

1. H. Maeda et al., "Fucoxanthin From Edible Seaweed, Undaria Pinnatifida, Shows Antiobesity Effect Through UCP1 Expression in White Adipose Tissues," *Biochemical and Biophysical Research Communications* 332, no. 2 (July 1, 2005): 392–397.

2. H. Maeda et al., "Fucoxanthin and Its Metabolite, Fucoxanthinol, Suppress Adipocyte Differentiation in 3T3-L1 Cells," *Internal Journal of Molecular Medicine* 18, no. 1 (July 2006): 147–152.

3. Medical Research News, "Brown Seaweed with Anti-Obesity Potential," September 12, 2006, http://www.news-medical.net/?id=20082 (accessed September 2, 2008).

4. Yorkshire-Forward.com, "Seaweed 'Fights Fat,' Scientists Reveal," September 12, 2006, http://www.yorkshire-forward.com/www/view.asp?content_id=4283&parent_id=263 (accessed September 2, 2008).

5. Joanne Englash, "Weight Loss Supplements: 5 Myths!" eDiets.com, http://www.ediets.com/news/article.cfm/1/cmi_2310883/cid_1/code_30174 (accessed July 27, 2007).

6. Hal Bodley, "Medical Examiner: Ephedra a Factor in Bechler Death," March 13, 2003, http://www.usatoday.com/sports/baseball/al/orioles/2003-03-13-bechler-exam _x.htm (accessed August 27, 2007).

7. Sally Fallon and Mary G. Enig, PhD, "Vitamin A Saga," Weston A. Price Foundation, http://www.westonaprice.org/basicnutrition/vitaminasaga.html (accessed September 2, 2008).

CHAPTER 8 CLEANSE FOR YOUR IDEAL WEIGHT

1. S. Bengmark, "Ecological Control of the Gastrointestinal Tract. The Role of Probiotic Flora," *Gut* 42 (1998): 2–7.

2. Wikipedia.org, "Horace Fletcher," http://en.wikipedia.org/wiki/Horace_Fletcher (accessed September 3, 2008).

3. Claire Heald, "Going Ape," BBC News, January 11, 2007, http://news.bbc .co.uk/2/hi/uk_news/magazine/6248975.stm (accessed September 3, 2008).

CHAPTER 9 GET FIT FOR YOUR IDEAL WEIGHT

1. Charles Stuart Platkin, "Counting Steps With Pedometer Seems to Encourage Fitness," *Honolulu Advertiser*, March 24, 2004.

2. Al Sears, MD, *PACE: Rediscover Your Native Fitness* (Wellington, FL: Wellness Research & Consulting, Inc., 2006), 7.

3. Jeannine Stein, "The Amish Paradox," *Los Angeles Times*, January 12, 2004.

4. Jay Groves, EdD, "The Digital Pedometer," Diabetes Exercise and Sports Association, http://www.diabetes-exercise.org/Docs/jay_groves_practioners_article.asp (accessed September 3, 2008).

5. C. A. Gillette, R. C. Bullough, and C. L. Melby, "Post Exercise Energy Expenditure in Response to Acute Aerobic or Resistive Exercise," *International Journal of Sport Nutrition* 4, no. 4 (1994): 347–360.

6. Peter Jaret, "A Healthy Mix of Rest and Motion," *New York Times*, May 3, 2007.

7. Ibid.

8. Larry Trivieri Jr., *Alternative Medicine: The Definitive Guide* (Berkeley, CA: Celestial Arts, 2002), 37–38.

9. PowerAthletesMag.com, "Exclusive Interview with the 'Evil Russian' Pavel Tsatsouline," *Girevik* magazine, issue 1, http://www.powerathletesmag.com/archives/Girevik/First/interview. htm (accessed September 4, 2008).

10. J. T. Salonon et al., "Physical Activity and Risk of Myocardial Infarction, Cerebral Stroke, and Death: A Longitudinal Study in Eastern Finland," *American Journal of Epidemiology* 115, no. 4 (1982): 526–537.

11. Michael F. Roizen, MD, and Mehmet C. Oz, Mehmet, MD, *YOU: The Owner's Manual* (New York: Harper Collins, 2005), 122.

12. Nanci Hellmich, "Sleep Loss May Equal Weight Gain," *USA Today*, December 6, 2004, http://www.usatoday.com/news/health/2004-12-06-sleep-weight
-gain_x.htm (accessed August 29, 2007).

13. Milly Dawson, "The Quest for Sleep," *bp Magazine*, Spring 2006, as reprinted at National Alliance on Mental Illness, http://www.nami.org/template.cfm?template=/ContentManagement/ ContentDisplay.cfm&ContentID=32467&lstid=275 (accessed September 4, 2008); and Jacob Teitelbaum, MD, "Getting Eight to Nine Hours of Sleep—the Foundation of Pain Relief," TalkAboutSleep.com, http://www.talkabout
sleep.com/sleep-disorders/2005/04/fibromyalgia-eight-hours.htm (accessed September 4, 2008).

Chapter 10 Reduce Toxins for Your Ideal Weight

1. DietJokes.co.uk, "The Dieter's Psalm," http://www.dietjokes.co.uk/jokes/074.php (accessed September 4, 2008).

2. Liz Lipski, PhD, CCN, "Basics of Nutrition and Healthy Eating," WomentoWomen.com, http://www.womentowomen.com/nutritionandweightloss/
nutritionalbasics.asp (accessed September 4, 2008).

3. Denise Mann, "Are Artificial Sweeteners Safe?" WebMD.com, http://www.webmd .com/content/Article/102/106833.htm (accessed September 4, 2008).

4. Don Colbert, *Toxic Relief* (Lake Mary, FL: Siloam, 1999, 2003), 15.

5. Theo Colborn, *Our Stolen Future*, "About Phthalates," http://www .ourstolenfuture.org/NewScience/oncompounds/phthalates/phthalates.htm#health (accessed September 4, 2008).

6. AirBrains.org, "Perfumes and Scents," http://www.airbrains.org/SCENTS.htm (accessed September 4, 2008).

7. American Lung Association, "Indoor Air Quality," http://www.alaw.org/air_quality/ indoor_air_quality/ (accessed September 4, 2008).

8. Mindy Pennybacker, "Healthier Home Cleaning," *The Green Guide* magazine, September 8, 2003, http://www.thegreenguide.com/doc/98/clean (accessed September 4, 2008).

CHAPTER 11 THINK FOR YOUR IDEAL WEIGHT

1. Heinz von Foerster, "On Constructing a Reality," Readings That Matter to Me, http://grace.evergreen.edu/~arunc/texts/cybernetics/heinz/constructing/constructing.html (accessed September 4, 2008).

2. Sue Goetinck Ambrose, "A Cell Forgets," *Dallas Morning News*, reprinted in *San Diego Union-Tribune*, October 20, 2004, http://www.signonsandiego.com/uniontrib/20041020/news_z1c20cell.html (accessed September 4, 2008).

3. Ibid.

4. TheHealingCodes.com, "Interview with Bruce Lipton, PhD, Cellular Biologist and Author of *The Biology of Belief*," http://thehealingcodes.com/lipton_interview.htm (accessed September 18, 2007).

CHAPTER 12 TAKE WEIGHT OFF THE WORLD

1. Jim Robbins, "Think Global, Eat Local," *Los Angeles Times Magazine*, July 31, 2005, 9–10.

2. Elizabeth Weise, "Study: 90% of the Ocean's Edible Species May Be Gone by 2048," *USA Today*, http://www.usatoday.com/tech/science/discoveries/2006-11-02
-overfishing-threat_x.htm (accessed September 4, 2008).

3. *In Pink* magazine, Decatur, Georgia, Premiere Issue, 2007.

4. Elizabeth Weise, "Panel Calls Chemical a 'Likely Carcinogen,'" *USA Today*, June 29, 2005, http://www.usatoday.com/news/health/2005-06-29-teflon-usat_x.htm (accessed September 4, 2008).

CHAPTER 13 THE RESULTS ARE IN...

1. MensHealth.com, "The Best and Worst Cities for Men 2007," http://www
.menshealth.com/cda/article.do?site=MensHealth&channel=health&category=
metrogrades&conitem=84a7481031e48010VgnVCM200000cee793cd____ (accessed September 5, 2008).

INDEX

T

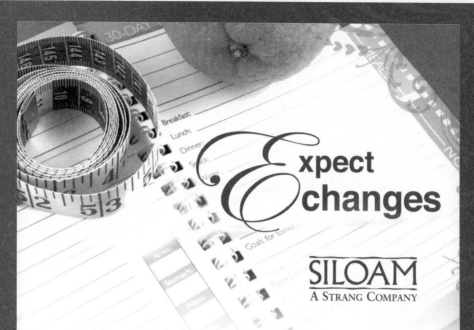
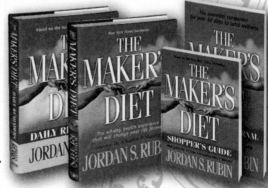

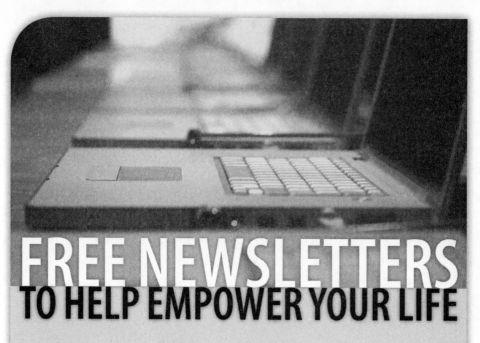

FREE NEWSLETTERS
TO HELP EMPOWER YOUR LIFE

Why subscribe today?

☐ **DELIVERED DIRECTLY TO YOU.** All you have to do is open your inbox and read.

☐ **EXCLUSIVE CONTENT.** We cover the news overlooked by the mainstream press.

☐ **STAY CURRENT.** Find the latest court rulings, revivals, and cultural trends.

☐ **UPDATE OTHERS.** Easy to forward to friends and family with the click of your mouse.

CHOOSE THE E-NEWSLETTER THAT INTERESTS YOU MOST:

- Christian news
- Daily devotionals
- Spiritual empowerment
- And much, much more

SIGN UP AT: **http://freenewsletters.charismamag.com**

8178